Dermatology

Visual Recognition and Case Reviews

Christine J. Ko

Dermatology

Visual Recognition and Case Reviews

Christine J. Ko MD

Professor of Dermatology and Pathology
Yale Medical School
New Haven, CT
USA

For additional online content visit ExpertConsult.com

ELSEVIER

Edinburgh   London   New York   Oxford   Philadelphia   St Louis   Sydney   Toronto   2017

ELSEVIER

Notices

Knowledge and best practice in this field are constantly changing. As new research and experience broaden our understanding, changes in research methods, professional practices, or medical treatment may become necessary.

Practitioners and researchers must always rely on their own experience and knowledge in evaluating and using any information, methods, compounds, or experiments described herein. In using such information or methods they should be mindful of their own safety and the safety of others, including parties for whom they have a professional responsibility.

With respect to any drug or pharmaceutical products identified, readers are advised to check the most current information provided (i) on procedures featured or (ii) by the manufacturer of each product to be administered, to verify the recommended dose or formula, the method and duration of administration, and contraindications. It is the responsibility of practitioners, relying on their own experience and knowledge of their patients, to make diagnoses, to determine dosages and the best treatment for each individual patient, and to take all appropriate safety precautions.

To the fullest extent of the law, neither the Publisher nor the authors, contributors, or editors, assume any liability for any injury and/or damage to persons or property as a matter of products liability, negligence or otherwise, or from any use or operation of any methods, products, instructions, or ideas contained in the material herein.

ISBN: 978-0-3233-7531-3

Content Strategist: Russell Gabbedy
Content Development Specialist: Fiona Conn
Project Manager: Anne Collett
Design: Christian Bilbow
Illustration Manager: Karen Giacomucci
Illustrator: MacPS LLC, Richard Tibbitts
Marketing Manager: Kristin McNally

ELSEVIER your source for books, journals and multimedia in the health sciences

www.elsevierhealth.com

  Working together to grow libraries in developing countries

www.elsevier.com • www.bookaid.org

The publisher's policy is to use paper manufactured from sustainable forests

Printed in China

Last digit is the print number: 9 8 7 6 5 4 3 2 1

Contents

To Peter, Dylan, and Owen

This atlas would not have been possible without the pre-existing body of work, published and unpublished, of numerous dermatologists. Extensive credit is due to all authors and editors whose excellent photographs and schematics are reproduced here, particularly those who worked on the third edition of *Dermatology* edited by Jean Bolognia, Joseph Jorizzo and Julie Schaffer (Saunders 2013), but also of other textbooks and journal articles. Every effort has been made to appropriately credit contributors, and any errors or omissions are unintentional. A special thanks is also due to the many patients who consented to photography of their presentations, allowing us to learn from them.

This atlas is meant to be used as an introduction to dermatology and dermatopathology and as a rich source of images that can hone the visual recognition skills of both the novice and expert in dermatology and/or pathology, as well as other specialties that examine the skin. The main purpose is to present classic visual clues that point to the correct diagnosis, as that is the important first step in proper management and care. Given the above goals, the minimal text and absence of treatment algorithms were deliberate, emphasizing the need to supplement this atlas with comprehensive textbooks and original articles.

Acknowledgments

Dermatology: Visual Recognition and Case Reviews came to fruition with the aid of various dermatology resources to enhance the key concepts, correlations and learnings within the text. Numerous figures from the following leading titles, collections and colleagues have been incorporated throughout the chapters and we gratefully acknowledge this volume of content and principally credit the following:

-Jean L. Bolognia, MD
-Julie V. Schaffer, MD
-Kalman Watsky, MD
-Karynne O. Duncan, MD
-Bolognia JL, Jorizzo JL, Schaffer JV, et al. *Dermatology*, 3rd ed. Philadelphia, PA: Elsevier Saunders, 2012.
-Bolognia JL, Schaffer JV, Duncan KO, Ko CJ. *Dermatology Essentials*. Philadelphia, PA: Elsevier Saunders, 2014.
-Yale Dermatology Residents' Slide Collection
-Yale Department of Dermatology faculty, including Jennifer M. McNiff, MD, Richard Antaya, MD, Irwin Braverman, MD, Brittany Craiglow, MD, Leonard Milstone, MD, and Jennifer N. Choi, MD (currently at Northwestern University).

-Other leading titles
Callen JP, Jorizzo JL. *Dermatological Signs of Internal Disease*, 4e. Philadelphia, PA: Elsevier Saunders, 2009.
Eichenfield LF, Frieden IJ, Zaenglein AL, Mathes E. *Neonatal and Infant Dermatology*, 3e. London: Saunders, 2014.
Elston D. Clinical image collection. *Dermatopathology*, 2e. London: Elsevier Saunders, 2014.
James WD, Berger T, Elston D. *Andrews' Diseases of the Skin*, 11e. Edinburgh: Saunders, 2011.
Patterson JW. *Weedon's Skin Pathology*, 4e. London: Churchill Livingstone, 2015.
Patterson JW. *Practical Skin Pathology*: A Diagnostic Approach. Philadelphia: Saunders, 2013.
Schachner LA, Hansen RE (Eds). *Pediatric Dermatology*, 4e. London: Elsevier Mosby, 2011.
Tyring SK, Lupi O, Hengge UR. *Tropical Dermatology*. London: Churchill Livingstone, 2005.
Weston WL, Lane AT, Morelli JG. *Color Textbook of Pediatric Dermatology*, 4e. St Louis: Mosby, 2007.

Many thanks as well to the Elsevier team, particularly Russell Gabbedy, Fiona Conn, and Anne Collett, for all their work on this project.

Key Concepts 1

INTRODUCTION

The "how" of coming to a diagnosis for visual specialties such as dermatology and dermatopathology is not transparent. Ultimately, the entire process is summed up with gestalt phrases such as "it just doesn't look like that" or "that's what it looks like to me" (*Table 1.1*). *You see it and you know it.* This is akin to being told that an elephant is an elephant by a parent or teacher, with the brain learning to recognize an elephant without necessarily being told that key features include the trunk, the large ears, the shape of the body and squat legs.

Breaking things down into key features can be useful in better training the eye and brain to see and recognize things more readily (*Table 1.2*). This chapter goes over basic concepts that are involved in such gestalt recognition in dermatology. Such cognitive knowledge of why things are different (how to separate or categorize) is integral to visual recognition, especially for things that have overarching similarities. For example, a leopard, a cheetah, and a jaguar are all large cats of similar height, but each animal's spots are distinctive; knowing this is key to rapid gestalt recognition of these unique animals. This chapter will cover body site/region, age, distribution, patterns, linear lesions, epidermal vs. dermal vs. deeper, acute vs. chronic eczematous, inflammatory cell types (epidermal and dermal), classic lesions, lesions with zones of color, lesional topography, types of scale, and color.

Table 1.1 Visual recognition in dermatology as related to cognitive psychology		
Dermatologic concepts		Cognitive psychology concepts
Overview ("from the doorway")	Close-up view (lesion itself)	Gestalt
Age Body site Distribution Pattern	Pattern Color Topography • Epidermal (including scale) • Dermal • Subcutaneous	Figure–ground separation Similarity Proximity Continuity Order Closure

Table 1.2 Visual recognition of three different big cats by their spots		
Cheetah spots	Leopard spots	Jaguar spots

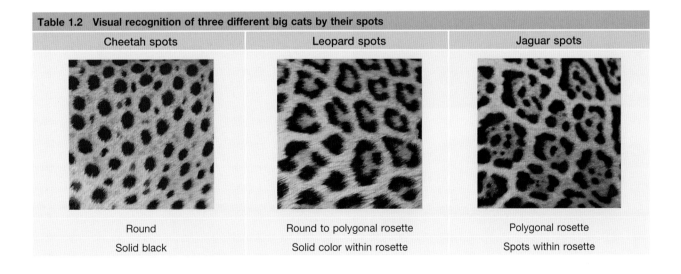

Round	Round to polygonal rosette	Polygonal rosette
Solid black	Solid color within rosette	Spots within rosette

BODY SITE/REGIONAL

Key Differences

- Scalp – numerous anagen hair follicles with bulbs (arrows) in the fat *(Fig. 1.1)*
- Ear – vellus hair follicles (arrows) and central cartilage (*) *(Fig. 1.2)*
- Face – prominent hair follicles and sebaceous glands within the dermis *(Fig. 1.3)*
- Eyelid – vellus hair follicles (arrows) and underlying skeletal muscle (*) *(Fig. 1.4)*
- Cutaneous lip – epidermis with keratin and a granular layer (arrows); skeletal muscle (*) *(Fig. 1.5)*
- Mucosal lip – pale epithelium that lacks a granular layer and does not keratinize *(Fig. 1.6)*
- Areola – acanthotic, pigmented epidermis with dermal smooth muscle bundles (arrows) *(Fig. 1.7)*
- Back – thick dermis *(Fig. 1.8)*
- Axilla – undulating epidermis with deep apocrine glands (arrows) *(Fig. 1.9)*
- Acral – thick stratum corneum with stratum lucidum (arrow) *(Fig. 1.10)*
- Nail – nail plate (arrow), nail matrix (black bar), and nail bed *(Fig. 1.11)*

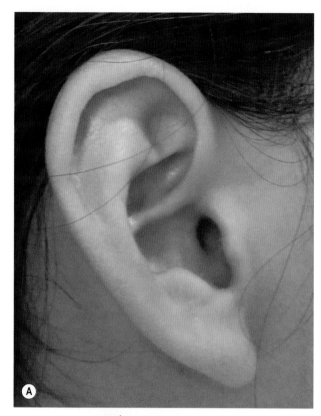

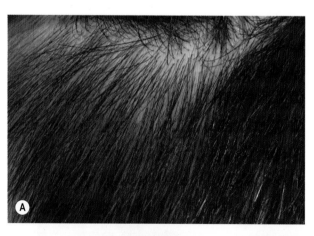

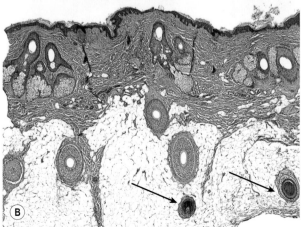

Fig. 1.1 Scalp.

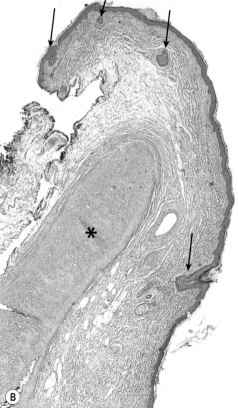

Fig. 1.2 Ear.

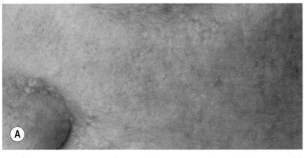

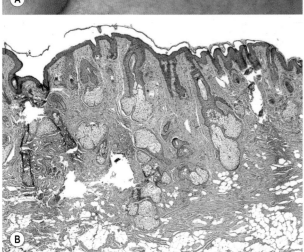

Fig. 1.3 Face.

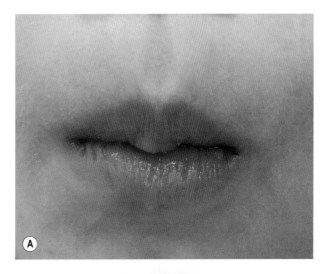

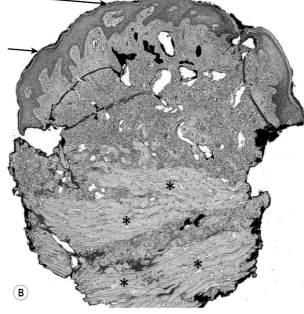

Fig. 1.5 Cutaneous lip.

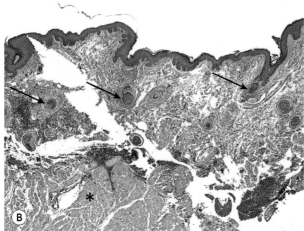

Fig. 1.4 Eyelid.

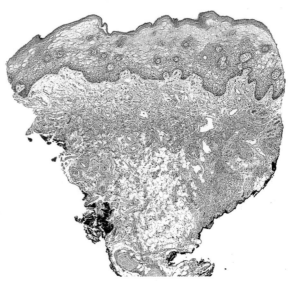

Fig. 1.6 Mucosal lip.

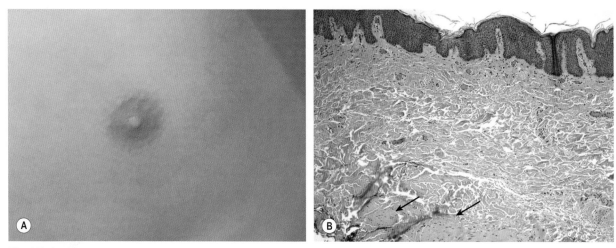

Fig. 1.7 Areola.

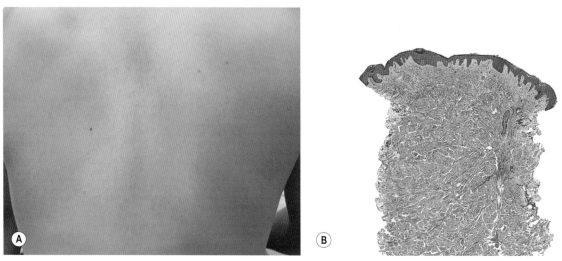

Fig. 1.8 Back.

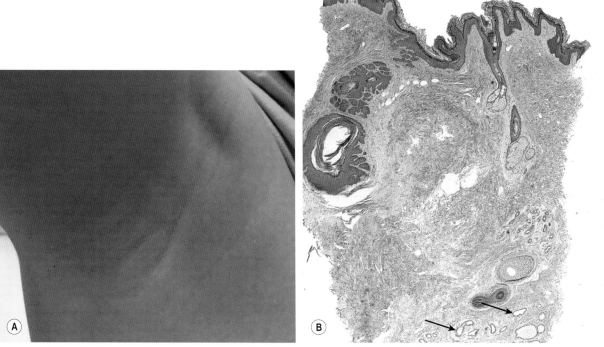

Fig. 1.9 Axilla.

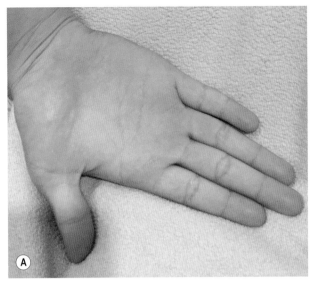

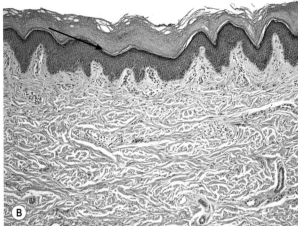

Fig. 1.10 Acral skin.

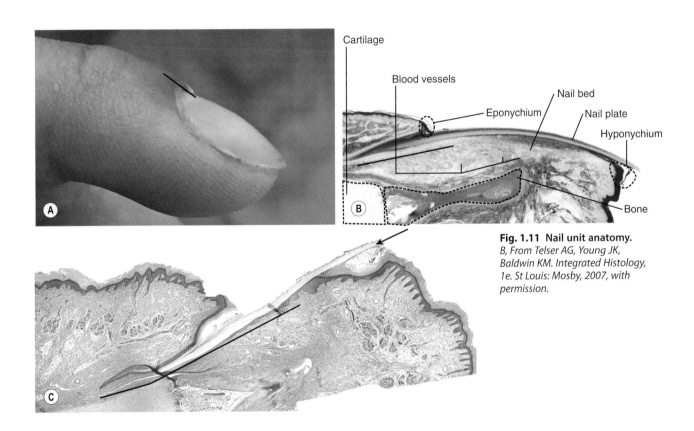

Cartilage

Blood vessels

Eponychium

Nail bed

Nail plate

Hyponychium

Bone

Fig. 1.11 Nail unit anatomy.
*B, From Telser AG, Young JK,
Baldwin KM. Integrated Histology,
1e. St Louis: Mosby, 2007, with
permission.*

AGE

- Young skin has small adnexal structures (arrows) and more compact dermis *(Figs 1.12, 1.13)*
- Sun-damaged skin has characteristic solar elastosis (arrows) *(Fig. 1.14)*

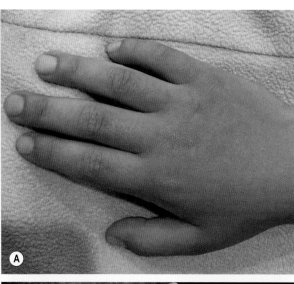

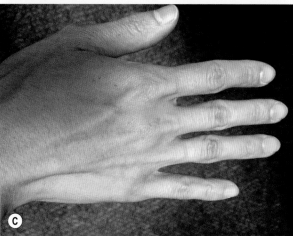

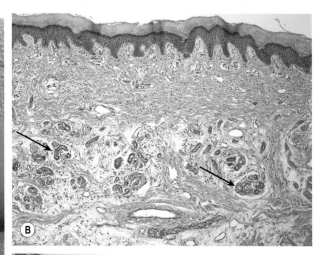

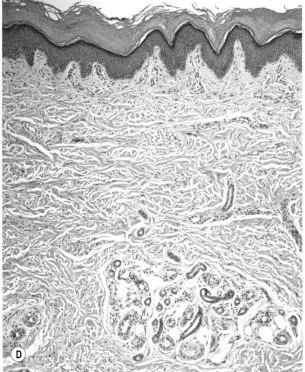

Fig. 1.12 Dorsal hand. A,B Child. **C,D** Adult.

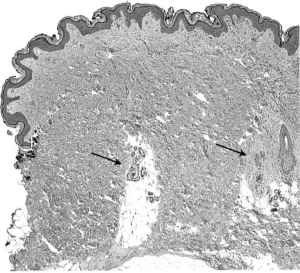

Fig. 1.13 Groin, 2-year-old.

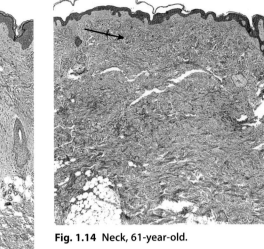

Fig. 1.14 Neck, 61-year-old.

DISTRIBUTION

Extensive – more than one body part affected with multiple lesions; may preferentially affect extensor surfaces (e.g. elbows/knees) vs flexor surfaces (e.g. antecubital/popliteal fossae) or ventral vs dorsal surfaces *(Fig. 1.15)*

Photodistribution – can vary depending on the type of clothing worn; sun-protected sites of the face/neck generally include the central upper cutaneous lip and submental area *(Fig. 1.16A; see Fig. 3.7)*

Double-covered areas – generally includes sites covered by undergarments *(Fig. 1.16B)*

Acral – hands/feet but also the tips of the ears/nose *(Fig. 1.16C)*

Body folds – inframammary/intertriginous *(Fig. 1.16D)*

Generalized – involving the majority of the cutaneous surface *(Fig. 1.17)*

Dermatomal – patterns of cutaneous innervation by spinal nerve roots *(Fig. 1.18A)*

Blaschkoid – follows patterns of embryonic cell migration; while the linear pattern on the extremities is similar to the dermatomal pattern, the V-shaped curves over the trunk and the S-shapes on the abdomen are characteristic *(Fig. 1.18B)*

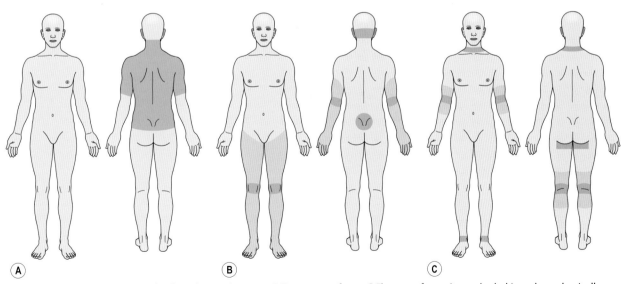

Fig. 1.15 Distribution. A Upper back and posterior arms. **B** Extensor surfaces. **C** Flexor surfaces. Areas shaded in red are classically involved; light pink areas may also be involved.

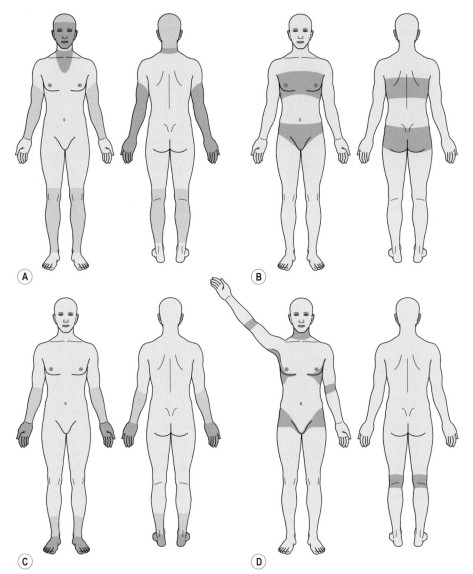

Fig. 1.16 Distribution. A Photodistribution. **B** Double-covered sites. **C** Acral. **D** Body folds. Areas shaded in red are classically involved; light pink areas may also be involved.

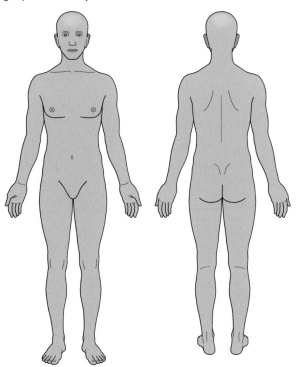

Fig. 1.17 Distribution – generalized.

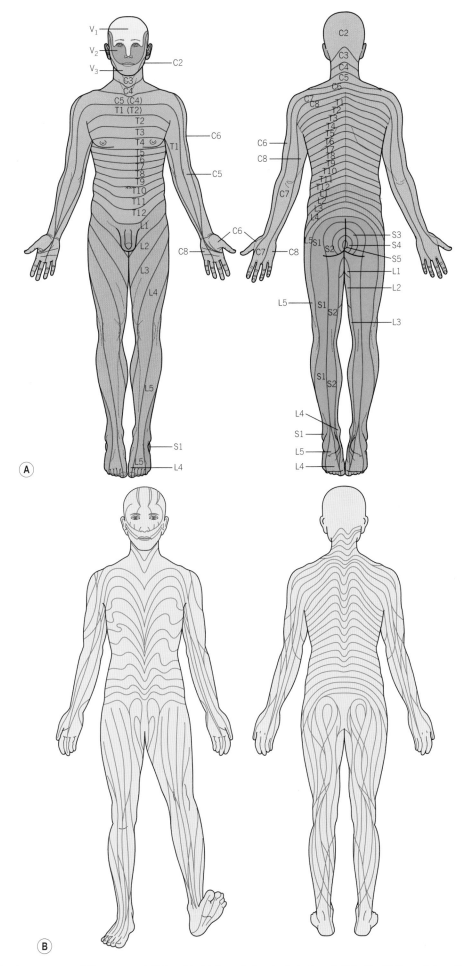

Fig. 1.18 Distribution patterns. A Dermatomal. **B** Blaschkoid. *From Bolognia JL, Jorizzo JL, Schaffer JV. Dermatology, 3e. London: Saunders, 2012, with permission.*

PATTERNS

Thin stripes – often corresponds to Blaschko's lines *(see Fig. 1.18B, Fig. 1.19)*
Rarer patterns of mosaicism include phylloid *(Fig. 1.20)* and checkerboard/segmental *(Fig. 1.21)*
Small net – regular with the "holes" of the net ~1 cm in size *(Fig. 1.22A,B)*
Large net – irregular with the "holes" of an incomplete net usually >1 cm in size *(see Fig. 1.22C,D)*

Annular/serpiginous *(Fig. 1.23A)*
Concentric rings *(Fig. 1.23B)*
Intersecting raised rings *(Fig. 1.24)*
Chinese letters *(Fig. 1.25)*
Exogenous – the shape corresponds to the contact area of the external contactant *(Fig. 1.26)*

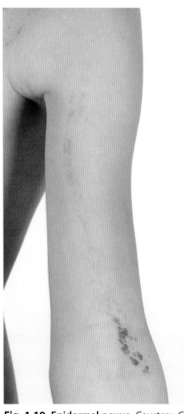

Fig. 1.19 Epidermal nevus. *Courtesy, Celia Moss, MD. From Bolognia JL, Jorizzo JL, Schaffer JV. Dermatology, 3e. London: Saunders, 2012, with permission.*

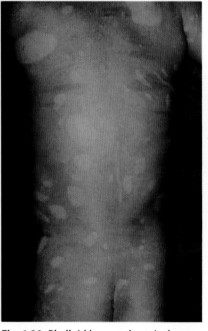

Fig. 1.20 Phylloid hypomelanosis due to mosaicism for trisomy 13. *Courtesy, Rudolf Happle, MD.*

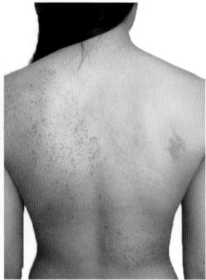

Fig. 1.21 Nevus spilus maculosa. *Courtesy, Jae Choi, MD.*

Pattern of livedo reticularis versus livedo racemosa

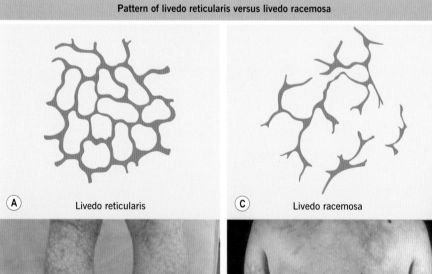

(A) Livedo reticularis

(C) Livedo racemosa

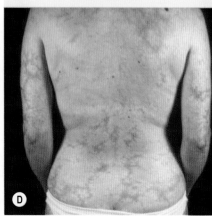

Fig. 1.22 Small and large nets. A,B Livedo reticularis. **C,D** Livedo racemosa. Sneddon syndrome in **D**. *D, Courtesy, Christopher Baker and Robert Kelly, MD. B, Courtesy, Peter Heald, MD. A,C,D, From Bolognia JL, Jorizzo JL, Schaffer JV. Dermatology, 3e. London: Saunders, 2012, with permission.*

(B)

(D)

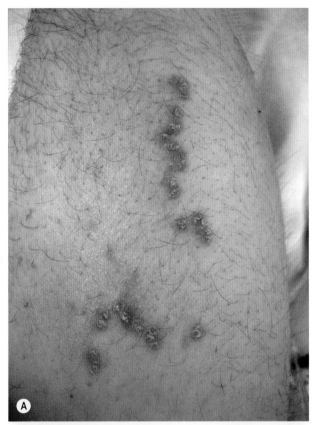

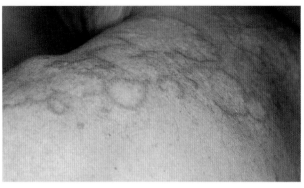

Fig. 1.24 Annular elastolytic giant cell granuloma. *Courtesy, Kalman Watsky, MD. From Bolognia JL, Jorizzo JL, Schaffer JV. Dermatology, 3e. London: Saunders, 2012, with permission.*

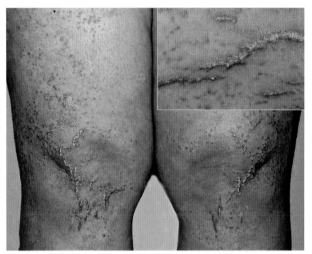

Fig. 1.25 Keratosis lichenoides chronica. *Courtesy, Kathryn Schwarzenberger, MD. From Bolognia JL, Jorizzo JL, Schaffer JV. Dermatology, 3e. London: Saunders, 2012, with permission.*

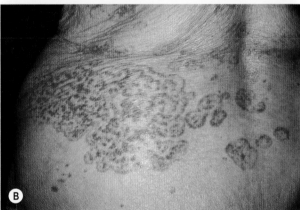

Fig. 1.23 A Elastosis perforans serpiginosa. **B** Erythema gyratum repens in a patient with breast carcinoma. *A, Courtesy, Yale Dermatology Residents' Slide Collection. B, Courtesy, Jeffrey Callen, MD. B, From Bolognia JL, Jorizzo JL, Schaffer JV. Dermatology, 3e. London: Saunders, 2012, with permission.*

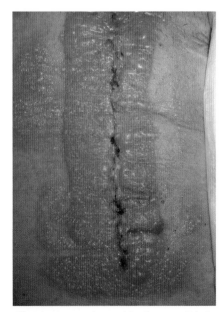

Fig. 1.26 Allergic contact dermatitis. *Courtesy, Yale Dermatology Residents' Slide Collection.*

LINEAR LESIONS

Inflammatory *(Fig. 1.27)*, mosaic *(Fig. 1.28)*, vascular *(Fig. 1.29)*, infectious, and externally-induced *(Fig. 1.30)* disorders can present with linear lesions. Lesions within a dermatome and koebnerized lesions can also be linear. In linear psoriasis, characteristic silvery scale is seen over red plaques; the presence of psoriatic lesions *(see Fig. 1.27A; arrow)* outside of the linear lesion distinguishes this clinically from inflammatory linear verrucous epidermal nevus. Linear lichen planus is typically composed of flat-topped purplish papules with Wickham's striae. Lichen striatus can have a similar appearance to lichen planus, but lesions are usually small (1–2 mm) with minimal scale. In incontinentia pigmenti, an initial vesicular stage becomes verrucous and hyperpigmented with late-stage hypopigmentation and absent adnexal structures *(see Fig. 1.28A)*. In Goltz syndrome, linear streaks are composed of yellowish papules (fat herniation), telangiectasias, hyperpigmented macules, atrophic foci, and hypopigmented splotches.

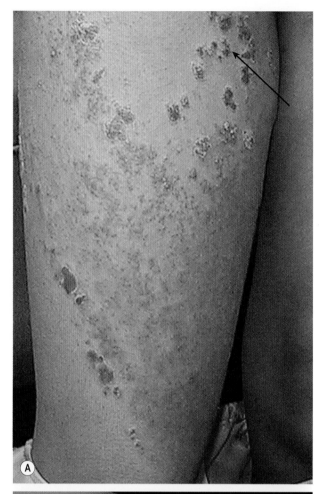

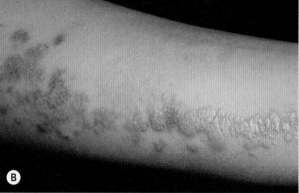

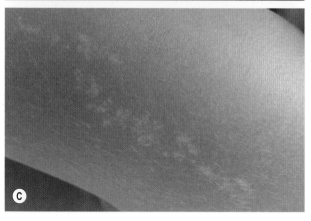

Fig. 1.27 Inflammatory. A Linear psoriasis. **B** Linear lichen planus. **C** Lichen striatus. *B, Courtesy, Joyce Rico, MD. From Bolognia JL, Jorizzo JL, Schaffer JV. Dermatology, 3e. London: Saunders, 2012, with permission. C, Courtesy, Brittany Craiglow, MD.*

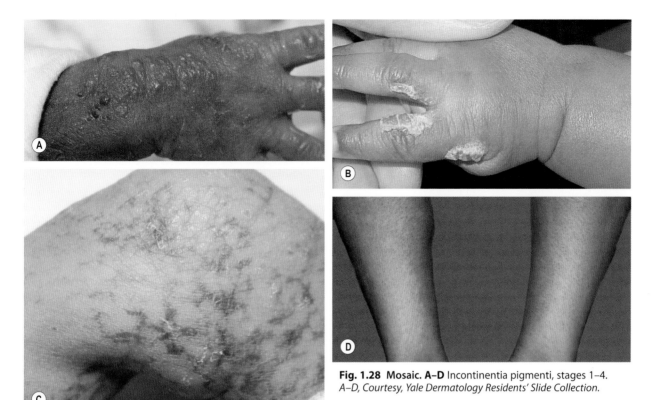

Fig. 1.28 Mosaic. A–D Incontinentia pigmenti, stages 1–4. *A–D, Courtesy, Yale Dermatology Residents' Slide Collection.*

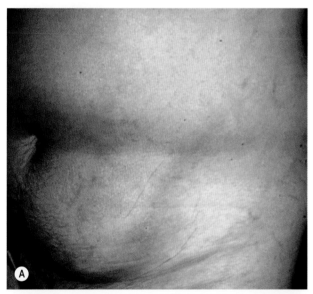

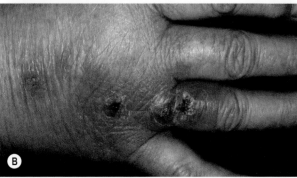

Fig. 1.29 Vascular. A Superficial thrombophlebitis in a patient with Behçet's disease. **B** Sporotrichoid spread of an atypical mycobacterial infection. *A, Courtesy, Samuel Moschella, MD. B, Courtesy, Yale Dermatology Residents' Slide Collection. A, From Bolognia JB, Jorizzo JL, Rapini RP. Dermatology, 2e. London: Saunders, 2008, with permission.*

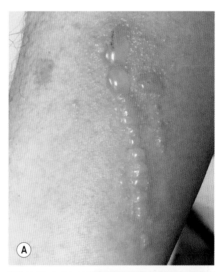

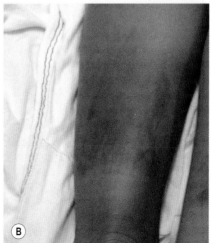

Fig. 1.30 Externally induced. A Poison ivy. **B** Phytophotodermatitis, postinflammatory pigmentary alteration. *A, Courtesy, Joyce Rico, MD. B, Courtesy, Yale Dermatology Residents' Slide Collection.*

EPIDERMAL VS DERMAL VS DEEP SOFT TISSUE

Tumors, inflammation, edema, or other deposits can affect the epidermis, dermis or deeper soft tissue *(Fig. 1.31)*. Inflammation of the epidermis is addressed in the next section. Inflammation affecting the epidermis can be follicular (e.g. folliculitis) or non-follicular (e.g. pustular psoriasis).

Basic Epidermal Patterns

*Eczematous/Spongiotic**

Clinical:
Crust, "wet" appearance and/or vesicles (circles), erythema (arrow) *(Fig. 1.32A)*

Microscopic:
Parakeratosis with serum, intercellular edema/vesicles (circles), perivascular inflammation and slightly dilated vessels (arrow) *(Fig. 1.32B)*

*Psoriasiform**

Clinical:
Silvery to white scaly (arrow) plaque (bar), sharp demarcation from normal skin, bright red erythema underlying scale *(Fig. 1.33A)*

Microscopic:
Dry parakeratosis (arrow), regular acanthosis (bar), often there are neutrophils in the epidermis *(Fig. 1.33B)*

Lichenoid[#]

Clinical:
Violaceous (arrow), lesions often flat-topped *(Fig. 1.34A)*

Microscopic:
Band-like lymphocytic infiltrate (arrow), pigment incontinence *(Fig. 1.34B)*

Vacuolar[#]

Clinical:
Thin lesions, may be dusky in color *(Fig. 1.35A)*

Microscopic:
Vacuoles in basal cells (arrows) *(Fig. 1.35B)*

---

*Can have overlapping features, especially in chronic spongiotic conditions

[#]Can have overlapping features; note that there is not a true clinical–pathologic correlate for the vacuolar pattern in the same way as there is for the other 3 basic patterns

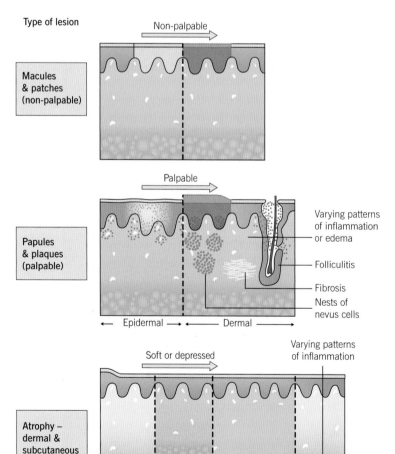

Type of lesion

Fig. 1.31 Epidermal vs dermal vs deep soft tissue involvement. *Adapted from Bolognia JL, Jorizzo JL, Schaffer JV. Dermatology, 3e. London: Saunders, 2012, with permission.*

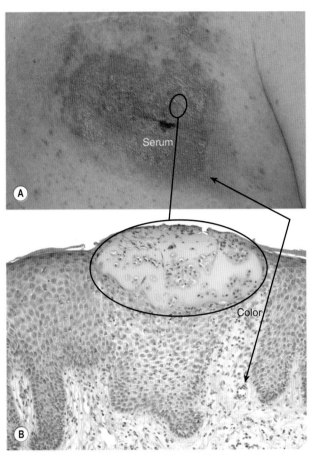

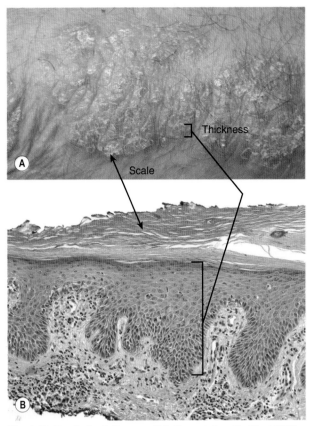

Fig. 1.32 Allergic contact dermatitis to adhesive. *A, Courtesy, Kalman Watsky, MD.*

Fig. 1.33 Psoriasis. *A, Courtesy, Yale Dermatology Residents' Slide Collection.*

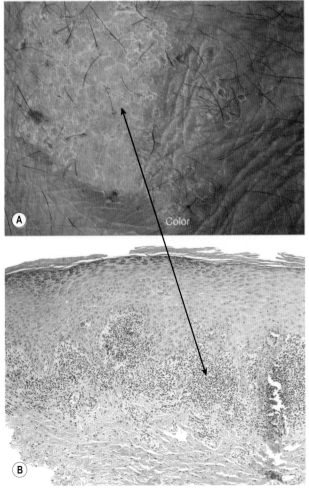

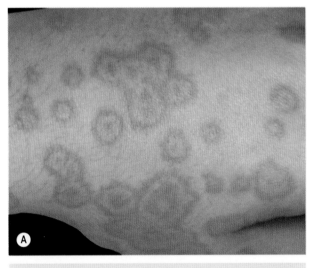

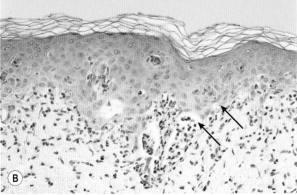

Fig. 1.34 Lichen planus. *A, Courtesy, Yale Dermatology Residents' Slide Collection.*

Fig. 1.35 Erythema multiforme. *A, Courtesy, Yale Dermatology Residents' Slide Collection. A, From Bolognia JL, Jorizzo JL, Schaffer JV. Dermatology, 3e. London: Saunders, 2012, with permission.*

ACUTE VS CHRONIC ECZEMATOUS/SPONGIOTIC

Acute Eczematous/Spongiotic Processes

Clinical:
Surface serum/crust ("weeping"/"boiling over") and/or vesicles (arrow), erythema *(Figs 1.36A, 1.37); can become impetiginized*

Microscopic:
Parakeratosis with serum/inflammatory cells and/or intraepidermal vesicles (arrow) and perivascular inflammation *(Fig. 1.36B)*

Chronic Eczematous/Spongiotic Processes

Clinical:
Thickened/lichenified (bar), scaly (arrow) plaques +/− erythema *(Figs 1.38A, 1.39)*

Microscopic:
Hyperkeratosis +/− parakeratosis (arrow), hypergranulosis, acanthosis (bar) and vertically streaked dermal collagen (asterisks), perivascular inflammation *(Fig. 1.38B)*

Other eczematous processes are illustrated in Figs 1.40–1.42.

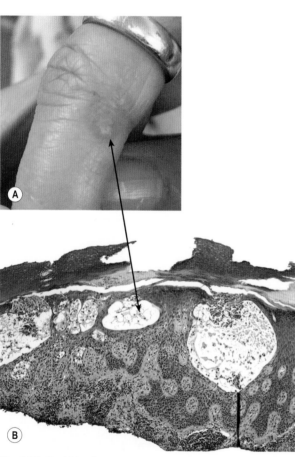

Fig. 1.36 Dyshidrotic eczema.

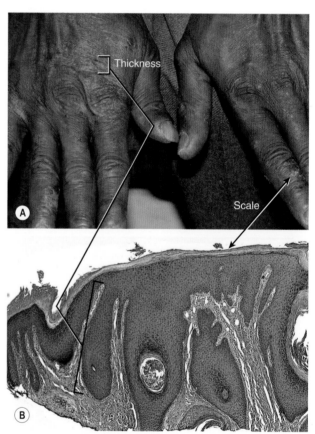

Fig. 1.38 Chronic dermatitis with lichenification. *A, Courtesy, Kalman Watsky, MD.*

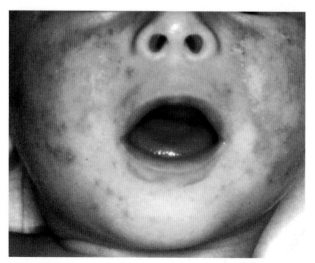

Fig. 1.37 Acute atopic dermatitis, infant. *Courtesy, Kalman Watsky, MD.*

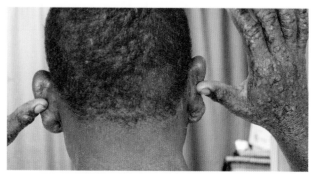

Fig. 1.39 Chronic atopic dermatitis. *Courtesy, Yale Dermatology Residents' Slide Collection.*

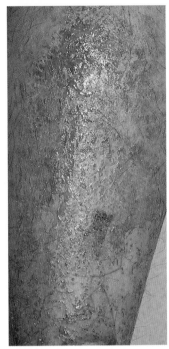

Fig. 1.40 Acute allergic contact dermatitis.

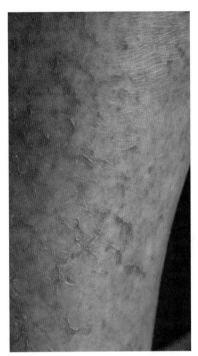

Fig. 1.41 Asteatotic eczema. *Courtesy, Yale Dermatology Residents' Slide Collection.*

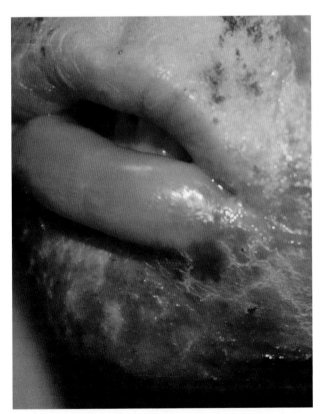

Fig. 1.42 Impetiginized atopic dermatitis. *Courtesy, Yale Dermatology Residents' Slide Collection.*

INFLAMMATORY CELL TYPES – EPIDERMAL

Neutrophils – often associated with pustules clinically *(Fig. 1.43)*

Eosinophils – may be associated with blistering/erosions clinically *(Fig. 1.44)*

Lymphocytes (arrows) – often present in spongiotic processes but can also represent cutaneous T-cell lymphoma *(Fig. 1.45)*

Langerhans cells (circle) – the prototype is Langerhans cell histiocytosis; small collections of Langerhans cells are also present in spongiotic processes *(Fig. 1.46)*

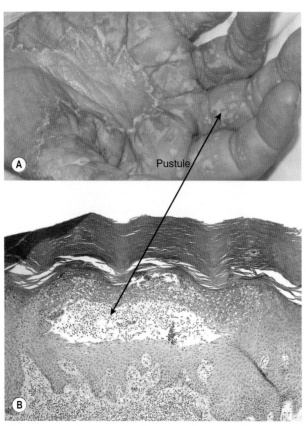

Fig. 1.43 Pustular psoriasis. *Courtesy, Yale Dermatology Residents' Slide Collection.*

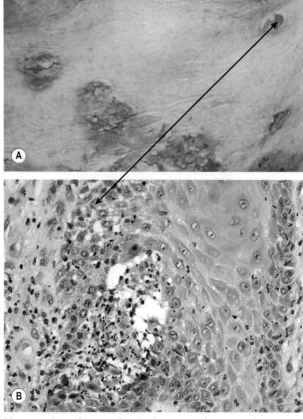

Fig. 1.44 Pemphigus vulgaris. *Courtesy, Yale Dermatology Residents' Slide Collection.*

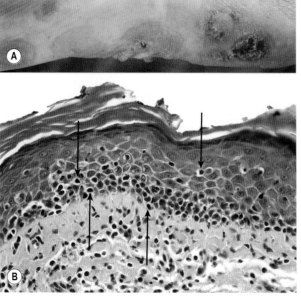

Fig. 1.45 Mycosis fungoides. *Courtesy, Yale Dermatology Residents' Slide Collection.*

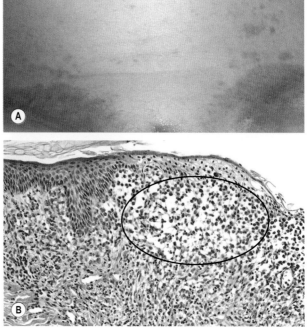

Fig. 1.46 Langerhans cell histiocytosis. *A, Courtesy, Irwin Braverman, MD.*

INFLAMMATORY CELL TYPES – DERMAL

The predominant type of dermal inflammatory cell can sometimes be predicted by the color of clinical lesions.

Langerhans cell histiocytosis – purpuric papules and plaques; Langerhans cells and extravasated erythrocytes in the dermis *(Fig. 1.46A,B)*

Granulomatous disorders – classically red–brown to pink with a yellowish tinge if lesions are pressed firmly with a glass slide; collections of histiocytes (granulomas) are in the dermis (circles) *(Fig. 1.47A,B)*

Mast cells – pink to red–brown and may blister with manipulation; mast cells classically have central nuclei with abundant slightly granular cytoplasm *(Fig. 1.47C,D)*

Dense pan-dermal neutrophilic infiltrates – deep, hot red to vesicular/translucent when acute and untreated *(Fig. 1.47E,F)*

Dense pan-dermal lymphocytic infiltrates – pink–red to purple firm papulonodule *(Fig. 1.47G,H)*

Sparse dermal lymphocytic infiltrates (may be admixed with neutrophils and/or eosinophils) – light pink *(Fig. 1.47I,J)*

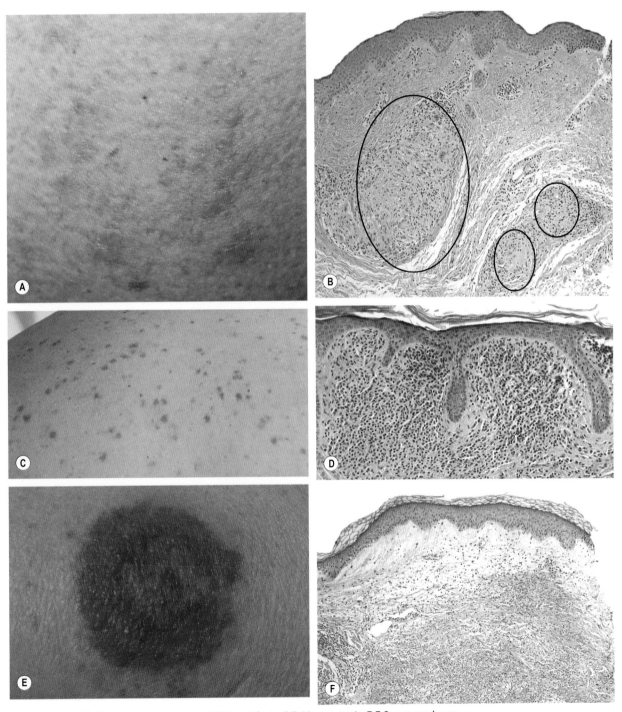

Fig. 1.47 Dermal inflammatory processes. A,B Sarcoidosis. **C,D** Mastocytosis. **E,F** Sweet syndrome.

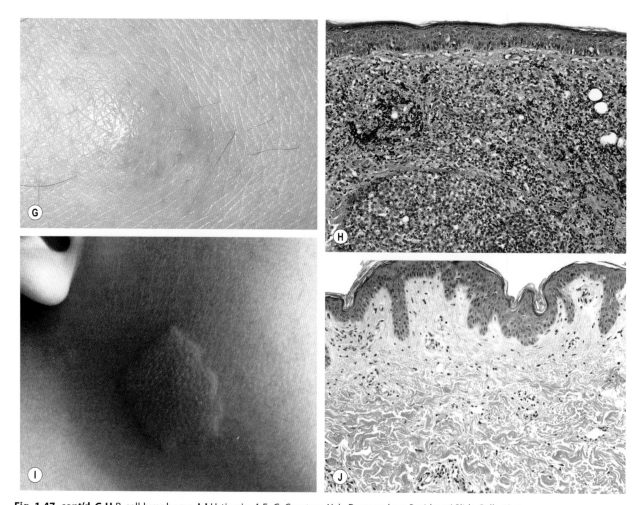

Fig. 1.47, cont'd G,H B-cell lymphoma. **I,J** Urticaria. *A,E–G, Courtesy, Yale Dermatology Residents' Slide Collection.*

CLASSIC LESIONS *(Fig. 1.48)*

	Term	Clinical features	Microscopic example	Clinical example
Related by size	Macule	• Flat, circumscribed, non-palpable • <1 cm in diameter • Often hypo- or hyperpigmented • Also other colors (e.g. pink, red, violet) • It can be round, oval, or irregular in shape • May be sharply marginated or blend into the surrounding skin		 Solar lentigines
	Patch	• Flat, circumscribed • >1 cm in diameter • Often hypo- or hyperpigmented • Also other colors (e.g. blue, violet)		 Vitiligo
Related by size	Papule	• Elevated, circumscribed • <1 cm in diameter • Elevation due to increased thickness of the epidermis and/or cells or deposits within the dermis • May have secondary changes (e.g. scale, crust) • Need to distinguish from vesicle or pustule • When viewed in profile, it may be flat-topped, dome-shaped, filiform, pedunculated, smooth, verrucous, or umbilicated		 Seborrheic keratoses
	Plaque	• Elevated, circumscribed • >1 cm in diameter • Elevation due to increased thickness of the epidermis and/or cells or deposits within the dermis • May have secondary changes (e.g. scale, crust, erosion) • May be a distinct lesion or formed by confluence of papules		 Psoriasis

Fig. 1.48 Classic lesions. *Adapted from Bolognia JL, Schaffer JV, Duncan KO, Ko CJ. Dermatology Essentials, 1e. Philadelphia: Saunders, 2014, with permission.*

Term	Clinical features	Microscopic example	Clinical example
Nodule	• Elevated, circumscribed • Larger volume than papule, often >1.5 cm in diameter • Involves the dermis and may extend to the subcutis • Greatest mass may be beneath the skin surface • Can be compressible, soft, rubbery, or firm to palpation		 Epidermal inclusion cysts
Vesicle	• Elevated, circumscribed • <1 cm in diameter • Fluid containing usually clear but may be hemorrhagic • May become pustular, umbilicated or an erosion		 Herpes zoster
Bulla	• Elevated, circumscribed • >1 cm in diameter • Fluid containing usually clear but may be hemorrhagic • May become an erosion or ulceration		 Bullous fixed drug eruption
Pustule	• Elevated, circumscribed • Usually <1 cm in diameter • Contains purulent material (neutrophils, eosinophils) • May be infectious or sterile		 Steroid folliculitis

Related by size →

Fig. 1.48, cont'd Classic lesions.

LESIONS WITH ZONES OF COLOR

Key Differences

- Typical target – 3 zones of color (middle zone is often edematous and pale; arrows), palpable *(Fig. 1.49A)*

- Atypical target – classically only 2 zones of color, irregular border, non-palpable unless there is a central blister *(Fig. 1.49B)*

- Annular, non-scaly – ring with unaffected center *(Fig. 1.49C,D)*

- Annular, scaly – scaly ring with unaffected center; scale on outer border in tinea *(Fig. 1.49E)*; scale on the inner border in erythema annulare centrifugum *(Fig. 1.49F)*

Fig. 1.49 Lesions with zones of color. A Erythema multiforme. **B** Toxic epidermal necrolysis. **C** Giant annular urticaria (urticaria multiforme). **D** Granuloma annulare. **E** Tinea corporis. **F** Erythema annulare centrifugum. *A, Courtesy, Kalman Watsky, MD; C–E, Courtesy, Yale Dermatology Residents' Slide Collection. B, From Callen JP, Jorizzo JL. Dermatological Signs of Internal Disease, 4e. Philadelphia: Saunders, 2009.*

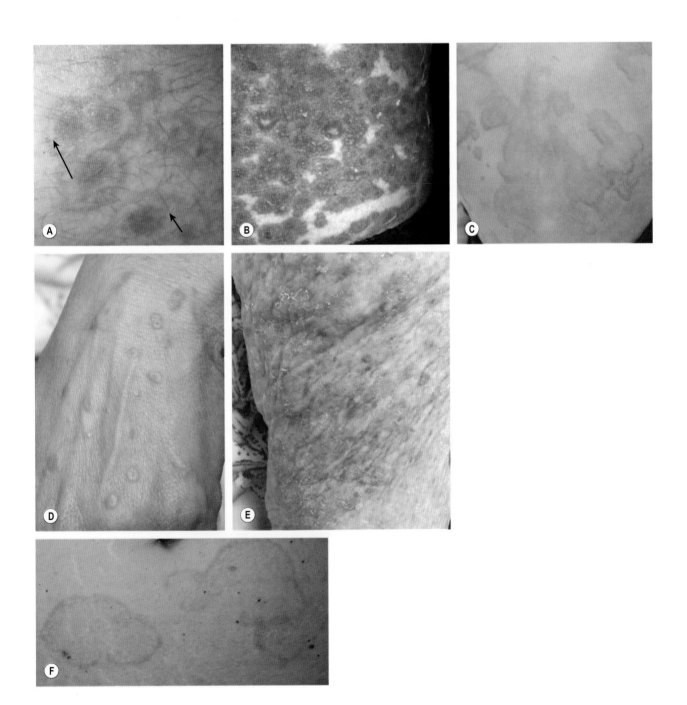

LESIONAL TOPOGRAPHY *(Fig. 1.50)*

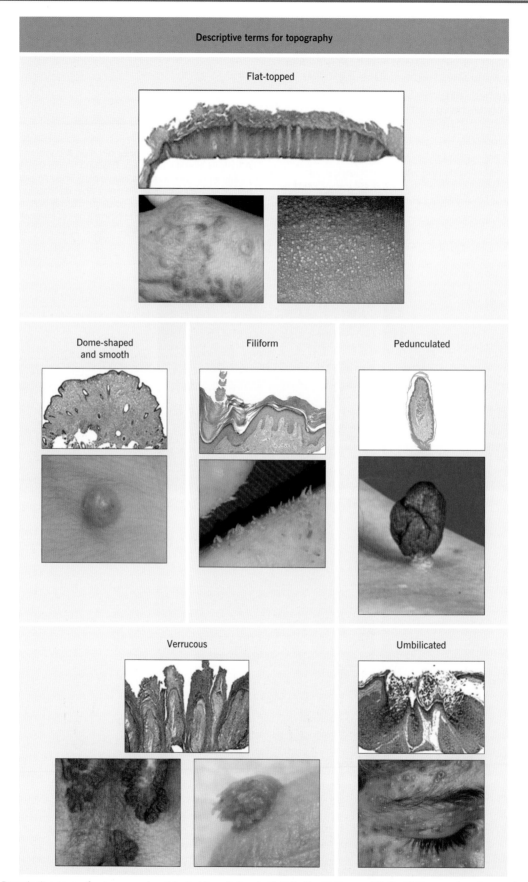

Fig. 1.50 Descriptive terms for topography. *Adapted from Bolognia JL, Schaffer JV, Duncan KO, Ko CJ. Dermatology Essentials, 1e. Philadelphia: Saunders, 2014, with permission.*

COLOR AS A CLUE

Color	Common causes		
	Endogenous		Exogenous
Pink to red to purple	• Erythrocytes • Inflammation • Vessels	Example: Kaposi sarcoma 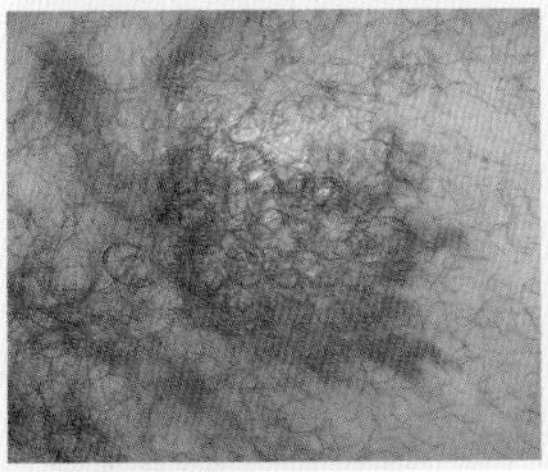 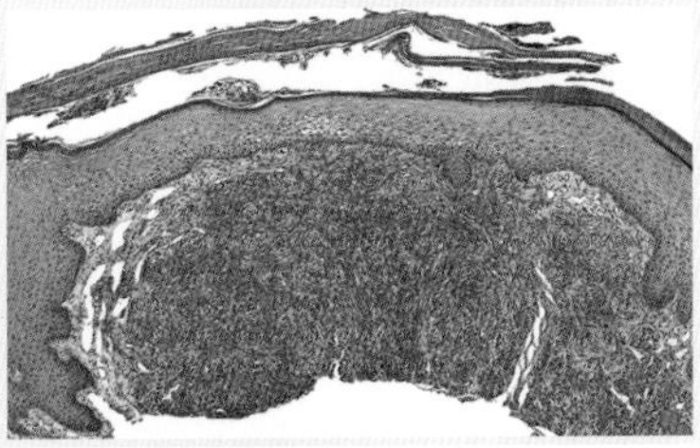	• Tattoo pigment
Black	• Melanin • Inflammation • Vessels (i.e. occlusion) • Necrosis	Example: Calciphylaxis 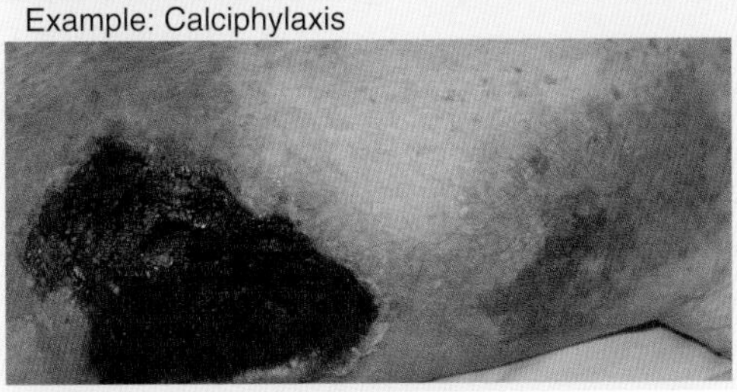	• Tattoo pigment • Poison ivy sap • Tick
Blue	• Melanin • Vessels	Example: Vascular malformation 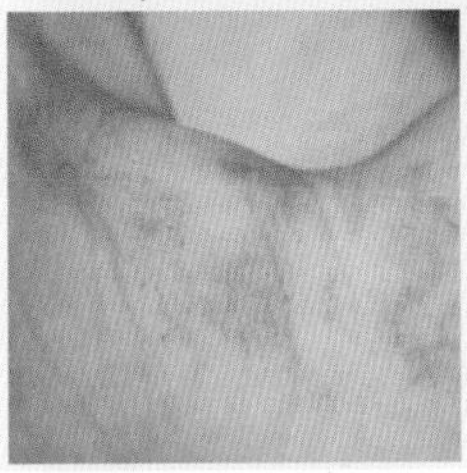 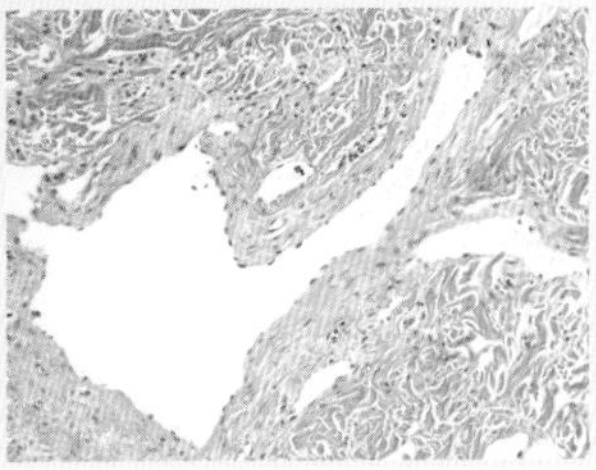	• Drug pigment (e.g. minocycline) • Heavy metals • Tattoo pigment
Yellow	• Lipid • Connective tissue (CT) • Deposition (e.g. urate in gout) • Keratin	Example: CT nevus 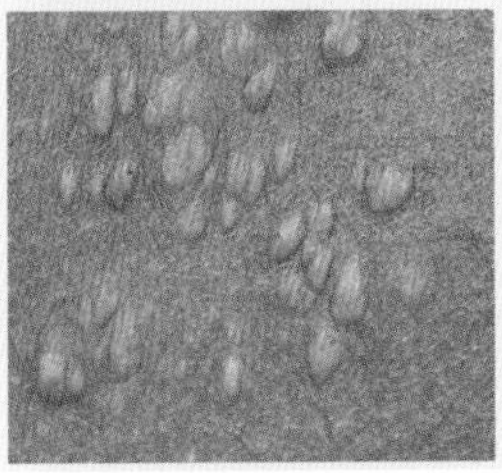 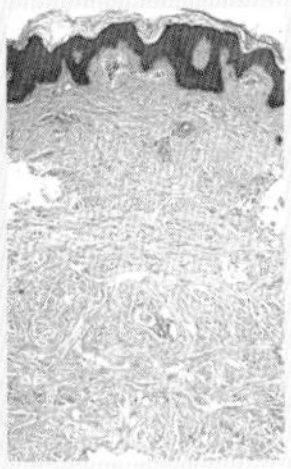	• Drug pigment
Brown	• Melanin • Hemosiderin • Cellular proliferation (e.g. dermatofibroma)	Example: Melasma 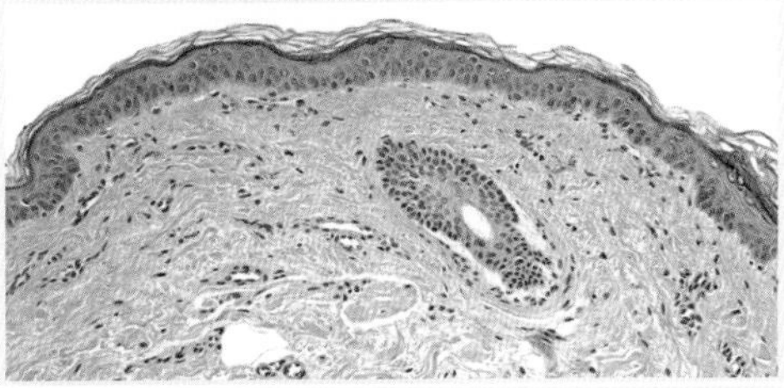	• Drug pigment
White	• Decreased melanin • Vasospasm • Deposition (e.g. calcium) • Keratin • Cellular proliferation (e.g. scar)	Example: Nevus anemicus 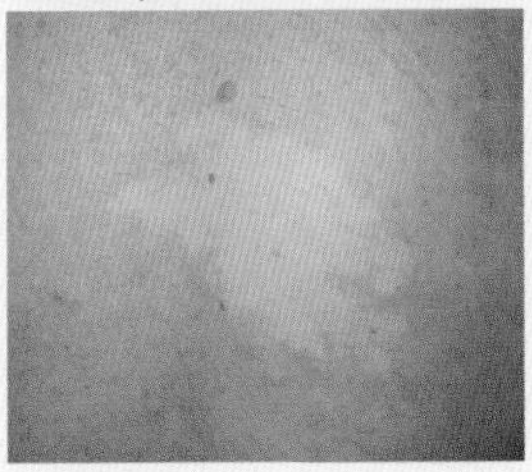	• Tattoo pigment

Fig. 1.51 Color as a clue to the clinical diagnosis. *Adapted from Bolognia JL, Jorizzo JL, Schaffer JV. Dermatology, 3e. London: Saunders, 2012, with permission.*

TYPES OF SCALE

Scale, Often Over Erythema

Key Differences (Fig. 1.52)

A. Psoriasis – silvery to white–yellow or micaceous

B. Pityriasis rosea – collarettes +/– central fine scale

C. Lichen planus – Wickham's striae

D. Seborrheic dermatitis – greasy

E. Nummular dermatitis – weeping

F. Lichen simplex chronicus – lichenified

G. Tinea versicolor – powdery (especially when lightly scraped)

H. Pemphigus foliaceus – cornflake-like

I. Erythema annulare centrifugum – trailing scale that is on the inner margin of the red, inflamed border

J. Tinea corporis – scale may be on the advancing, outer margin

Scale, Often Without Erythema

Epidermolytic hyperkeratosis – corrugated (arranged in parallel lines) *(Fig. 1.53A,B)*

Ichthyosis vulgaris – rectangular shapes with overlying fine white scale *(Fig. 1.53C,D)*

Lamellar – plate-like, lifting at edges *(Fig. 1.53E,F)*

X-linked – "dirty" appearance, preferentially affects the posterior neck and spares the body folds *(Fig. 1.53G,H)*

KERATODERMA

Diffuse – involving the entire palm or sole *(Fig. 1.54A)*

Focal – involving part of the palm or sole *(Fig. 1.54B)*

Punctate – small, discrete keratotic lesions on the palm or sole

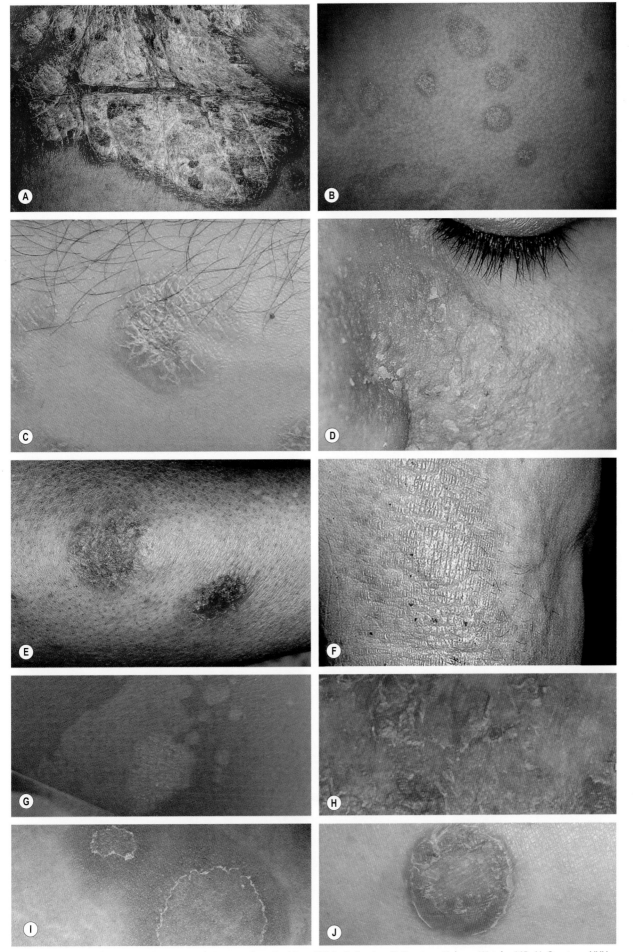

Fig. 1.52 Types of scale. *A,B,F, Courtesy, Yale Dermatology Residents' Slide Collection; E, Courtesy, Kalman Watsky, MD; H, Courtesy, NYU Slide Collection. A-F,H, From Bolognia JL, Jorizzo JL, Schaffer JV. Dermatology, 3e. London: Saunders, 2012, with permission. I, From Schwarzenberger K, Werchniak AE, Ko C. General Dermatology. London: Saunders, 2009.*

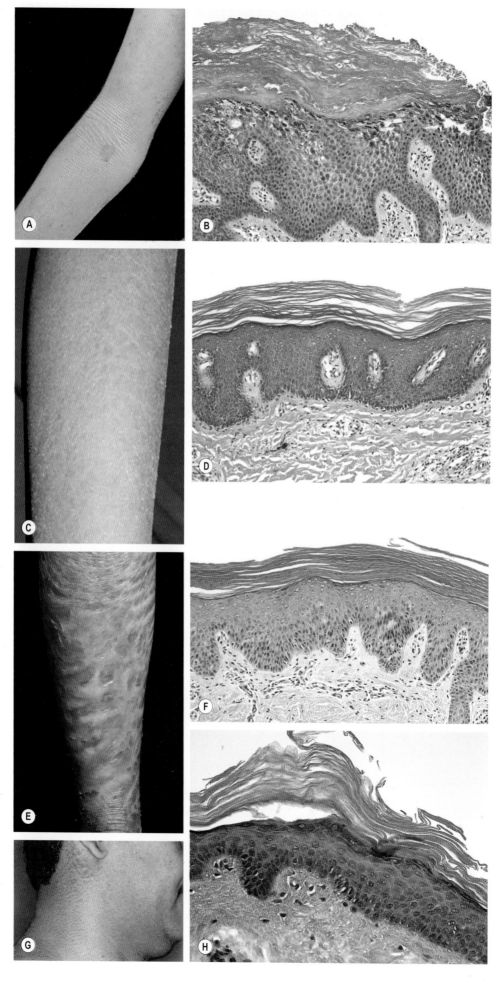

Fig. 1.53 Scale – often without erythema. A,B Epidermolytic ichthyosis. **C,D** Ichthyosis vulgaris. **E,F** Lamellar ichthyosis. **G,H** X-linked ichthyosis. *A,E Courtesy, Britt Craiglow, MD; C, Courtesy, Julie V Schaffer, MD; G, Courtesy, Gabriele Richard, MD and Franziska Ringpfeil, MD; H, From Fernandes NF, Janniger CK, Schwartz RA. X-linked ichthyosis: an oculocutaneous genodermatosis. J Am Acad Dermatol. 2010;62:480–85, © Elsevier.*

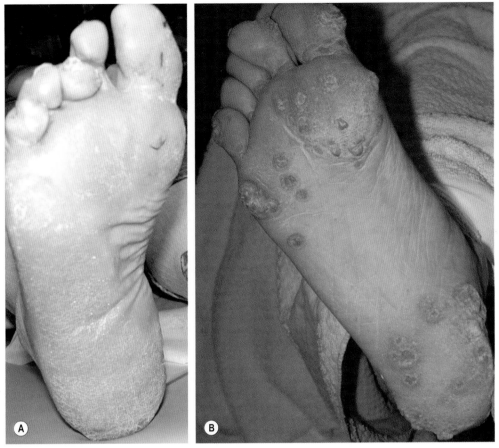

Fig. 1.54 Keratoderma. A Diffuse. **B** Focal. *Courtesy, Yale Dermatology Residents' Slide Collection.*

Differential Diagnosis for Given Body Sites and Morphology

2

While an elephant is easily recognizable given its distinctive features, larger cats are harder to tell apart, especially since we see them infrequently and rarely, if ever, see them side by side. However, there are distinguishing features, even just in the morphology of their spots. Knowing the concept is aided by seeing the spots side-by-side (see Table 1.2). In this vein, this chapter addresses disorders that can present on a given body site with a particular morphology, emphasizing key differences. Body sites include facial, body folds, acral, and truncal.

FACIAL

Multiple Papules, White–Yellow

Key Differences (Fig. 2.1)

- Cowden syndrome – verrucous (arrow) or smooth surfaced, may involve ears
- Birt-Hogg-Dubé syndrome – smooth, monomorphous, often on ears and neck as well as central face
- Syringomas – often clustered over eyelids
- Sebaceous hyperplasia – often umbilicated, yellowish papules

- Sebaceous tumors (especially sebaceous adenomas) – yellow to red papulonodules
- Milia/comedones – smooth, shiny papules; when punctured, keratin can be expressed
- Trichoepitheliomas – predilection for central face

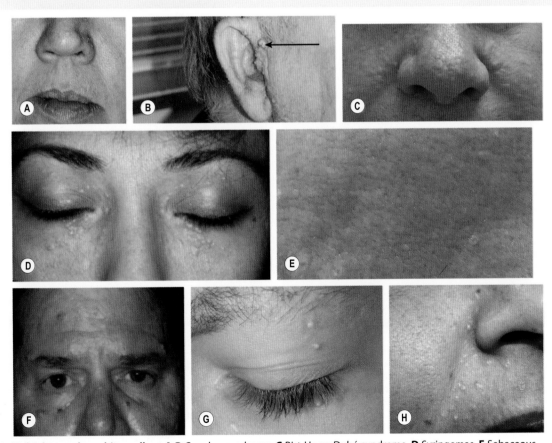

Fig. 2.1 Multiple papules, white–yellow. A,B Cowden syndrome. **C** Birt-Hogg-Dubé syndrome. **D** Syringomas. **E** Sebaceous hyperplasia. **F** Sebaceous adenomas in Muir–Torre syndrome. **G** Milia. **H** Multiple trichoepitheliomas. *A, Courtesy, Kalman Watsky, MD; B, Courtesy, Jennifer Choi, MD; C, Courtesy, Barry Goldberg, MD; D,G, Courtesy, Yale Dermatology Residents' Slide Collection; F, Courtesy, Dan Ring, MD; H, Courtesy, Sean Christensen, MD, PhD. A,F,G, From Bolognia JL, Jorizzo JL, Schaffer JV. Dermatology, 3e. London: Saunders, 2012, with permission.*

Multiple Papules, Red–Pink to Brown

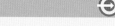

- Acne vulgaris – comedones and/or pustules present as well
- Acne rosacea – absent comedones, telangiectasias and/or crusting often evident
- Granulomatous rosacea – brown–pink discrete papules

- Angiofibromas of tuberous sclerosis – firm papules clustered near nose/nasolabial folds
- Trichoepitheliomas and/or cylindromas – nose/nasolabial folds or other parts of face, other stigmata of tuberous sclerosis absent

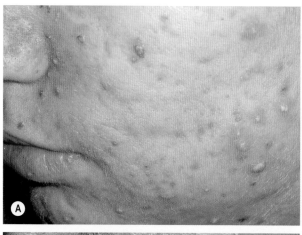

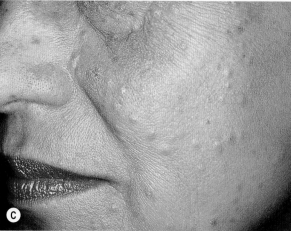

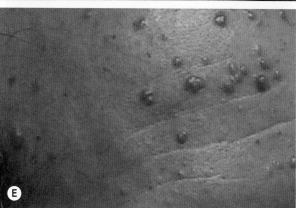

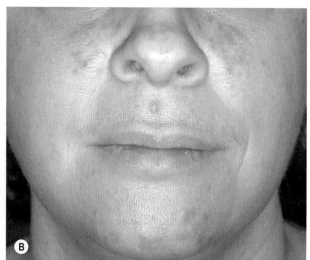

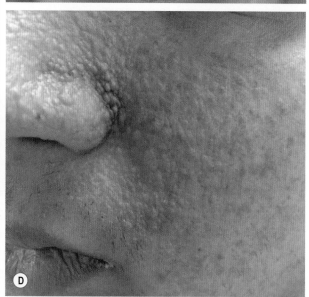

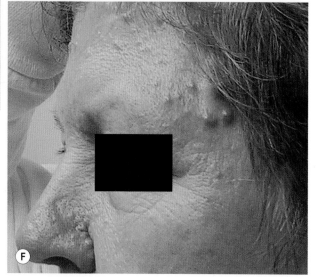

Fig. 2.2 Multiple papules, red–pink to brown. A Acne vulgaris. **B** Acne rosacea. **C** Granulomatous rosacea. **D** Angiofibromas of tuberous sclerosis. **E** Multiple familial trichoepitheliomas. **F** Multiple cylindromas. *A, Courtesy, Andrea L Zaenglein, MD and Diane Thiboutot, MD; B,C, Courtesy, Yale Dermatology Residents' Slide Collection; D, Courtesy, Brian Shuch, MD. A,C, From Bolognia JL, Jorizzo JL, Schaffer JV. Dermatology, 3e. London: Saunders, 2012, with permission.*

Acneiform Lesions

Key Differences (Fig. 2.3)

- Acne vulgaris – presence of open and closed comedones

- Steroid-induced rosacea – erythematous papules and papulopustules, absent comedones

- Periorificial dermatitis – monomorphous papules, confluent around the mouth

- Keratosis pilaris rubra – "grain-like" follicular papules on a background of erythema

- Trichostasis spinulosa – often on the nose, follicular orifices contain vellus hairs and keratinous debris that can be extruded with pressure

- Pseudofolliculitis barbae – follicular-based papules over the beard area

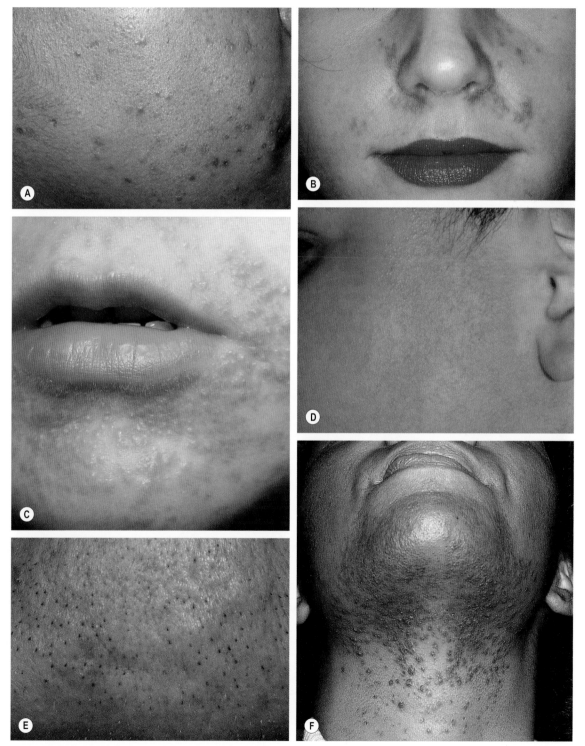

Fig. 2.3 Acneiform lesions. A Comedonal acne vulgaris. **B** Steroid rosacea. **C** Periorificial dermatitis. **D** Keratosis pilaris rubra. **E** Trichostasis spinulosa. **F** Pseudofolliculitis barbae. *A, Courtesy, Andrea L Zaenglein, MD and Diane Thiboutot, MD; B, Courtesy, Kalman Watsky, MD; C, Courtesy, Yale Dermatology Residents' Slide Collection; D, Courtesy, Julie V Schaffer, MD; E, Courtesy, Judit Stenn, MD; F, Courtesy, A Paul Kelly, MD. A,B,D–F, From Bolognia JL, Jorizzo JL, Schaffer JV. Dermatology, 3e. London: Saunders, 2012, with permission.*

Pustules

Pustules (see Chapter 7) may be sterile or due to an infectious agent, in which case culture studies and/or biopsy may be necessary for a definitive diagnosis.

Key Differences (Fig. 2.4)

- Acne vulgaris – comedones often present
- Acne rosacea – absent comedones, background erythema/telangiectasias

- Fungal or bacterial infection – erythematous plaque studded with pustules
- Herpes virus infection – clustered vesicles and/or pustules, base may be erythematous

---

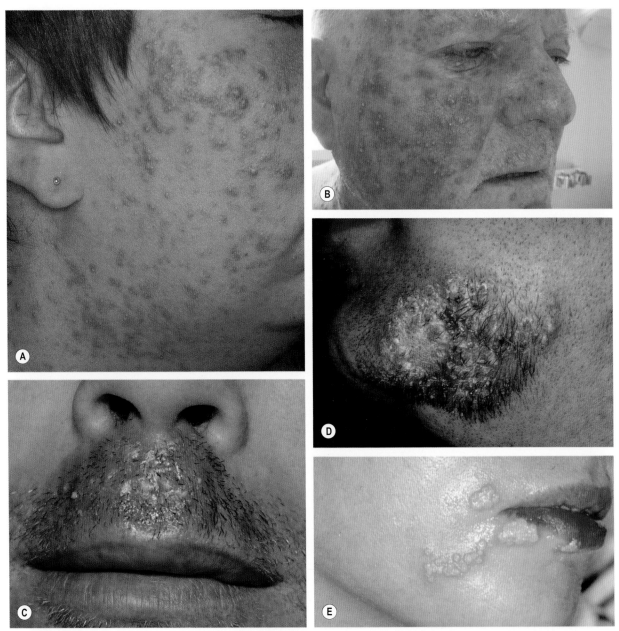

Fig. 2.4 Pustules. A Acne vulgaris. **B** Acne rosacea. **C** Fungal infection. **D** Staphylococcal folliculitis. **E** Herpes simplex virus infection. *A,C, Courtesy, Kalman Watsky, MD; B, Courtesy Uwe Wollina, MD; D, Courtesy, Yale Dermatology Residents' Slide Collection; E, Courtesy, Dirk Elston, MD. A,C,D, From Bolognia JL, Jorizzo JL, Schaffer JV. Dermatology, 3e. London: Saunders, 2012, with permission. B, From Wollina U. Rosacea and rhinophyma in the elderly. Clin Dermatol. 2011;29:61–8. E, From Elston D. Clinical image collection. Dermatopathology, 2e. London: Saunders, 2014.*

"Telangiectasia"

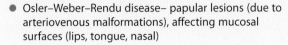

Key Differences (Fig. 2.5)

- CREST syndrome (limited scleroderma) – mat-like (squared-off) telangiectasias
- Osler–Weber–Rendu disease– papular lesions (due to arteriovenous malformations), affecting mucosal surfaces (lips, tongue, nasal)
- Rosacea – overlaps with dermatoheliosis in later stages
- Dermatoheliosis – telangiectasias and erythema over facial prominences

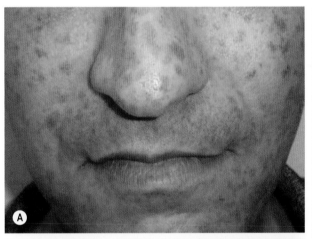

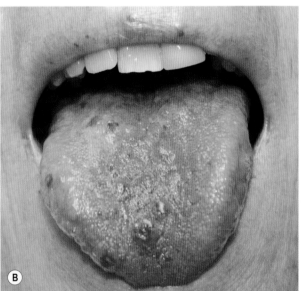

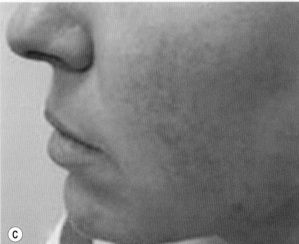

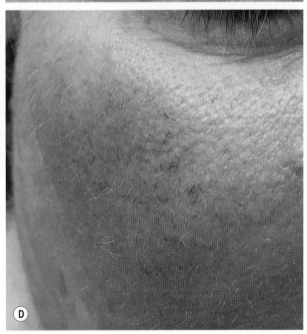

Fig. 2.5 Telangiectasia. A CREST syndrome. **B** Hereditary hemorrhagic telangiectasia (Osler–Weber–Rendu disease). **C** Erythematotelangiectatic rosacea. **D** Dermatoheliosis. *A, Courtesy, M Kari Connolly, MD; B, Courtesy, Yale Dermatology Residents' Slide Collection; C, From Two AM, Wu W, Gallo RL. Hata TR Rosacea : Part I. Introduction, categorization, histology, pathogenesis, and risk factors. J Am Acad Dermatol 2015; 72: 749–758, with permission. A, From Bolognia JL, Jorizzo JL, Schaffer JV. Dermatology, 3e. London: Saunders, 2012, with permission.*

Malar Erythema

Key Differences (Fig. 2.6)

- Rosacea – erythema is often fixed, telangiectasias in more advanced disease
- Acute lupus erythematosus – sparing of nasolabial folds, small erosions, scale may be present
- Dermatomyositis – involvement of eyelids and nasolabial folds
- Allergic contact dermatitis – edema and weeping lesions
- Pemphigus erythematosus – plaques with scale-crust and obvious erosions
- Seborrheic dermatitis – greasy scale, often accentuated in nasolabial folds

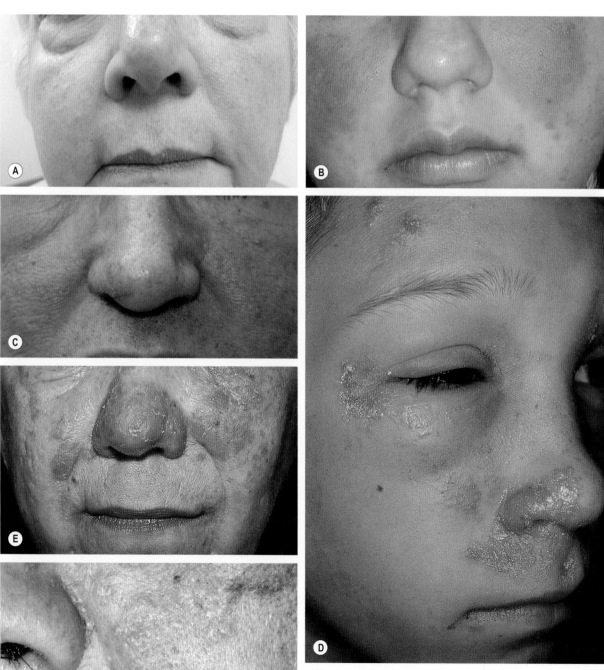

Fig. 2.6 Malar erythema. A Erythematotelangiectatic rosacea, early. **B** Lupus erythematosus, malar rash. **C** Dermatomyositis. **D** Allergic contact dermatitis, acute, secondary to poison ivy. **E** Pemphigus erythematosus. **F** Seborrheic dermatitis. *B,C, Courtesy, Yale Dermatology Residents' Slide Collection; D, Courtesy, Jean L Bolognia, MD; E, Courtesy, Ronald P Rapini, MD; F, Courtesy, Dirk Elston, MD. D,E, From Bolognia JL, Jorizzo JL, Schaffer JV. Dermatology, 3e. London: Saunders, 2012, with permission. F, From Elston D. Clinical image collection. Dermatopathology, 2e. London: Saunders, 2014.*

Juicy Papules/Plaques/Nodules

The infiltrate may be lymphocytic, mixed, neutrophilic, or granulomatous.

Key Differences (Fig. 2.7)

Lymphocytic

- Lymphoma:
  - Folliculotropic mycosis fungoides – infiltrated plaque with loss of eyebrow hair
  - B-cell lymphoma – pink–red to purple papulonodules
- Lupus tumidus – pink–violet plaques
- Lymphocytic infiltrate of Jessner – often annular, absent scale
- Polymorphous light eruption – edematous pink lesions, occur minutes to hours after sun exposure in spring and early summer

Mixed

- Granuloma faciale – red–brown plaque with prominent follicular orifices

Neutrophilic

- Sweet's syndrome – crusted bright red papulonodules

Granulomatous

- Sarcoidosis – often affects the nose, infiltrated violaceous to red–brown plaque

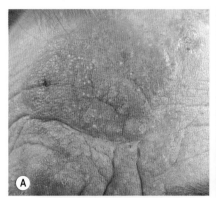
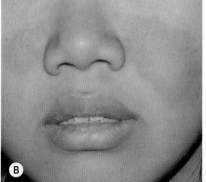
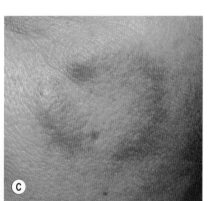
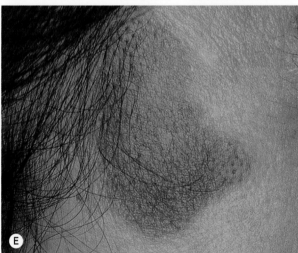
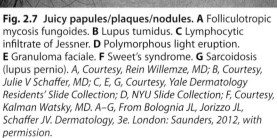
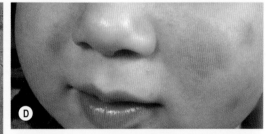
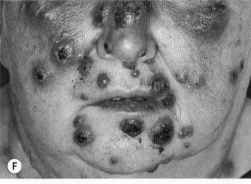
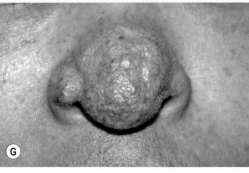

Fig. 2.7 Juicy papules/plaques/nodules. A Folliculotropic mycosis fungoides. **B** Lupus tumidus. **C** Lymphocytic infiltrate of Jessner. **D** Polymorphous light eruption. **E** Granuloma faciale. **F** Sweet's syndrome. **G** Sarcoidosis (lupus pernio). *A, Courtesy, Rein Willemze, MD; B, Courtesy, Julie V Schaffer, MD; C, E, G, Courtesy, Yale Dermatology Residents' Slide Collection; D, NYU Slide Collection; F, Courtesy, Kalman Watsky, MD. A–G, From Bolognia JL, Jorizzo JL, Schaffer JV. Dermatology, 3e. London: Saunders, 2012, with permission.*

Flat Brown Patch

May be secondary to increased melanocytes, increased melanin, and/or dermal pigment.

Key Differences (Fig. 2.8)

- Lentigo maligna (melanoma *in situ*) – irregular with color variation
- Melasma – evenly light brown with an irregular border
- Hori nevus – light brown to blue–gray macules clustering into patches, on cheeks, typically in Asian women

- Ochronosis – brown to black patches secondary to topical hydroquinone

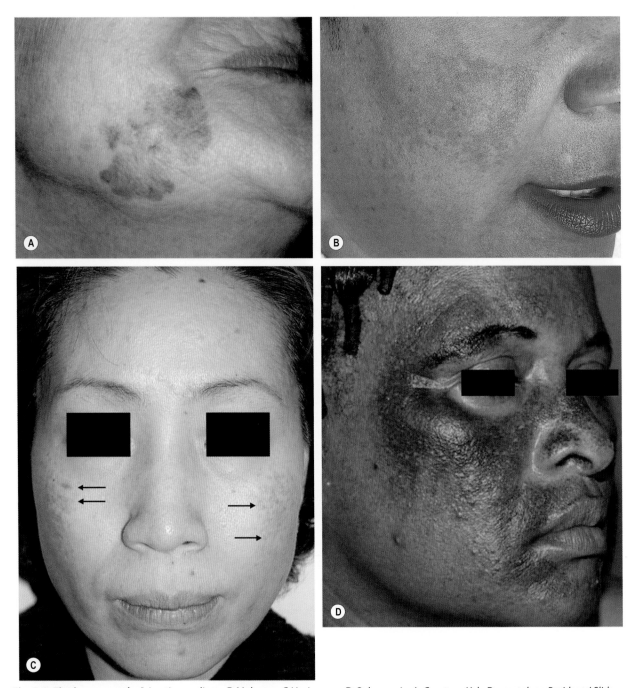

Fig. 2.8 Flat brown patch. A Lentigo maligna. **B** Melasma. **C** Hori nevus. **D** Ochronosis. *A, Courtesy, Yale Dermatology Residents' Slide Collection. B, Courtesy, NYU Slide Collection. D, Courtesy, Regional Dermatology Training Centre, Moshi, Tanzania. A,B, From Bolognia JL, Jorizzo JL, Schaffer JV. Dermatology, 3e. London: Saunders, 2012, with permission. C From, Park JM, Tsao H, Tsao S. Acquired bilateral nevus of Ota-like macules (Hori nevus). J Am Acad Dermatol. 2009;61:88–93. D, From Bolognia JL, Schaffer JV, Duncan KO, Ko CJ. Dermatology Essentials, 1e. Philadelphia: Saunders, 2014, with permission.*

Annular or Serpiginous

Key Differences (Fig. 2.9)

- Tinea faciei – scale may be minimal, pustules may be present
- Seborrheic dermatitis, petaloid – abundant scale

- Annular elastolytic giant cell granuloma – central clearing, pink–red rim with minimal scale
- Lymphocytic infiltrate of Jessner – absent scale (*see Fig. 2.7C*)

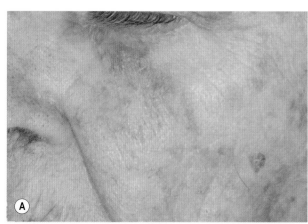

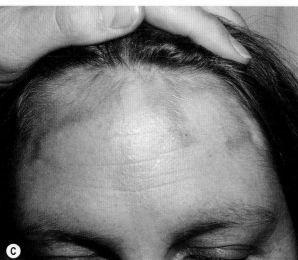

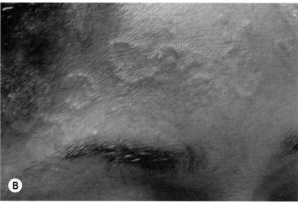

Fig. 2.9 Annular or serpiginous. A Tinea faciei. **B** Seborrheic dermatitis. **C** Annular elastolytic giant cell granuloma (actinic granuloma). *A, Courtesy, Jean L Bolognia, MD. From Bolognia JL, Jorizzo JL, Schaffer JV. Dermatology, 3e. London: Saunders, 2012, with permission. C, From James WD, Berger T, Elston D. Andrews' Diseases of the Skin, 11e. Edinburgh: Saunders, 2011, with permission.*

Lip Swelling

May be secondary to edema, an infiltrative process, or a tumor.

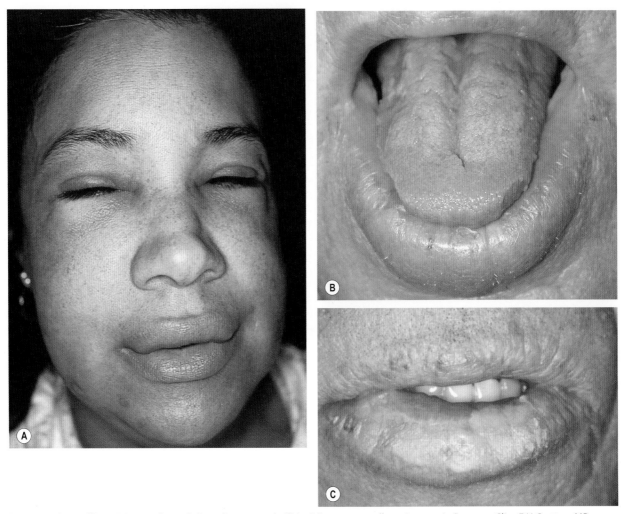

Fig. 2.10 Lip swelling. A Angioedema. **B** Granulomatous cheilitis. **C** Squamous cell carcinoma. *A, Courtesy, Clive E H Grattan, MD; B, Courtesy, Yale Dermatology Residents' Slide Collection; C, Courtesy, H Peter Sawyer, MD. A,C, From Bolognia JL, Jorizzo JL, Schaffer JV. Dermatology, 3e. London: Saunders, 2012, with permission.*

Tongue

Key Differences (Fig. 2.11)

- Geographic tongue – well-delineated erythema with white serpiginous borders
- Fissured (scrotal) tongue – furrows and grooves
- Amyloidosis – macroglossia (impressions of teeth may be evident on lateral borders)
- Hairy tongue – elongated, discolored papillae
- Median rhomboid glossitis – diamond to oval area of erythema and atrophy, often due to local overgrowth of *Candida*

- Thrush – solid white plaques in random distribution
- Oral hairy leukoplakia – shaggy white plaques on lateral tongue
- Lichen planus – erosions, lacy white plaques, and/or scarring

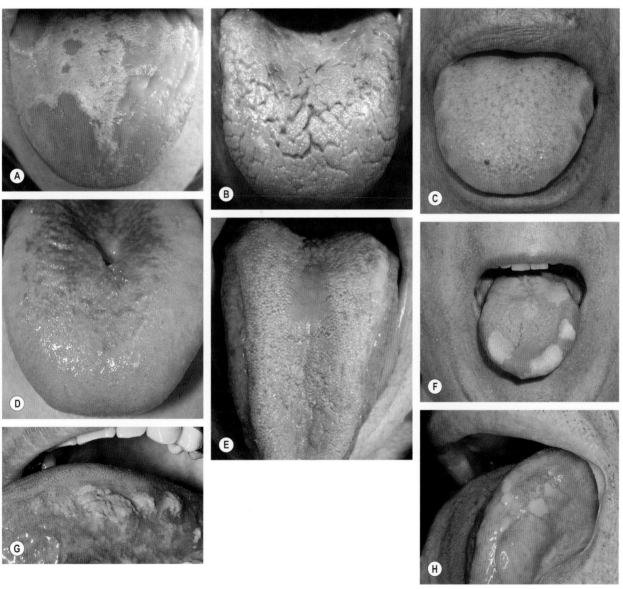

Fig. 2.11 Tongue. A Geographic tongue. **B** Fissured tongue. **C** Amyloidosis (macroglossia). **D** Hairy tongue. **E** Median rhomboid glossitis. **F** Thrush. **G** Oral hairy leukoplakia. **H** Lichen planus. *A–D, Courtesy, Yale Dermatology Residents' Slide Collection; E, Courtesy, NYU Slide Collection; G, Courtesy, Carl M Allen, MD, and Charles Camisa, MD; H, Courtesy, Louis A Fragola, Jr, MD. E,G, From Bolognia JL, Schaffer JV, Duncan KO, Ko CJ. Dermatology Essentials, 1e. Philadelphia: Saunders, 2014, with permission. F,H, From Bolognia JL, Jorizzo JL, Schaffer JV. Dermatology, 3e. London: Saunders, 2012, with permission.*

Gingiva

- Desquamative (erosive) gingivitis – erythema and erosions, associated with blistering disorders like cicatricial pemphigoid and pemphigus vulgaris

- Gingival hyperplasia – due to medications (e.g. phenytoin, cyclosporine), mouth breathing, poor hygiene, infiltrative processes

- Strawberry gums – red–purple gingiva, resembling strawberries

- Cobblestoning – numerous papules

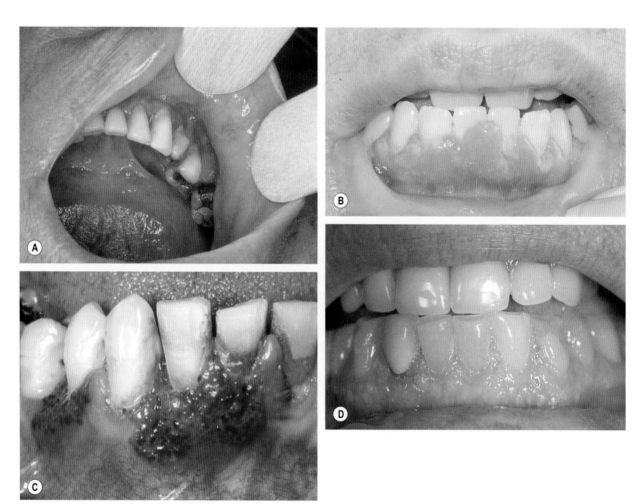

Fig. 2.12 Gingiva. A Desquamative gingivitis. **B** Gingival hyperplasia. **C** Strawberry gums in Wegener's granulomatosis. **D** Gingival cobblestoning in Cowden syndrome. *A,B, Courtesy, Yale Dermatology Residents' Slide Collection; C, Courtesy Carl M Allen, MD, and Charles Camisa, MD. D, Courtesy, Jeffrey Callen, MD. A,C,D, From Bolognia JL, Jorizzo JL, Schaffer JV. Dermatology, 3e. London: Saunders, 2012, with permission.*

Buccal Mucosa

Key Differences (Fig. 2.13)

- Morsicatio buccarum – shaggy white plaque along bite line

- Lichen planus – lacy white plaques, erosions may be evident
- Thrush – cottage cheese-like

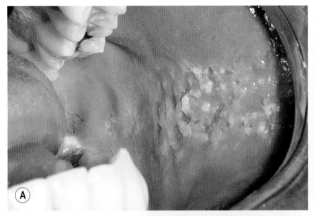

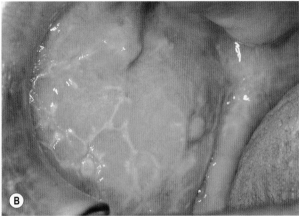

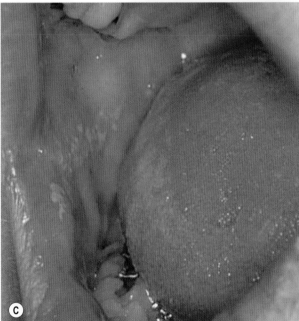

Fig. 2.13 Buccal mucosa. A Morsicatio buccarum. **B** Lichen planus. **C** Thrush. *A, Courtesy Carl M Allen, MD, and Charles Camisa, MD; B, Courtesy, Yale Dermatology Residents' Slide Collection; C, Courtesy, Judit Stenn, MD. A–C, From Bolognia JL, Jorizzo JL, Schaffer JV. Dermatology, 3e. London: Saunders, 2012, with permission.*

BODY FOLDS

Diaper Area (Infants)

Key Differences (Fig. 2.14)

- Irritant contact dermatitis – spares folds
- Candidiasis – bright red erythema, satellite papulopustules (arrows)
- Seborrheic dermatitis – moist/scaly plaques, involving folds
- Psoriasis – well-demarcated, uniformly pink plaques, psoriatic lesions outside of body folds
- Langerhans cell histiocytosis – petechiae, erosions/ulcers

Perineum/Groin of Adults

Key Differences (Fig. 2.15)

- Intertrigo – moist appearance
- Inverse psoriasis – well-demarcated uniformly pink–red patches
- Tinea – often spares scrotum, annular border
- Candidiasis – often involves scrotum, satellite papulopustules
- Erythrasma – pink to brown scaly patches, pink fluorescence under Wood's lamp
- Hailey–Hailey disease – irregularly cracked appearance of linear erosions
- Extramammary Paget's disease – white hyperkeratosis intermixed with red eroded foci
- Langerhans cell histiocytosis – petechiae and erosions

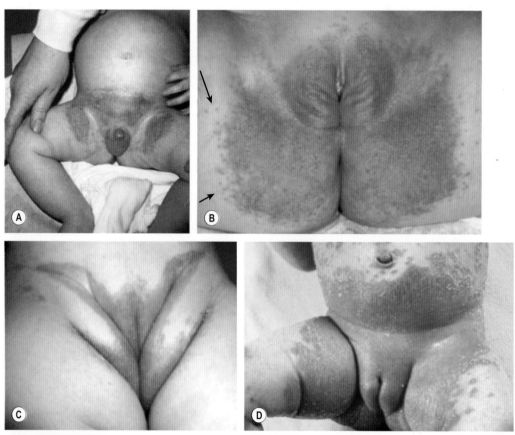

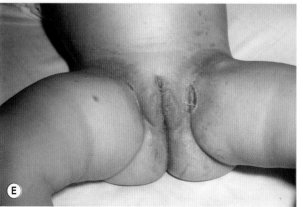

Fig. 2.14 Diaper area (infants). A Irritant contact dermatitis. **B** Candidiasis. **C** Seborrheic dermatitis. **D** Psoriasis. **E** Langerhans cell histiocytosis. *A–D, From Schachner LA, Hansen RE. Pediatric Dermatology, 4e. London: Mosby, 2011, with permission. E, Courtesy, Irwin Braverman, MD.*

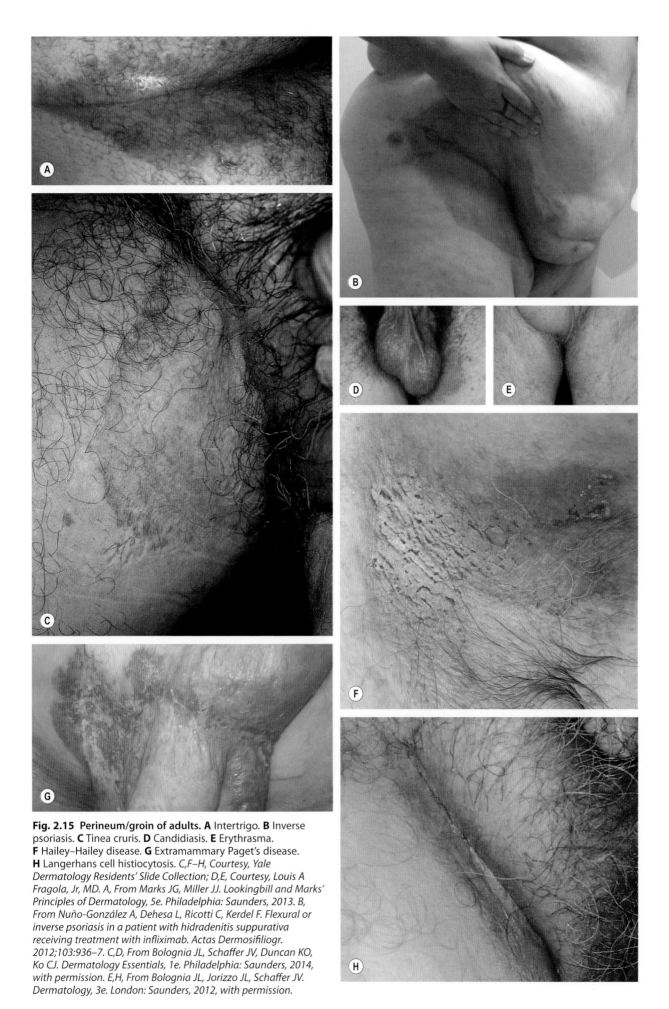

Fig. 2.15 Perineum/groin of adults. A Intertrigo. **B** Inverse psoriasis. **C** Tinea cruris. **D** Candidiasis. **E** Erythrasma. **F** Hailey–Hailey disease. **G** Extramammary Paget's disease. **H** Langerhans cell histiocytosis. *C,F–H, Courtesy, Yale Dermatology Residents' Slide Collection; D,E, Courtesy, Louis A Fragola, Jr, MD. A, From Marks JG, Miller JJ. Lookingbill and Marks' Principles of Dermatology, 5e. Philadelphia: Saunders, 2013. B, From Nuño-González A, Dehesa L, Ricotti C, Kerdel F. Flexural or inverse psoriasis in a patient with hidradenitis suppurativa receiving treatment with infliximab. Actas Dermosifiliogr. 2012;103:936–7. C,D, From Bolognia JL, Schaffer JV, Duncan KO, Ko CJ. Dermatology Essentials, 1e. Philadelphia: Saunders, 2014, with permission. E,H, From Bolognia JL, Jorizzo JL, Schaffer JV. Dermatology, 3e. London: Saunders, 2012, with permission.*

Vulvar Rash

- Lichen sclerosus – initially affects the clitoral hood and the perineal body, petechiae may be evident; shiny ivory–white plaque is classic; late stage with scarring
- Lichen planus – lacy white hyperkeratosis (arrow) may be evident, erosions often present on mucosal surfaces, late stage with scarring
- Lichen simplex chronicus – thickening (lichenification) +/– erythema
- Psoriasis – red plaques that may be well-demarcated
- Hailey–Hailey disease – irregularly cracked appearance of linear erosions

Perianal Rash

- Perianal streptococcal disease – sharply demarcated bright, moist erythema extending from the anal verge
- Lichen sclerosus – ivory–white foci (arrow)
- Psoriasis – well-demarcated uniformly pink–red
- Irritant contact dermatitis (erosive perianal eruption) – often due to frequent stooling and/or diarrhea in young babies, favors convex surfaces
- Hand, foot, and mouth disease – circular erosions and papulovesicles
- Zinc deficiency – perianal weepy plaques with peripheral crusting

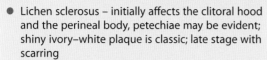

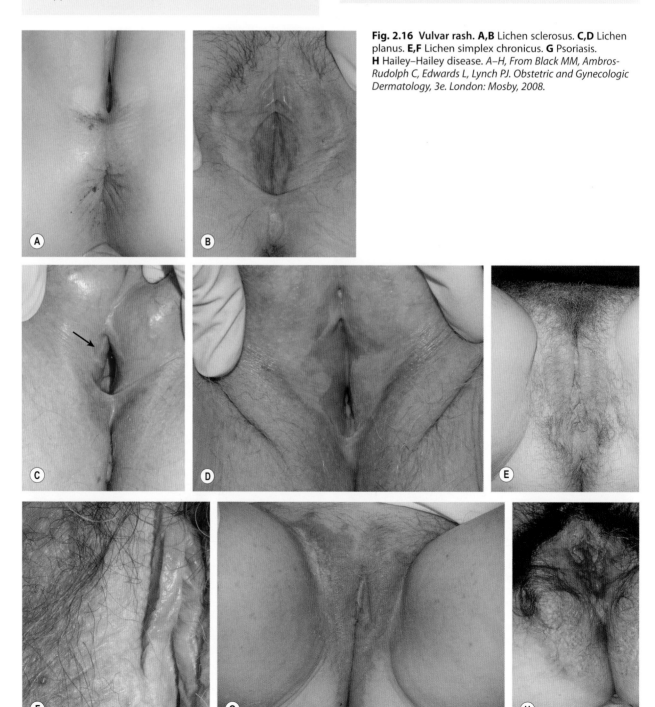

Fig. 2.16 Vulvar rash. **A,B** Lichen sclerosus. **C,D** Lichen planus. **E,F** Lichen simplex chronicus. **G** Psoriasis. **H** Hailey–Hailey disease. *A–H, From Black MM, Ambros-Rudolph C, Edwards L, Lynch PJ. Obstetric and Gynecologic Dermatology, 3e. London: Mosby, 2008.*

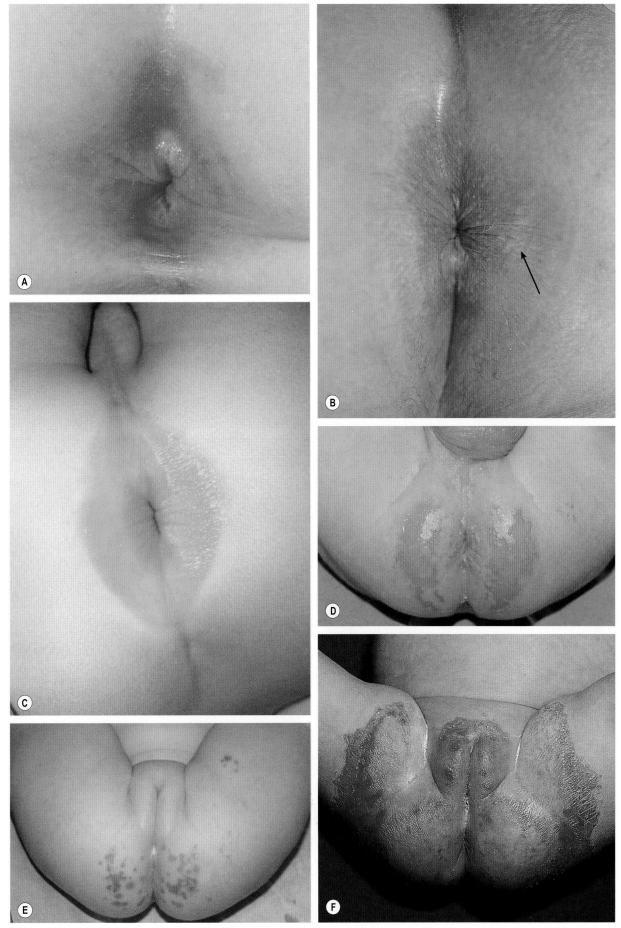

Fig. 2.17 Perianal rash. A Perianal streptococcal disease. **B** Lichen sclerosus. **C** Psoriasis. **D** Irritant contact dermatitis. **E** Hand, foot, and mouth disease. **F** Zinc deficiency. *B, Courtesy, Susan M Cooper, MD. A, Courtesy, Julie V Schaffer, MD. A,B, From Bolognia JL, Jorizzo JL, Schaffer JV. Dermatology, 3e. London: Saunders, 2012, with permission. C–F, From Eichenfield LF, Frieden IJ, Zaenglein AL, Mathes E. Neonatal and Infant Dermatology, 3e. London: Saunders, 2014.*

Palmar Rash

Key Differences (Fig. 2.18)

- Atopic dermatitis – weeping lesions, often with foci of lichenification
- Dyshidrosis – deep-seated vesicles on lateral surfaces of fingers
- Psoriasis – adherent, dry white–yellow scale over erythema

- Tinea – scale accentuated in creases, one hand may be spared
- Contact dermatitis – irritant and allergic forms can be indistinguishable; patch testing is important
- Crusted scabies – prominent hyperkeratosis over hands and subungually

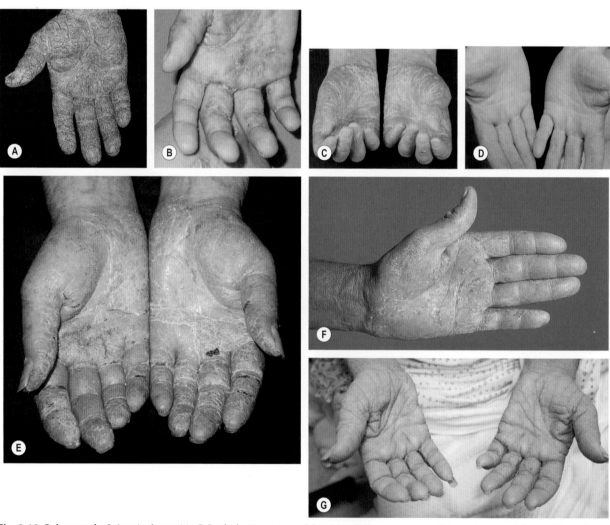

Fig. 2.18 **Palmar rash. A** Atopic dermatitis. **B** Dyshidrotic eczema. **C** Psoriasis. **D** Tinea manuum. **E** Irritant contact dermatitis. **F** Allergic contact dermatitis to chromate found in cement. **G** Crusted scabies. *A,D,G, Courtesy, Yale Dermatology Residents' Slide Collection; B, Courtesy, Dirk Elston, MD; C, Courtesy, Peter C M van de Kerkhof, MD; E, Courtesy, Kalman Watsky, MD; F, Courtesy, Peter S Friedmann, MD, and Mark Wilkinson, MD. A,C–F, From Bolognia JL, Jorizzo JL, Schaffer JV. Dermatology, 3e. London: Saunders, 2012, with permission. B, From Schachner LA, Hansen RE. Pediatric Dermatology, 4e. London: Mosby, 2011.*

Palmar Macules

- Erythema multiforme – target lesions with 3 zones; central zone may be vesicular
- Syphilis, secondary – brown–red macules, sometimes with a collarette of scale

Discrete Palmar Keratotic Lesions

- Dyshidrotic eczema – deep-seated vesicles (discrete spheres), often on the lateral fingers
- Scabies – linear burrows
- Keratolysis exfoliativa – annular white scale

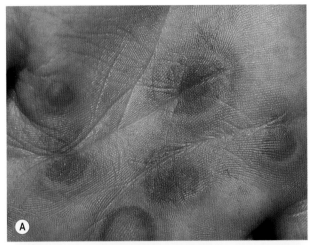

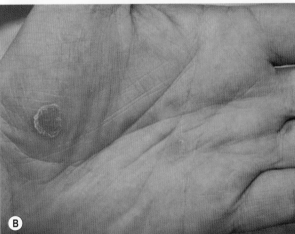

Fig. 2.19 Palmar macules. A Erythema multiforme. **B** Secondary syphilis. *A, Courtesy, William Weston, MD; B, Courtesy, Yale Dermatology Residents' Slide Collection. A, From Bolognia JL, Jorizzo JL, Schaffer JV. Dermatology, 3e. London: Saunders, 2012, with permission.*

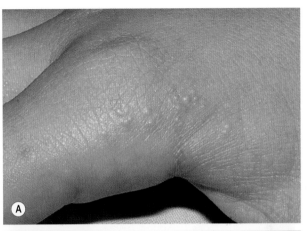

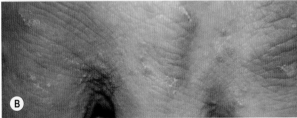

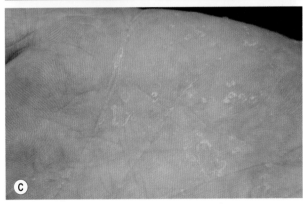

Fig. 2.20 Discrete palmar keratotic lesions. A Dyshidrotic eczema. **B** Scabies. **C** Keratolysis exfoliativa. *A, Courtesy, Anne Lucky, MD; B,C, Courtesy, Yale Dermatology Residents' Slide Collection. A, From Schachner LA, Hansen RE. Pediatric Dermatology, 4e. London: Mosby, 2011.*

Lower Leg Rash

Key Differences (Fig. 2.21)

- Stasis dermatitis – erythema, wet scale, often bilateral
- Lipodermatosclerosis – warm erythema when acute, tight skin, begins above the medial malleolus
- Cellulitis – warm, tender, often unilateral, expansion without treatment; associated fever and elevated white blood cell count
- Necrobiosis lipoidica – yellowish center, often with telangiectasia

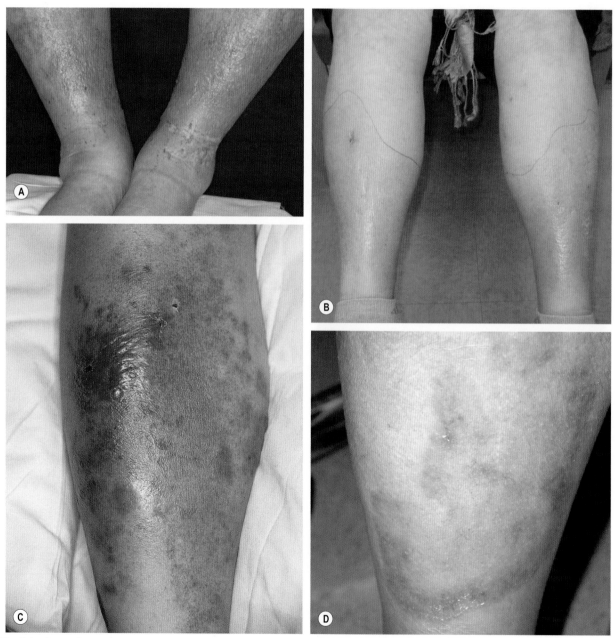

Fig. 2.21 Lower leg rash. A Stasis dermatitis. **B** Lipodermatosclerosis. **C** Cellulitis. **D** Necrobiosis lipoidica. *C,D, Courtesy, Yale Dermatology Residents' Slide Collection. A, From Elston D. Clinical image collection. Dermatopathology, 2e. London: Saunders, 2014. C, From Bolognia JL, Jorizzo JL, Schaffer JV. Dermatology, 3e. London: Saunders, 2012, with permission.*

Plantar Keratotic Lesions

Key Differences (Fig. 2.22)

- Pitted keratolysis – punched-out craters, favor pressure points
- Punctate keratoderma – discrete foci of hyperkeratosis

- Plantar warts – black dots, representing thrombosed capillaries

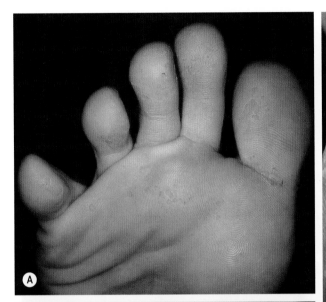

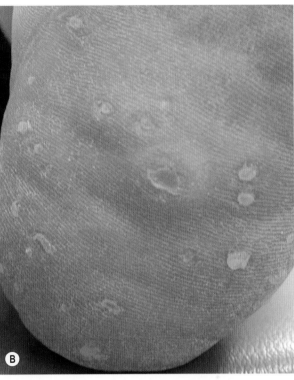

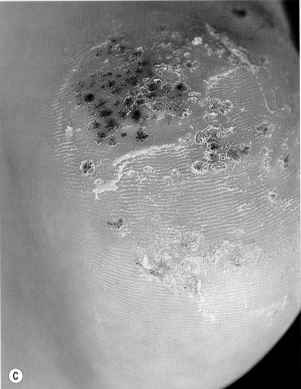

Fig. 2.22 Plantar keratotic lesions. A Pitted keratolysis.
B Punctate keratoderma. **C** Plantar warts. *A, Courtesy, Kalman Watsky, MD; B, Courtesy, Yale Dermatology Residents' Slide Collection; C, Courtesy, Reinhard Kimabuer, MD, and Petra Lenz, MD. A,C, From Bolognia JL, Jorizzo JL, Schaffer JV. Dermatology, 3e. London: Saunders, 2012, with permission.*

Plantar Rash

Key Differences (Fig. 2.23)

- Tinea pedis – fine scale, hand or nails may be infected as well; pustules may be present
- Psoriasis – well-demarcated plaques with adherent thick scale

- Contact dermatitis – patch testing often necessary, distribution may give clue to the contactant
- Juvenile plantar dermatosis – glazed appearance

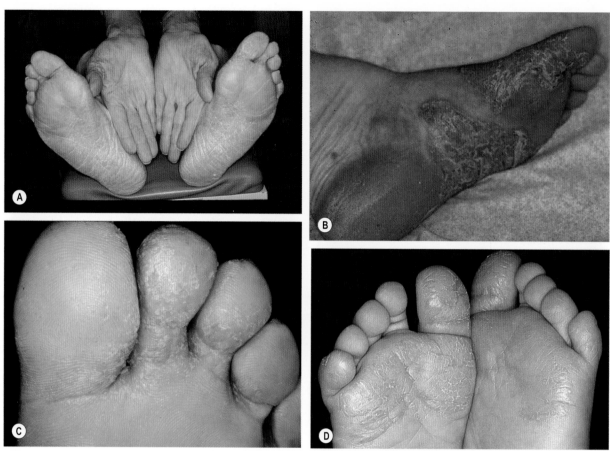

Fig. 2.23 Plantar rash. A Tinea pedis. **B** Psoriasis. **C** Contact dermatitis. **D** Juvenile plantar dermatosis. *A, Courtesy, Yale Dermatology Residents' Slide Collection; C, Courtesy, Louis A Fragola, Jr, MD; D, Courtesy, Kalman Watsky, MD. A,C,D, From Bolognia JL, Jorizzo JL, Schaffer JV. Dermatology, 3e. London: Saunders, 2012, with permission. B, From Menter A, Korman NJ, Elmets CA, et al. Guidelines of care for the management of psoriasis and psoriatic arthritis. J Am Acad Dermatol. 2011:65:137–74.*

TRUNCAL

May be due to an infiltrative process (i.e. mast cells, histiocytes, granulomatous diseases) or a tumor.

Red–Brown to Pink Papules

Key Differences (Fig. 2.24)

- Mastocytosis – evenly pigmented red–brown papules, can blister with stroking
- Histiocytosis – discrete red–brown papules
- Benign nevi – brown papules and macules
- Leiomyoma (pilar) – linear papules, often clustered
- Neurofibromas – soft, skin-colored to pinkish-tan, dome-shaped or polypoid, well-demarcated papules and nodules of various sizes, ill-defined violaceous lesions

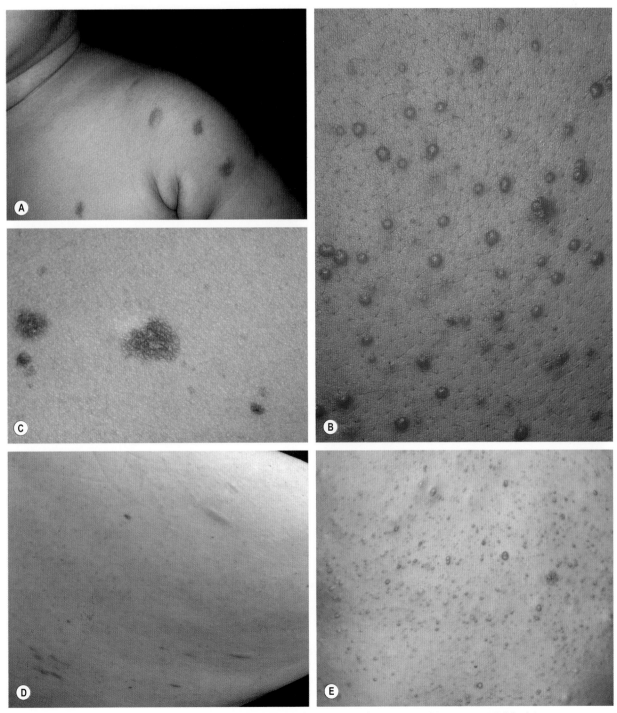

Fig. 2.24 Red–brown to pink papules. A Mastocytosis. **B** Generalized eruptive histicytoma. **C** Benign nevi. **D** Pilar leiomyomas. **E** Neurofibromas. *A, Courtesy, Michael Tharp, MD; B, Courtesy, Yale Dermatology Residents' Slide Collection; C, Courtesy, Jean L Bolognia, MD; E, Courtesy, Julie V Schaffer, MD. A,B,E, From Bolognia JL, Jorizzo JL, Schaffer JV. Dermatology, 3e. London: Saunders, 2012, with permission.*

Rash on the Back, Hospitalized Patient

⊕→

Key Differences (Fig. 2.25)

- Drug eruption – confluent pink macules and papules that extend beyond the back

- Grover's disease – eroded pink papules, often sparing the buttocks
- Folliculitis – follicular papulopustules

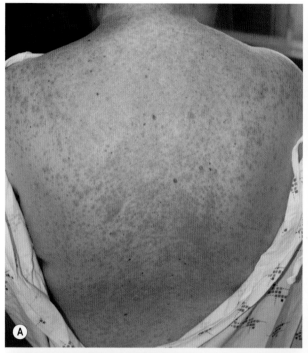

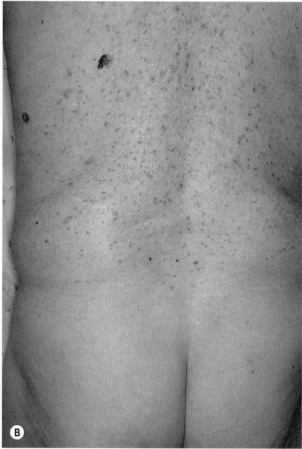

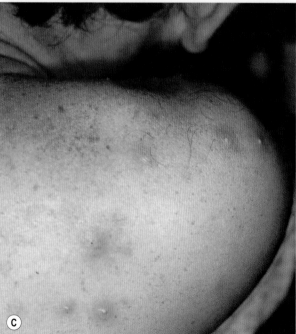

Fig. 2.25 Rash on the back, hospitalized patient. A Drug eruption to vemurafenib. **B** Grover's disease. **C** Folliculitis. *A,C, Courtesy, Yale Dermatology Residents' Slide Collection; B, Courtesy, Jean L Bolognia, MD. B,C, From Bolognia JL, Jorizzo JL, Schaffer JV. Dermatology, 3e. London: Saunders, 2012, with permission.*

Pigment Change on Upper Back

Key Differences (Fig. 2.26)

- Macular/biphasic amyloidosis – rippled pattern of hyperpigmentation

- Scleroderma – salt and pepper pattern of pigment loss

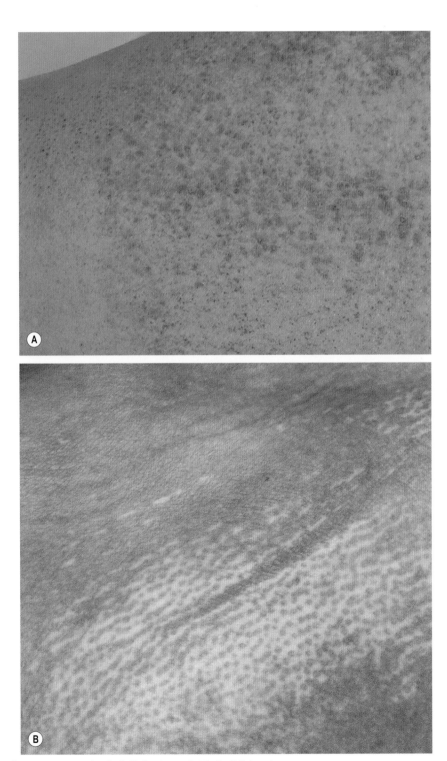

Fig. 2.26 **Pigment change on upper back.** **A** Biphasic amyloidosis. **B** Scleroderma.

Distribution – Specific Differentials | 3

This chapter covers three major patterns of involvement: erythroderma, photodistribution, and mosaic (linear) lesions. Solitary pigmented lesions are also addressed, as visual recognition of melanoma and its mimics is important.

ERYTHRODERMA (GENERALIZED ERYTHEMA)

Erythroderma (generalized erythema) can be due to many different diseases. The color of the erythema, the presence/absence and quality of scale, and particular associated clues are helpful in separating these diseases *(Table 3.1; Figs 3.1–3.4)*. History and laboratory findings may also be useful.

Atopic dermatitis and other eczematous processes as well as other diseases can also present with erythroderma *(Figs 3.5–3.6)*.

Table 3.1 Erythroderma (generalized erythema)

Selected entities	Clinical	Salient clues, if present
Pityriasis rubra pilaris	• Salmon-pink to orange color • Fine scale	• Islands of sparing *(Fig. 3.1A)* • Follicular papules *(Fig. 3.1B)* • Waxy palmoplantar keratoderma *(Fig. 3.1C)* • Nails: thickened • History of cephalocaudal spread
Psoriasis	• Pink–red color *(Fig. 3.2A)* • Silvery to white thick adherent scale, when present *(Fig. 3.2B)*	• Pustules • Nails: pitting or other changes • History of plaque-type psoriasis
Congenital ichthyosiform erythroderma (autosomal recessive congenital ichthyosis)	• Red–pink color *(Fig. 3.3A–D)* • Fine scale (may also have focal lamellar scales) *(Fig. 3.3 A–C)*	• Ectropion • History of collodion membrane at birth
Erythrodermic mycosis fungoides	• Bright red color • Variable scale	• Lymphadenopathy • History of mycosis fungoides
Sézary syndrome *(Fig. 3.4)*		• Distinguished from erythrodermic mycosis fungoides by circulating abnormal lymphocytes

Note: Not uncommonly, erythroderma can also be drug-induced or of unknown cause (idiopathic), or due to other disorders. *(See also Figs 3.5, 3.6.)*

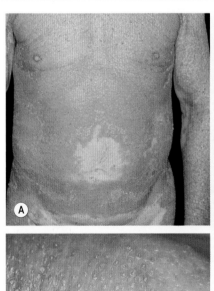

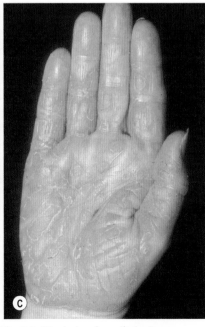

Fig. 3.1 Pityriasis rubra pilaris. *From Schwarzenberger K, Werchniak AE, Ko C. General Dermatology. London: Saunders, 2009.*

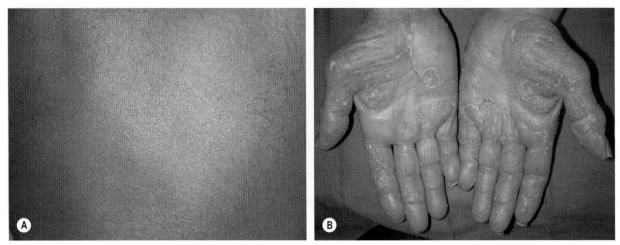

Fig. 3.2 Psoriasis, erythrodermic. *Courtesy, Yale Dermatology Residents' Slide Collection.*

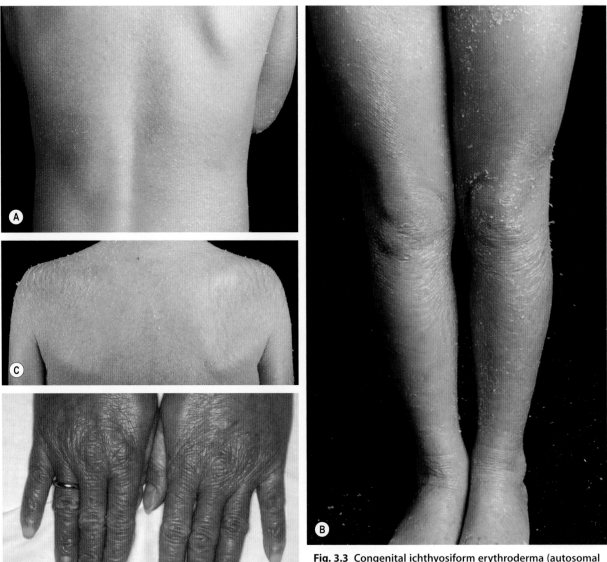

Fig. 3.3 Congenital ichthyosiform erythroderma (autosomal recessive congenital ichthyosis). *A–C, Courtesy, Britt Craiglow, MD; D, Courtesy, Leonard Milstone, MD.*

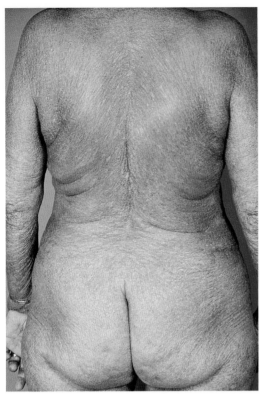

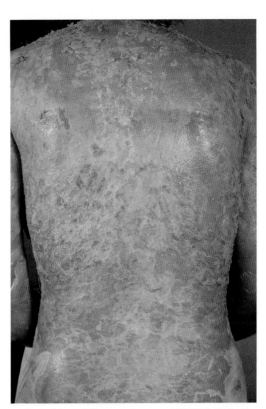

Fig. 3.4 Sézary syndrome. *Courtesy, Rein Willemze, MD. From Bolognia JL, Jorizzo JL, Schaffer JV. Dermatology, 3e. London: Saunders, 2012, with permission.*

Fig. 3.5 Pemphigus foliaceus. *Courtesy, NYU Slide Collection. From Bolognia JL, Jorizzo JL, Schaffer JV. Dermatology, 3e. London: Saunders, 2012, with permission.*

Fig. 3.6 Toxic epidermal necrolysis-like presentation of acute lupus erythematosus (acute syndrome of apoptotic pan-epidermolysis [ASAP]). *Courtesy, Yale Dermatology Residents' Slide Collection. From Bolognia JL, Jorizzo JL, Schaffer JV. Dermatology, 3e. London: Saunders, 2012, with permission.*

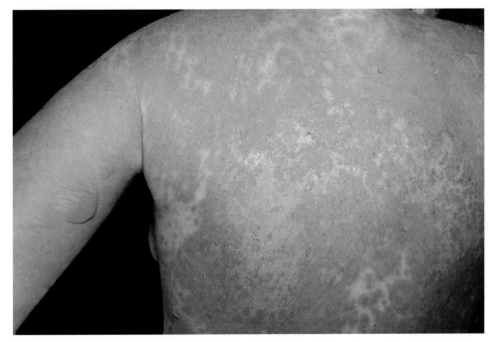

PHOTODISTRIBUTION

Once a photodistribution is determined *(see Fig. 1.16A, Fig. 3.7)*, the primary involvement of the epidermis versus dermis and the morphology of primary lesions aid in narrowing the differential; for example, epidermal reactions including acute to chronic eczematous/ spongiotic changes *(Fig. 3.8)*, epidermal vesiculation *(Fig. 3.9)*, erythematous papules and plaques *(Fig. 3.10)*, and pigmented patches *(Fig. 3.11)*.

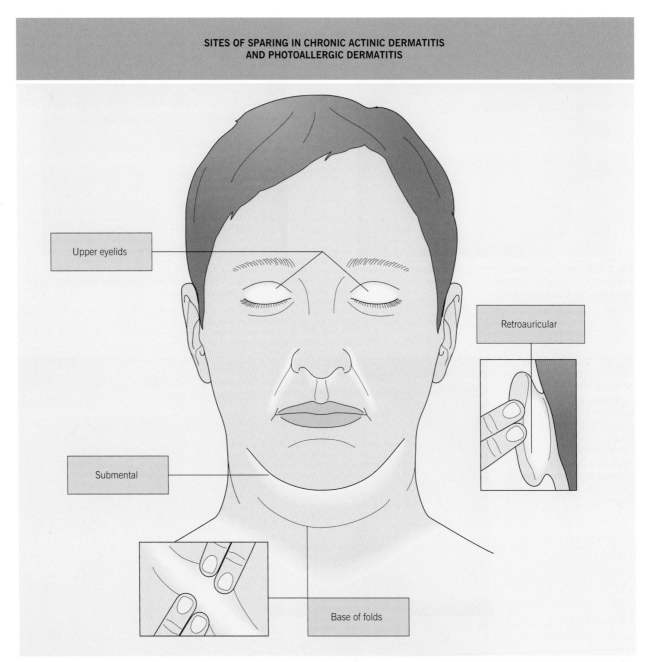

SITES OF SPARING IN CHRONIC ACTINIC DERMATITIS AND PHOTOALLERGIC DERMATITIS

Upper eyelids

Retroauricular

Submental

Base of folds

Fig. 3.7 Sites of sparing in chronic actinic dermatitis and photoallergic dermatitis. Relatively sun-protected sites include the upper eyelids, the nasolabial folds, the retroauricular areas, the submental region and the deepest portion of skin furrows. *From Bolognia JL, Jorizzo JL, Schaffer JV. Dermatology, 3e. London: Saunders, 2012, with permission.*

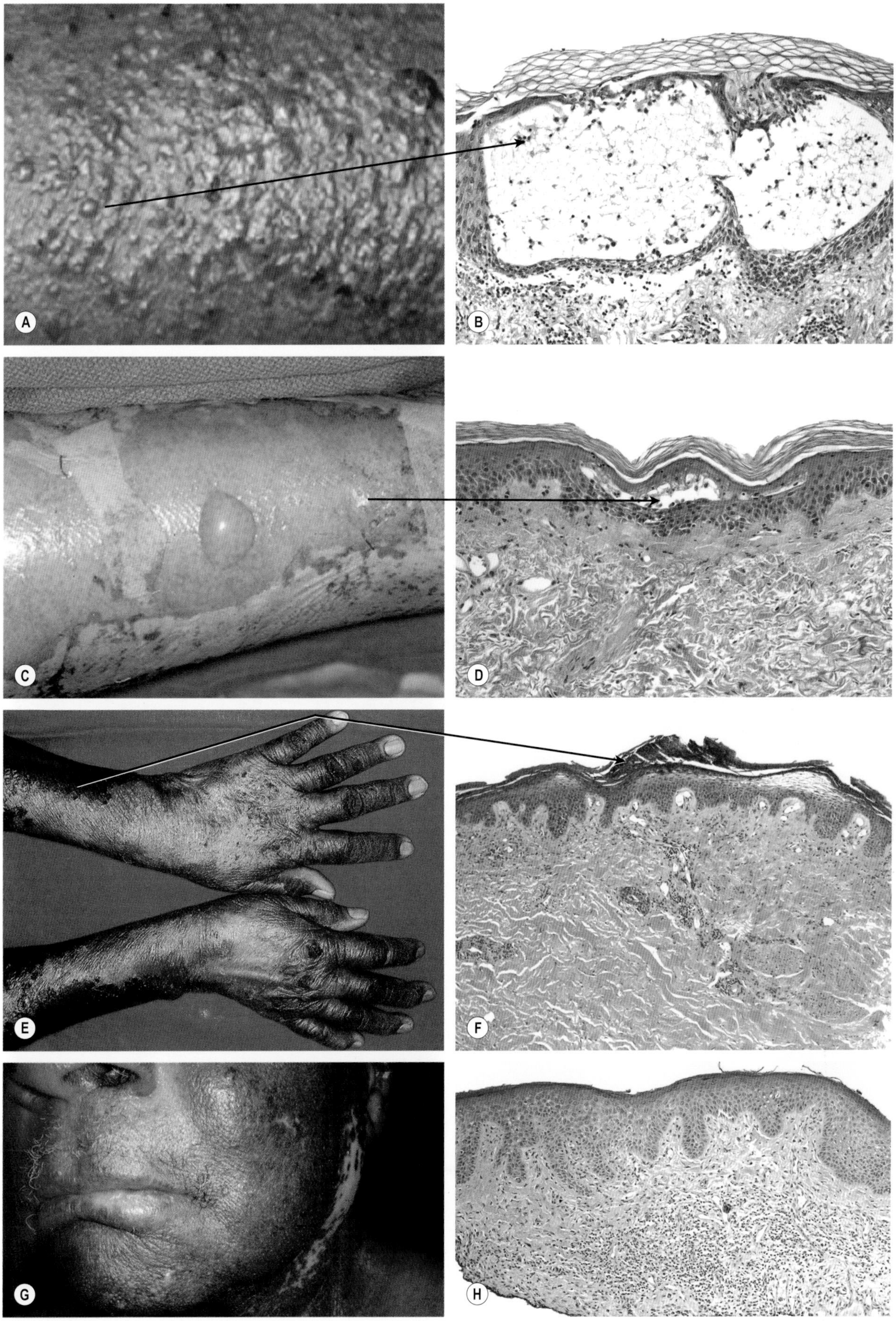

Fig. 3.8 Photoreactions. A,B Photoallergic reaction. **C,D** Phototoxic reaction. **E,F** Pellagra (niacin deficiency). **G,H** Chronic actinic dermatitis. *B, Courtesy, Lorenzo Cerroni, MD; E, Courtesy, Yale Dermatology Residents' Slide Collection. G, Courtesy, Henry Lim, MD. A,C, From Schwarzenberger K, Werchniak AE, Ko C. General Dermatology. London: Saunders, 2009. B,E,G, From Bolognia JL, Jorizzo JL, Schaffer JV. Dermatology, 3e. London: Saunders, 2012, with permission.*

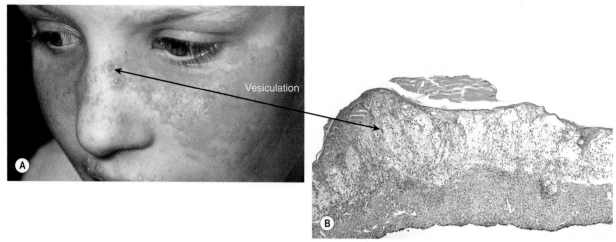

Vesiculation

Fig. 3.9 Hydroa vacciniforme. *Courtesy, John L M Hawk, MD. From Bolognia JL, Jorizzo JL, Schaffer JV. Dermatology, 3e. London: Saunders, 2012, with permission.*

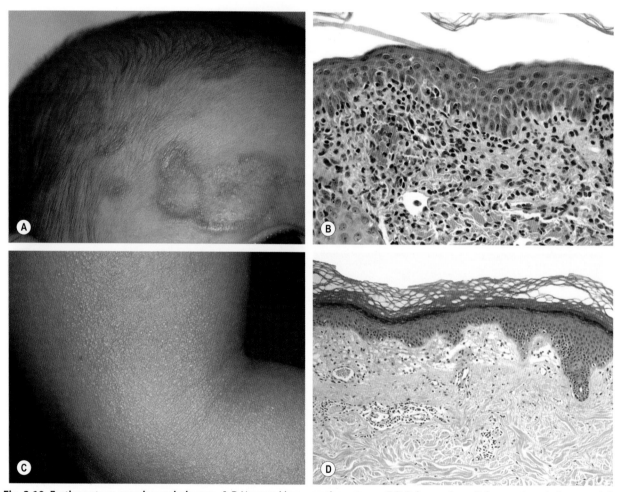

Fig. 3.10 Erythematous papules and plaques. A,B Neonatal lupus erythematosus. **C,D** Polymorphous light eruption. *A, Courtesy, Julie V Schaffer, MD; C, Courtesy, Yale Dermatology Residents' Slide Collection. A,C, From Bolognia JL, Jorizzo JL, Schaffer JV. Dermatology, 3e. London: Saunders, 2012, with permission.*

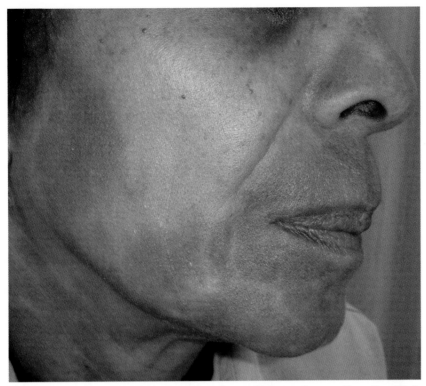

Fig. 3.11 Drug-induced photosensitivity and hyperpigmentation due to diltiazem. *Courtesy, Henry Lim, MD. From Bolognia JL, Jorizzo JL, Schaffer JV. Dermatology, 3e. London: Saunders, 2012, with permission.*

Table 3.2 Photoreactions		
Entity	Morphology	Histopathology
Epidermal photoreactions		
Photoallergic reaction	• Acute spongiotic/eczematous process	• Vesicles • Eosinophils
Phototoxic reaction (e.g. sunburn)	• Depending on severity, erythema to blistering	• Necrotic keratinocytes
Pellagra	• Flaky paint scale and erythema	• Parakeratosis and/or necrosis of the upper epidermis
Chronic actinic dermatitis	• Lichenification and erythema	• Mild spongiosis, acanthosis, hyperkeratosis
Hydroa vacciniforme	• Vesicles and erythema	• Reticular degeneration
Dermal photoreactions		
Neonatal lupus erythematosus	• Annular erythematous plaques	• Interface vacuolar change • Dermal lymphocytes
Polymorphous light eruption	• Erythematous, edematous papules and plaques	• Papillary dermal edema • Perivascular lymphocytes
Drug-induced pigmentary alteration	• Pigment change in sun-exposed skin	• Dermal deposition of pigment

MOSAIC DISTRIBUTION

A mosaic distribution of lesions *(see Fig. 1.18B)* can be specific for particular genodermatoses *(Fig. 3.12)*; lesions may be due to epidermal *(Fig. 3.13)* or dermal processes *(Fig. 3.14)*.

Key Differences

- Epidermal nevus – brown papules, clustered in linear arrays
- Inflammatory linear verrucous epidermal nevus – erythematous scaly papules and plaques, resembling psoriasis

- Linear porokeratosis – pink, linear lesions with raised, scaly borders on careful examination
- Incontinentia pigmenti – scalloped or reticulated arrangement of erythema and vesicles, sometimes admixed with verrucous lesions and/or hyperpigmented, lace-like patterns

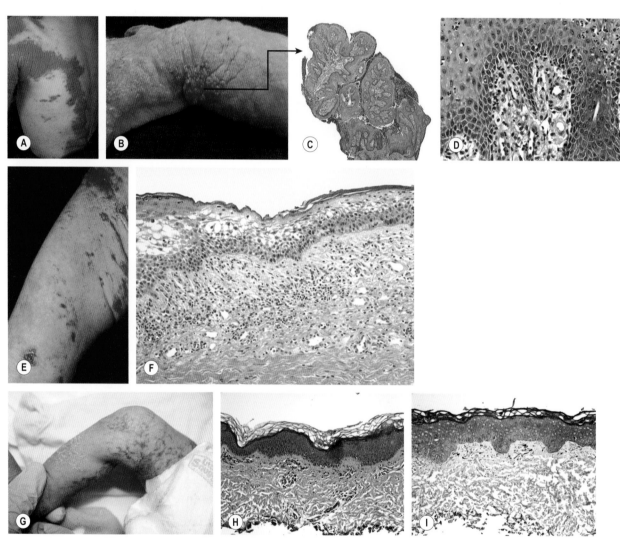

Fig. 3.12 Linear distribution. A–D CHILD syndrome (verruciform xanthoma on biopsy of the friable red nodule). Unilateral, thick pink plaques. **E,F** Goltz syndrome with characteristic atrophy and telangiectasias. **G–I** Incontinentia pigmenti, stage 3 (hyperpigmentation), with characteristic scalloped borders. Prominent pigment incontinence (H) highlighted with Fontana Masson staining (I). *A,B, Courtesy, Leonard Milstone, MD; E,G, Courtesy, Yale Dermatology Residents' Slide Collection. E, From Bolognia JL, Jorizzo JL, Schaffer JV. Dermatology, 3e. London: Saunders, 2012, with permission.*

Fig. 3.13 Linear distribution. A,B Epidermal nevus. Acanthosis and hyperkeratosis resembling a seborrheic keratosis (B). **C,D** Inflammatory linear verrucous epidermal nevus. Alternating ortho- and parakeratosis (D). **E,F** Linear porokeratosis. Cornoid lamella (column of parakeratosis; F). **G,H** Incontinentia pigmenti. Eosinophilic spongiosis with necrotic keratinocytes (arrow; H). *A,C,E, Courtesy, Yale Dermatology Residents' Slide Collection; H, Courtesy, Laura B Pincus, MD. A,E,G, From Bolognia JL, Jorizzo JL, Schaffer JV. Dermatology, 3e. London: Saunders, 2012, with permission. C, From Bolognia JL, Schaffer JV, Duncan KO, Ko CJ. Dermatology Essentials, 1e. Philadelphia: Saunders, 2014, with permission.*

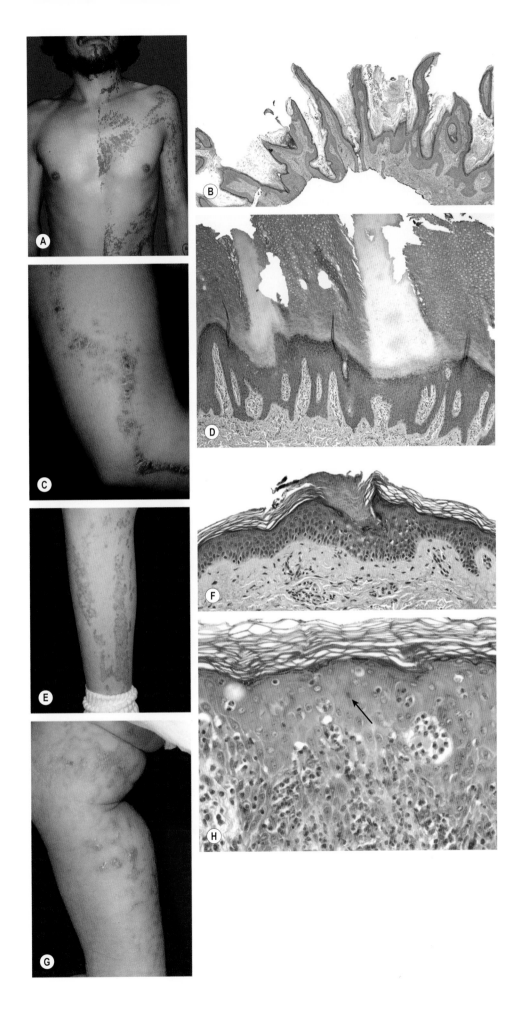

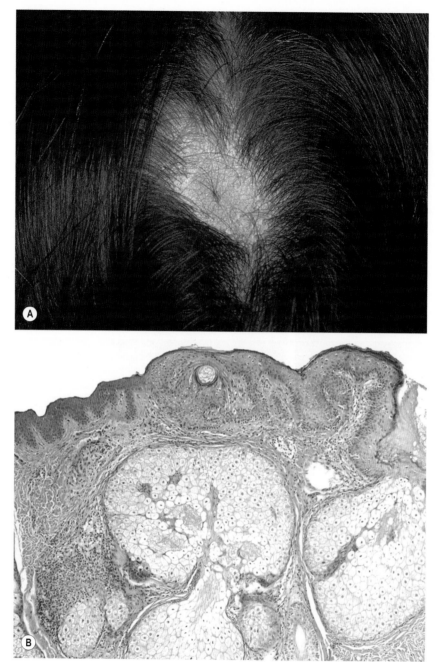

Fig. 3.14 Nevus sebaceus. A,B Mammillated, yellow–pink plaque, often oval or linear in configuration. The scalp is a typical site. Histopathologic findings include acanthosis of the epidermis and sebaceous glands connecting to the epidermal surface. *A, Courtesy, Yale Dermatology Residents' Slide Collection. A, From Bolognia JL, Jorizzo JL, Schaffer JV. Dermatology, 3e. London: Saunders, 2012, with permission.*

LOCALIZED PIGMENTED TUMORS

Key Differences (Fig. 3.15)

A. Angiokeratoma – red–black lacunas clearly visible as well-demarcated roundish structures; histopathology: dilated vessels in the superficial dermis containing erythrocytes

B. Malignant melanoma – asymmetry of color and structure, blue–white structures, and irregular streaks at the periphery; histopathology: asymmetric arrangement of melanocytic nests, with single melanocytes trailing off to one periphery

C. Nodular malignant melanoma – predominant blue–white veil with irregular black to brown dots, globules,

and blotches; histopathology: prominent dermal collections of atypical melanocytes

D. Pigmented basal cell carcinoma – leaf-like areas (islands of blue–gray color) at the periphery and a small erosion of reddish color; histopathology: basaloid islands containing melanin pigment

E. Seborrheic keratosis with typical milia-like cysts (white shining globules) and comedo-like openings (black targetoid globules); histopathology: acanthosis of the epidermis with pseudohorn cysts

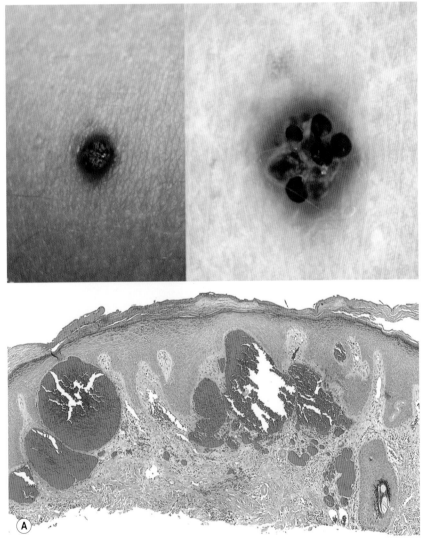

Fig. 3.15 (cont. on next page) Localized pigmented tumors. **A** Angiokeratoma.

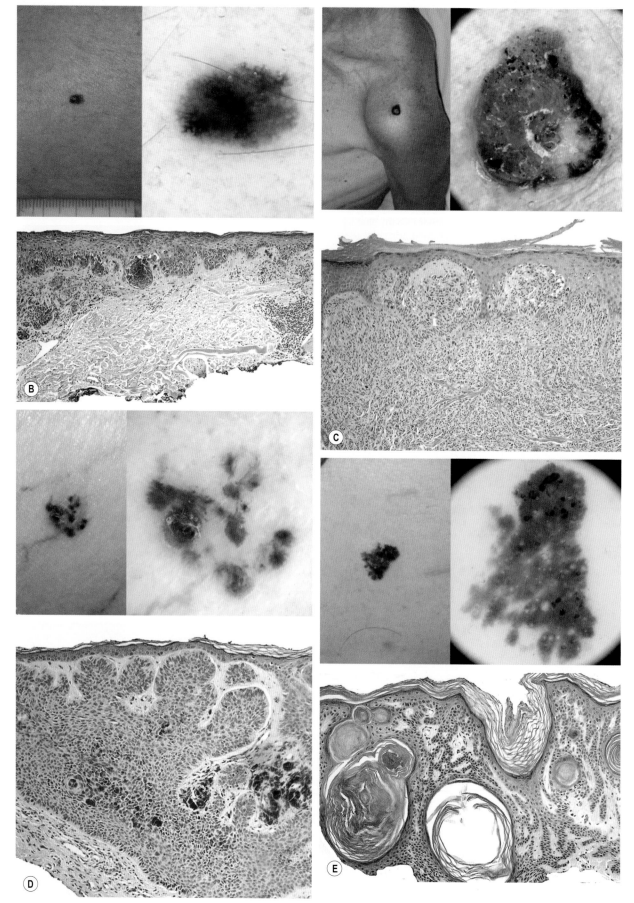

Fig. 3.15, cont'd Localized pigmented tumors. B Malignant melanoma. **C** Nodular malignant melanoma. **D** Pigmented basal cell carcinoma. **E** Seborrheic keratosis. Clinical and dermoscopic photos, *Courtesy, Giuseppe Argenziano, MD, and Iris Zalaudek, MD. From Bolognia JL, Schaffer JV, Duncan KO, Ko CJ. Dermatology Essentials, 1e. Philadelphia: Saunders, 2014, with permission.*

Psoriasiform Rashes 4

The term "psoriasiform" is used to mean "psoriasis-like", and therefore psoriasis is the prototype for these disorders, which generally have dry scale over erythematous plaques and papules. Some experts use "papulosquamous" for similar lesions (see Fig. 8.10). It is important to remember that this chapter is not all-inclusive, and other rashes can be psoriasiform (e.g. drug eruptions). This chapter covers psoriasis, pityriasis rubra pilaris, chronic eczematous dermatitis and pemphigus foliaceus.

PSORIASIS – CLASSIC PLAQUE TYPE

Often Symmetric
- Typically on the elbows/knees/scalp/lower back *(Fig. 4.1)*
- May be more generalized *(Fig. 4.2)*

Well-demarcated erythematous (circles) plaques (bar) *(Fig. 4.3A)*
Well-developed scale is silvery (arrow) *(Fig. 4.4)*

Histopathology:
Silvery scale corresponds to dry parakeratosis lacking serum (arrow) *(Fig. 4.3B)*

Hyperplastic/thickened epidermis (bar) with a diminished granular cell layer
Prominent vessels in the papillary dermis (circles)

Psoriasis – Clues

Lesions may koebnerize (linear arrays) *(Fig. 4.5)*
Nail changes – distal onycholysis (blue arrows), pitting (orange arrows), subungual hyperkeratosis (green arrow) *(Fig. 4.6)*, oil spots, thickening/yellow discoloration *(Fig. 4.7)*

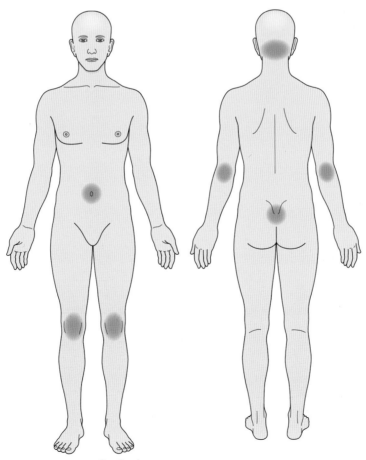

Fig. 4.1 Psoriasis, plaque type, most common distribution.

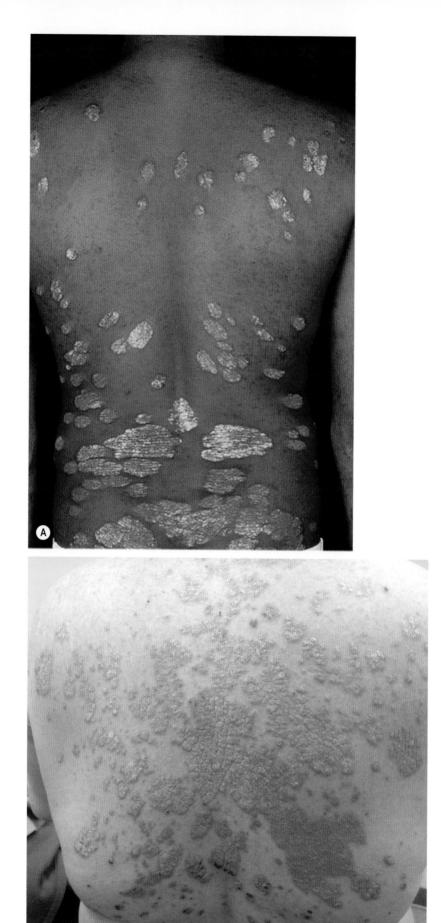

Fig. 4.2 Psoriasis, plaque type. *A, Courtesy, Peter C M van de Kerkhof, MD. From Bolognia JB, Jorizzo JL, Rapini RP. Dermatology, 2e. London: Saunders, 2008, with permission.*

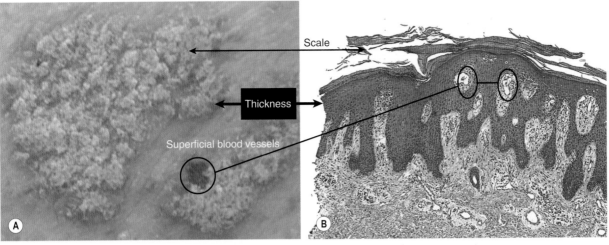

Fig. 4.3 Psoriasis. *A, From Bolognia JL, Jorizzo JL, Schaffer JV. Dermatology, 3e. London: Saunders, 2012, with permission.*

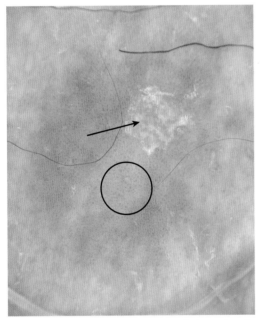

Fig. 4.4 Psoriasis (dermoscopy). Silvery scale (arrow) and prominent regular dotted vessels (circle). *Courtesy, Giuseppe Argenziano, MD, and Iris Zalaudek, MD. From Bolognia JL, Jorizzo JL, Schaffer JV. Dermatology, 3e. London: Saunders, 2012, with permission.*

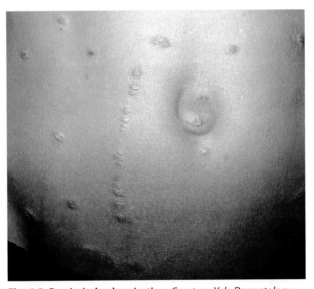

Fig. 4.5 Psoriasis, koebnerization. *Courtesy, Yale Dermatology Residents' Slide Collection. From Bolognia JL, Jorizzo JL, Schaffer JV. Dermatology, 3e. London: Saunders, 2012, with permission.*

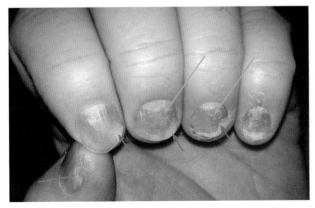

Fig. 4.6 Psoriatic nails.

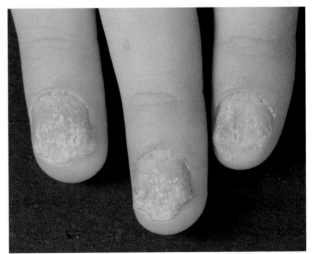

Fig. 4.7 Psoriatic nails. *Courtesy, Peter CM van de Kerkhof, MD, and Frank O Nestlé, MD. From Bolognia JL, Jorizzo JL, Schaffer JV. Dermatology, 3e. London: Saunders, 2012, with permission.*

PSORIASIS VARIANTS

Guttate (see Chapter 5) – small lesions with characteristic scale, generally <1 cm in size *(Fig. 4.8)*
Palmoplantar (see Chapter 2) – lesions with typical scale; underlying skin in these sites may not be erythematous *(Fig. 4.9)*
Inverse (see Chapter 2) – minimal scale over thin, pink plaques *(Fig. 4.10)*
Pustular (see Chapter 7) – erythema and pustules; pustules may form "lakes of pus" *(Fig. 4.11)*
Erythrodermic (see Chapter 3)
Linear (see Chapter 1)

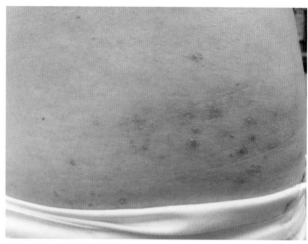

Fig. 4.8 Guttate psoriasis.

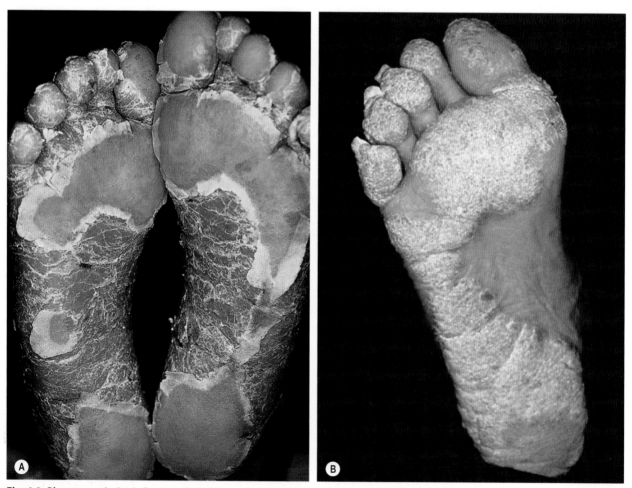

Fig. 4.9 Plantar psoriasis. *A, Courtesy, Peter CM van de Kerkhof, MD. B, Courtesy, Yale Dermatology Residents' Slide Collection. From Bolognia JL, Jorizzo JL, Schaffer JV. Dermatology, 3e. London: Saunders, 2012, with permission.*

Fig. 4.10 Inverse psoriasis. *Courtesy, Ronald P Rapini, MD. From Bolognia JL, Jorizzo JL, Schaffer JV. Dermatology, 3e. London: Saunders, 2012, with permission.*

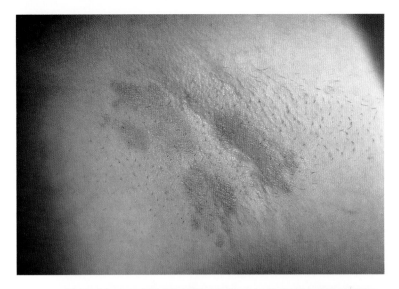

Fig. 4.11 Pustular psoriasis. On the finger, this is termed acrodermatitis continua of Hallopeau. *Courtesy, Yale Dermatology Residents' Slide Collection. From Bolognia JL, Schaffer JV, Duncan KO, Ko CJ. Dermatology Essentials, 1e. Philadelphia: Saunders, 2014, with permission.*

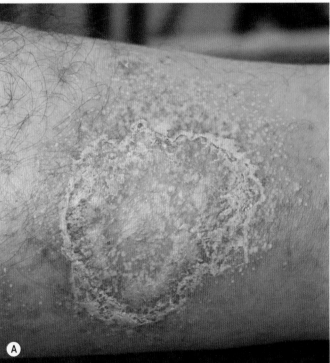

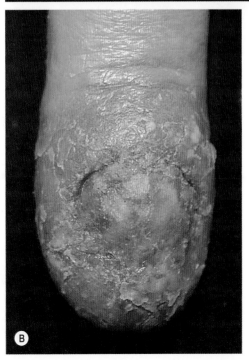

PITYRIASIS RUBRA PILARIS (CLASSIC TYPE)

Once well-developed, easily recognizable *(Figs 4.12, 4.13, see Fig. 3.1)*. Early lesions can resemble psoriasis *(Fig. 4.14A)*.

Classic adult/juvenile – salmon to orange erythroderma with islands of sparing (large or small in size) and follicular papules

Histopathology:
Checkerboard pattern of orthokeratosis and parakeratosis, acanthosis, and perivascular lymphocytes; follicular plugging *(see Fig. 4.14; arrow)*

Pityriasis Rubra Pilaris – Clues
Orange (arrow) to pink waxy keratoderma *(Fig. 4.15)*
Thickened nails
Islands of sparing (arrows) *(Fig. 4.16)*
Follicular papules *(Fig. 4.17)*

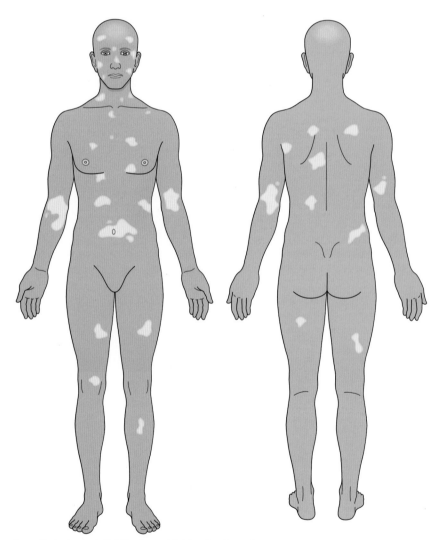

Fig. 4.12 Pityriasis rubra pilaris, typical distribution with islands of sparing.

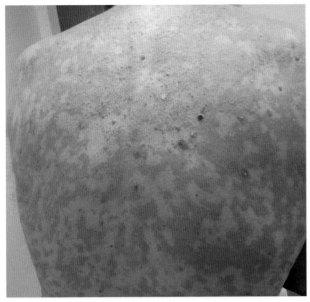

Fig. 4.13 Pityriasis rubra pilaris. *Courtesy, Brett King, MD*

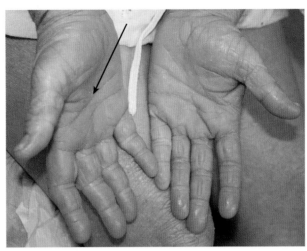

Fig. 4.15 Waxy keratoderma. *Courtesy, Evelyn Lilly, MD.*

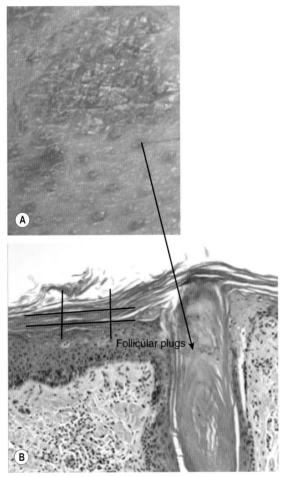

Follicular plugs

Fig. 4.14 Pityriasis rubra pilaris.

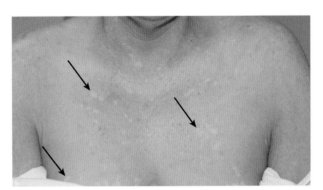

Fig. 4.16 Islands of sparing. *Courtesy, Evelyn Lilly, MD.*

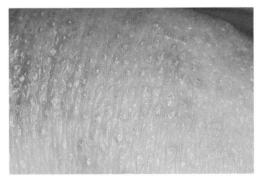

Fig. 4.17 Follicular hyperkeratosis *From Schwarzenberger K, Werchniak AE, Ko C. General Dermatology. London: Saunders, 2009.*

CHRONIC ECZEMATOUS DERMATITIS

Atopic dermatitis typically shows chronic changes post-infancy, in typical sites *(Fig. 4.18)*.
Thickened skin with accentuated skin markings (lichenification) *(Figs 4.19, 4.20)*
Excoriations are common

Histopathology:
Parakeratosis, minimal spongiosis, acanthosis, preserved granular layer *(Fig. 4.20B)*
There are many clues and associated features of atopic dermatitis *(Figs 4.21–4.27)*.

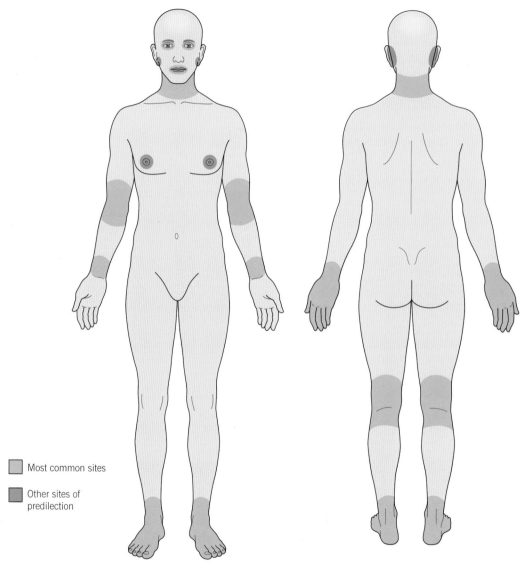

Most common sites

Other sites of predilection

Fig. 4.18 Atopic dermatitis, common sites affected post-infancy. *From Bolognia JL, Schaffer JV, Duncan KO, Ko CJ. Dermatology Essentials, 1e. Philadelphia: Saunders, 2014, with permission.*

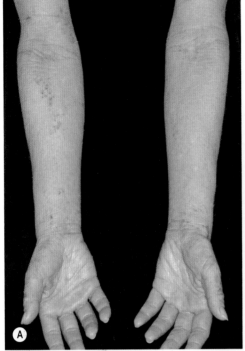

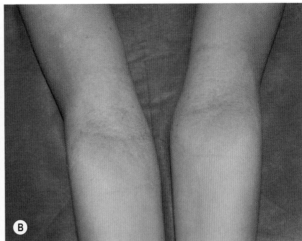

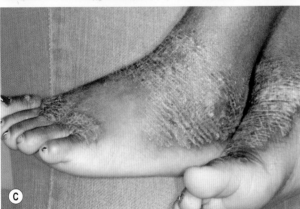

Fig. 4.19 Chronic atopic dermatitis. *A, Courtesy, Thomas Bieber, MD, and Caroline Bussmann, MD. B, Courtesy, Dirk Elston, MD; C, Courtesy Anne Lucky, MD. A, From Bolognia JL, Jorizzo JL, Schaffer JV. Dermatology, 3e. London: Saunders, 2012, with permission. B, From Elston D. Clinical image collection. Dermatopathology, 2e. London: Saunders, 2014. C, From Schachner LA, Hansen RE. Pediatric Dermatology, 4e. London: Mosby, 2011.*

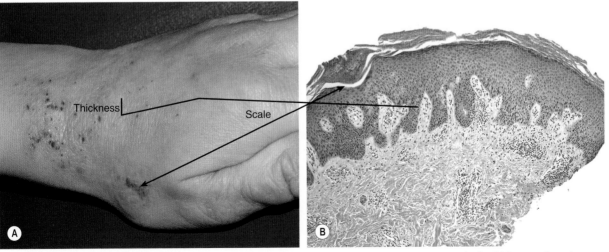

Fig. 4.20 Chronic atopic dermatitis. *A, Courtesy, Julie V Schaffer, MD. A, From Bolognia JL, Jorizzo JL, Schaffer JV. Dermatology, 3e. London: Saunders, 2012, with permission.*

Associated features of atopic dermatitis

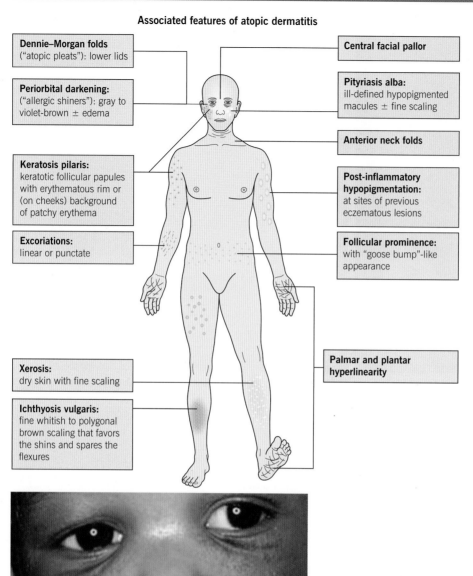

Dennie–Morgan folds
("atopic pleats"): lower lids

Periorbital darkening:
("allergic shiners"): gray to
violet-brown ± edema

Keratosis pilaris:
keratotic follicular papules
with erythematous rim or
(on cheeks) background
of patchy erythema

Excoriations:
linear or punctate

Xerosis:
dry skin with fine scaling

Ichthyosis vulgaris:
fine whitish to polygonal
brown scaling that favors
the shins and spares the
flexures

Central facial pallor

Pityriasis alba:
ill-defined hypopigmented
macules ± fine scaling

Anterior neck folds

**Post-inflammatory
hypopigmentation:**
at sites of previous
eczematous lesions

Follicular prominence:
with "goose bump"-like
appearance

**Palmar and plantar
hyperlinearity**

**Fig. 4.21 Associated features of
atopic dermatitis.** *From Bolognia
JL, Schaffer JV, Duncan KO, Ko CJ.
Dermatology Essentials, 1e.
Philadelphia: Saunders, 2014, with
permission.*

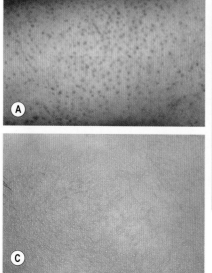

Fig. 4.22 Dennie–Morgan folds on the lower lids. *From
Bolognia JL, Schaffer JV, Duncan KO, Ko CJ. Dermatology Essentials,
1e. Philadelphia: Saunders, 2014, with permission.*

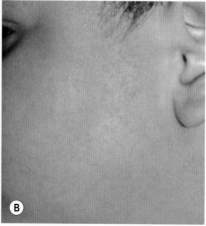

Fig. 4.23 A Keratosis pilaris. **B,C** Keratosis pilaris rubra on the face. *A, Courtesy, Yale
Dermatology Residents' Slide Collection; B,C, Courtesy, Julie V Schaffer, MD. From Bolognia
JL, Schaffer JV, Duncan KO, Ko CJ. Dermatology Essentials, 1e. Philadelphia: Saunders, 2014,
with permission.*

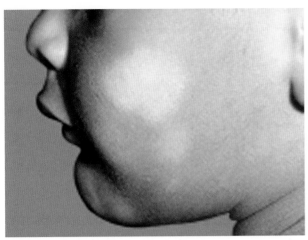

Fig. 4.24 Pityriasis alba. *Courtesy, Anthony J Mancini, MD. From Bolognia JL, Schaffer JV, Duncan KO, Ko CJ. Dermatology Essentials, 1e. Philadelphia: Saunders, 2014, with permission.*

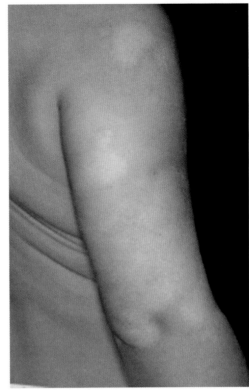

Fig. 4.25 Postinflammatory hypopigmentation. *Courtesy, Thomas Bieber, MD and Caroline Bussman, MD. From Bolognia JL, Schaffer JV, Duncan KO, Ko CJ. Dermatology Essentials, 1e. Philadelphia: Saunders, 2014, with permission.*

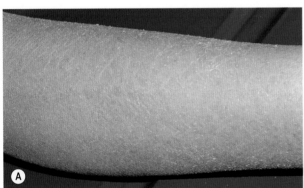

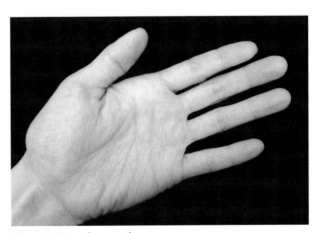

Fig. 4.27 Hyperlinear palm.

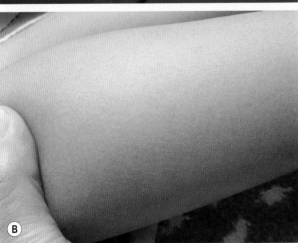

Fig. 4.26 Ichthyosis vulgaris versus mild xerosis. A Ichthyosis vulgaris. **B** Xerosis, mild. *A, Courtesy, Julie V Schaffer, MD. A, From Bolognia JL, Schaffer JV, Duncan KO, Ko CJ. Dermatology Essentials, 1e. Philadelphia: Saunders, 2014, with permission.*

PEMPHIGUS FOLIACEUS

Favors the scalp/face/upper trunk *(Fig. 4.28)* but may become generalized (see Chapter 3)
Erosions are a major clue *(arrows; Fig. 4.29)*

Histopathology:

Individual lesions are thickened (bar), red, with cornflake-like scale *(arrow; Fig. 4.30A)*
Scale and erosions correlate with subcorneal blistering *(arrow; Fig. 4.30B)*

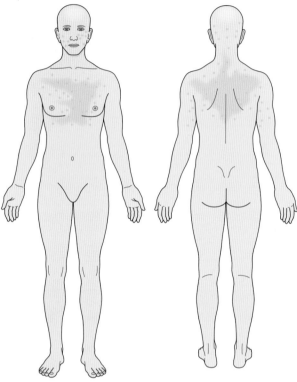

Fig 4.28 Pemphigus foliaceus. The distribution often favors the central face, scalp, and upper trunk.

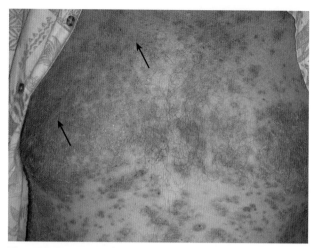

Fig. 4.29 Pemphigus foliaceus.

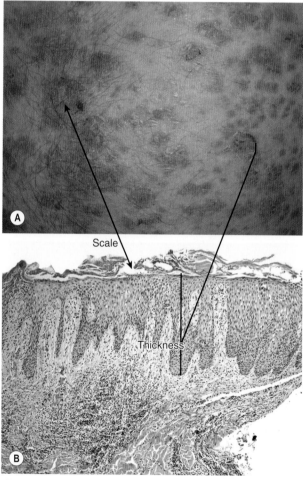

Fig. 4.30 Pemphigus foliaceus. Superficial erosions overlying pink plaques of thickened epidermis.

Key Differences (Fig. 4.31)

A. Psoriasis – adherent, white to silvery scale over bright red erythematous, well-demarcated papules and plaques

B. Pityriasis rubra pilaris – fine scale over pink–orange erythema, follicular papules

C. Chronic atopic dermatitis – accentuated skin markings (thickening), excoriations, ill-defined plaques

D. Pemphigus foliaceus – erosions and cornflake-like scale

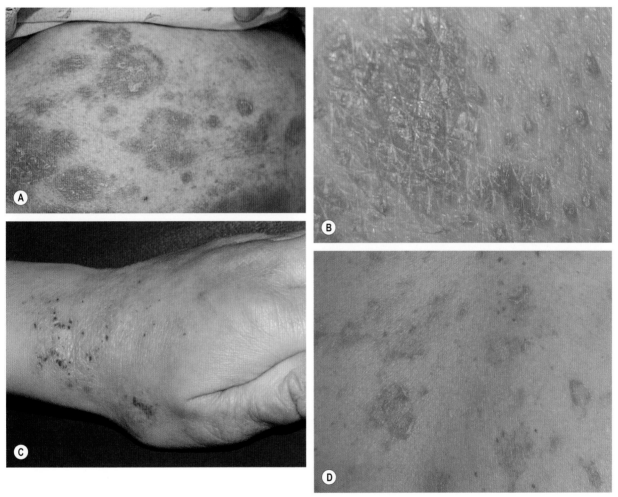

Fig. 4.31 **Psoriasiform rashes.** *C, Courtesy, Julie V Schaffer, MD. C, From Bolognia JL, Jorizzo JL, Schaffer JV. Dermatology, 3e. London: Saunders, 2012, with permission.*

Small, Scaly Lesions 5

This chapter includes guttate psoriasis, pityriasis rosea, lichen planus, pityriasis lichenoides, tinea versicolor, secondary syphilis, small plaque parapsoriasis, and Darier disease.

GUTTATE PSORIASIS

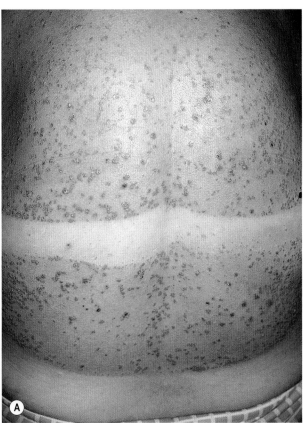

Pink to red papules *(Fig. 5.1)* with adherent white scale *(arrow; Fig. 5.2)*, generally <1 cm in diameter scattered over the trunk and extremities

Histopathology:
Slight acanthosis and mounds of parakeratosis that often contain neutrophils *(arrow; Fig. 5.2)*
Dilated papillary dermal vessels may be present *(circles; see Fig. 5.2)*

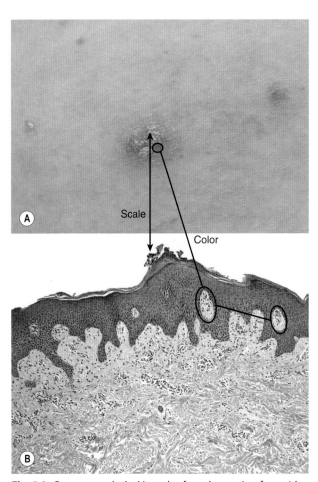

Fig. 5.2 Guttate psoriasis. Mounds of parakeratosis, often with neutrophils.

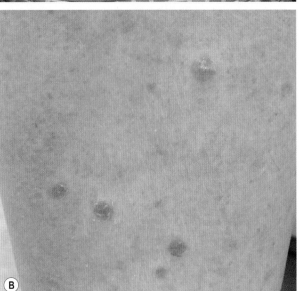

Fig. 5.1 Guttate psoriasis. Lesions in (**A**) developed after a sunburn (Koebner phenomenon). *A, Courtesy, Ronald Rapini, MD. A, From Bolognia JL, Jorizzo JL, Schaffer JV. Dermatology, 3e. London: Saunders, 2012, with permission.*

PITYRIASIS ROSEA

Classically starts with a herald patch (often the largest lesion)

- Precedes development of a widespread, symmetric eruption (see below)

Once well developed, widespread and symmetric (*Fig. 5.3*)

- Proximal extremities and trunk
- Follow Langer's lines, forming a "Christmas tree" pattern on the back

Fine white central scale (arrow) with collarettes overlying round to oval thin salmon-colored (circle) papules/plaques (*Figs 5.4, 5.5*)

Histopathology:
Mounds of parakeratosis *(arrow; see Fig. 5.5)*, generally without neutrophils

Mild spongiosis, mild perivascular lymphocytic infiltrate with extravasated erythrocytes *(circle; see Fig. 5.5)*

Pityriasis Rosea – Variants

Inverse (Fig. 5.6A)
- Tends to affect body folds (axillae, groin)
- Long axis of lesions along Langer's lines (*see Fig. 5.3*)

In Pigmented Skin (Fig. 5.6B)
- May have follicular prominence
- May be hyperpigmented centrally

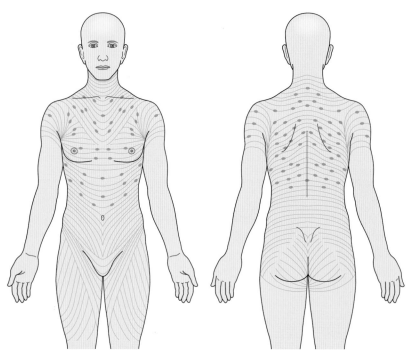

Fig. 5.3 Pityriasis rosea. The typical distribution, with lesions oriented with long axes parallel to the red lines (Langer's lines). *From Bolognia JL, Schaffer JV, Duncan KO, Ko CJ. Dermatology Essentials, 1e. Philadelphia: Saunders, 2014, with permission.*

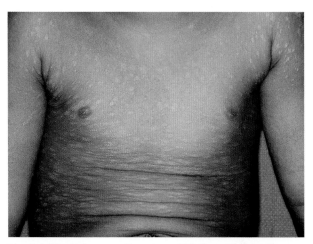

Fig. 5.4 Pityriasis rosea. *From James WD, Berger T, Elston D. Andrews' Diseases of the Skin, 11e. Edinburgh: Saunders, 2011.*

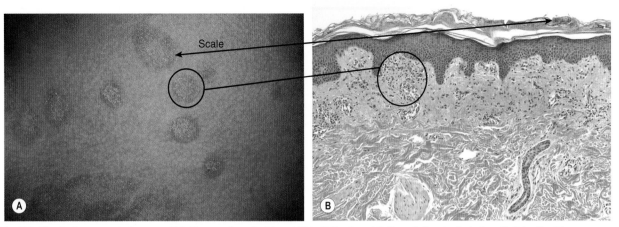

Fig. 5.5 Pityriasis rosea. *A, Courtesy, Yale Dermatology Residents' Slide Collection. A,B, From Bolognia JL, Jorizzo JL, Schaffer JV. Dermatology, 3e. London: Saunders, 2012, with permission.*

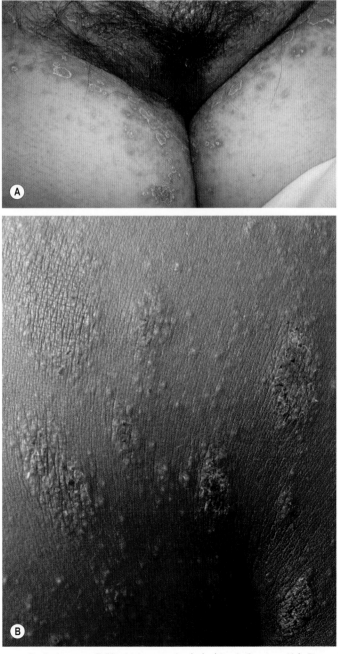

Fig. 5.6 Pityriasis rosea. A Inverse pityriasis rosea. **B** Pityriasis rosea in dark skin. *A, Courtesy, Yale Dermatology Residents' Slide Collection. B, Courtesy, Aisha Sethi, MD. B, From Bolognia JL, Schaffer JV, Duncan KO, Ko CJ. Dermatology Essentials, 1e. Philadelphia: Saunders, 2014, with permission.*

LICHEN PLANUS

Often Symmetric

- Classically on the wrists/forearms, ankles/shins, dorsal hands/feet, genital area *(Fig. 5.7)*
- May be more generalized

Flat-topped violaceous (circle) papules/plaques *(Figs 5.8, 5.9A)*

Classic scale is interconnecting white lines (Wickham's striae) (arrow), possibly corresponding to hyperkeratosis/hypergranulosis (arrow) *(Figs 5.9, 5.10)*

Histopathology:

Hyperplastic epidermis (hyperkeratotic and hypergranulotic) and lichenoid inflammation (circle) with pigment incontinence (orange arrows) *(Fig. 5.9B)*

Lichen Planus – Clues

Nail changes *(Fig. 5.11)* – atrophy and loss of nails, longitudinal fissuring, violaceous color periungually, pterygium (extension of skin onto nail bed), trachyonychia

Oral findings – lacy white plaques *(arrows; Fig. 5.12)*, erosions/ulcers

Koebnerization – lesions secondary to trauma, often in a linear configuration *(Fig. 5.13A)*

Thicker lesions or bullous lesions, particularly on the shins *(Fig. 5.13A; see Figs 13.13, 24.12)*

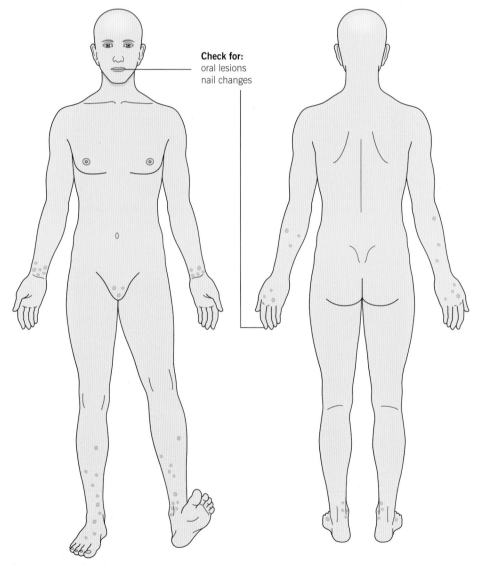

Check for:
oral lesions
nail changes

Fig. 5.7 Lichen planus, typical distribution.

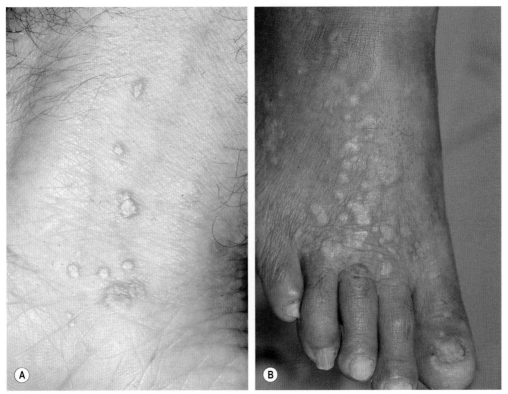

Fig. 5.8 Lichen planus. *From Schwarzenberger K, Werchniak AE, Ko C. General Dermatology. London: Saunders, 2009.*

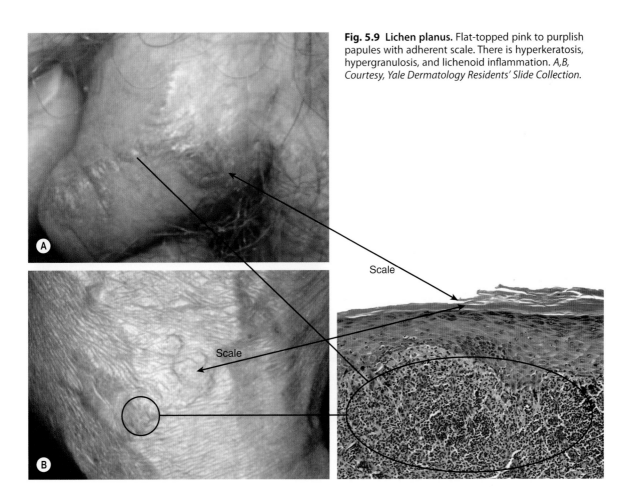

Fig. 5.9 Lichen planus. Flat-topped pink to purplish papules with adherent scale. There is hyperkeratosis, hypergranulosis, and lichenoid inflammation. *A,B, Courtesy, Yale Dermatology Residents' Slide Collection.*

Scale

Scale

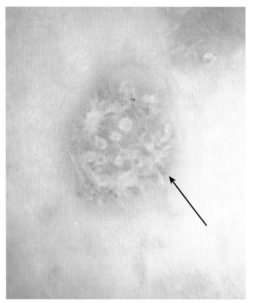

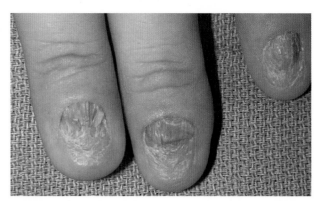

Fig. 5.11 Lichen planus of the nails. *Courtesy, Yale Dermatology Residents' Slide Collection.*

Fig. 5.10 Lichen planus, dermoscopy. *Courtesy, Iris Zalaudek, MD. From Bolognia JL, Jorizzo JL, Schaffer JV. Dermatology, 3e. London: Saunders, 2012, with permission.*

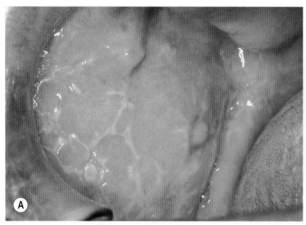

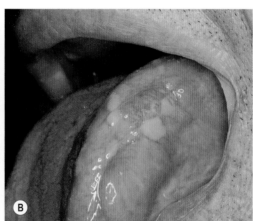

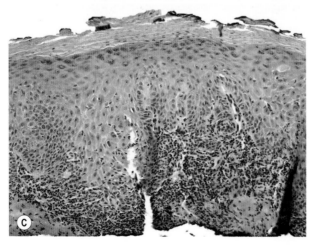

Fig. 5.12 Lichen planus, oral. Oral lesions include lacy white plaques (**A**) and erosions (**B**). Histopathologic findings are similar to those seen in Fig. 5.9. *A, Courtesy, Yale Dermatology Residents' Slide Collection; B, Courtesy, Louis A Fragola, Jr, MD. A,B, From Bolognia JL, Jorizzo JL, Schaffer JV. Dermatology, 3e. London: Saunders, 2012, with permission.*

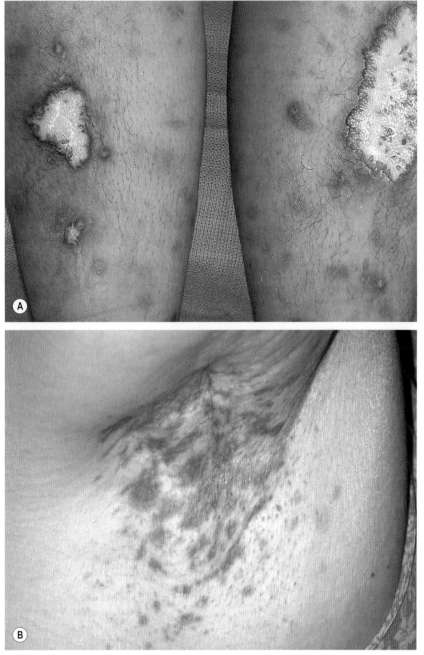

Fig. 5.13 Lichen planus – variants. A Hypertrophic lichen planus. **B** Lichen planus pigmentosus inversus. *Courtesy, Yale Dermatology Residents' Slide Collection.*

The acute and chronic forms exist on a spectrum.

Pityriasis Lichenoides et Varioliformis Acuta *(Fig. 5.14A,B)*

Pink to red papules with scale, some eroded or crusted, and vesicles
Lesions appear in crops and heal with scarring

Histopathology:
Parakeratosis above an epidermis with exocytosis of lymphocytes and interface change, superficial and deep perivascular inflammation

Pityriasis Lichenoides Chronica *(Fig. 5.14C-E)*

Red–brown to pink papules, sometimes with scale
Lesions appear in crops

Histopathology:
Exocytosis of lymphocytes with sparse perivascular inflammation

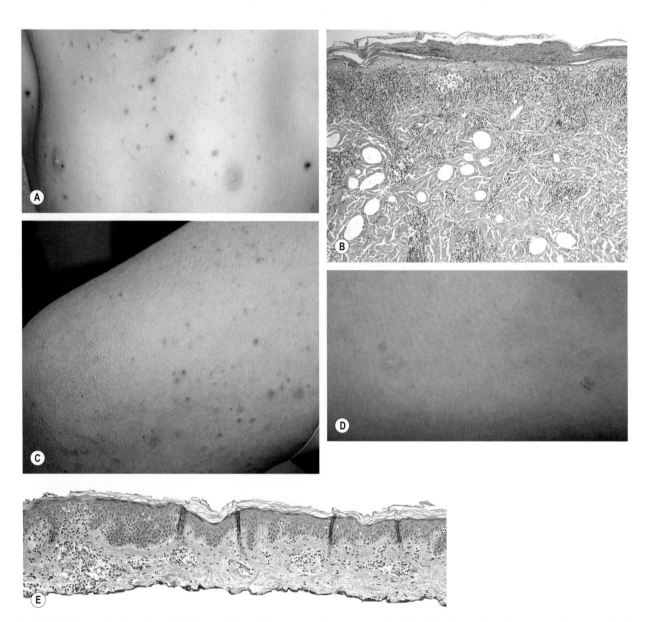

Fig. 5.14 Pityriasis lichenoides. A,B Pityriasis lichenoides et varioliformis acuta. **C–E** Pityriasis lichenoides chronica. *A, Courtesy, Julie V Schaffer, MD. C,D, Courtesy, Yale Dermatology Residents' Slide Collection. A, From Bolognia JL, Schaffer JV, Duncan KO, Ko CJ. Dermatology Essentials, 1e. Philadelphia: Saunders, 2014, with permission.*

TINEA VERSICOLOR

Superficial infection (*Malassezia* spp.)
Symmetric round to oval macules/patches to thin papules/plaques; color is variable (pink to brown or hypopigmented in dark skin); subtle powdery scale *(arrow; Fig. 5.15)*

Histopathology:
Round yeast and elongated hyphal forms in clusters in the stratum corneum *(short arrows; Fig. 5.15D)*; epidermis otherwise appears normal

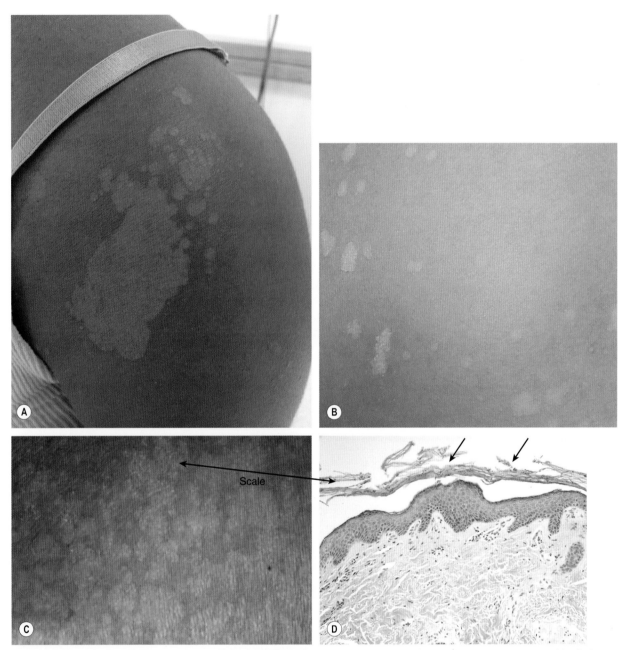

Fig. 5.15 Tinea versicolor. A,B Hypopigmented thin papules and plaques. **C,D** Fine, powdery scale containing yeast and hyphal forms. *A, Courtesy, Yale Dermatology Residents' Slide Collection. C, From Bolognia JL, Jorizzo JL, Schaffer JV. Dermatology, 3e. London: Saunders, 2012, with permission.*

SYPHILIS, SECONDARY

Thin pink plaques or red–brown papules and plaques with scale, often on the trunk *(Fig. 5.16)*

Histopathology:
Psoriasiform hyperplasia with lichenoid and perivascular lymphoplasmacytic inflammation *(see Fig. 5.16)*

Syphilis – Clues
Red–brown papules/plaques, sometimes with collarettes of scale, on palms/soles *(Fig. 5.17)*

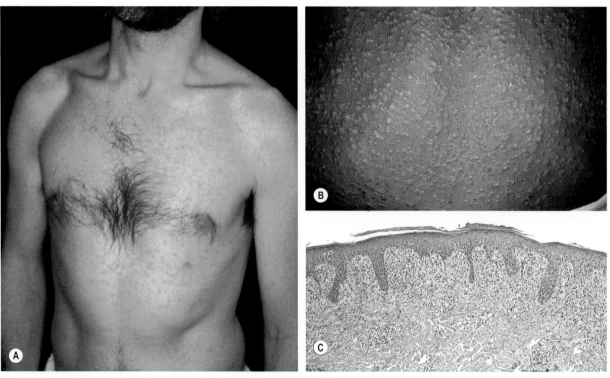

Fig. 5.16 Secondary syphilis. *A,B, Courtesy, Yale Dermatology Residents' Slide Collection. A,B, From Bolognia JL, Schaffer JV, Duncan KO, Ko CJ. Dermatology Essentials, 1e. Philadelphia: Saunders, 2014, with permission.*

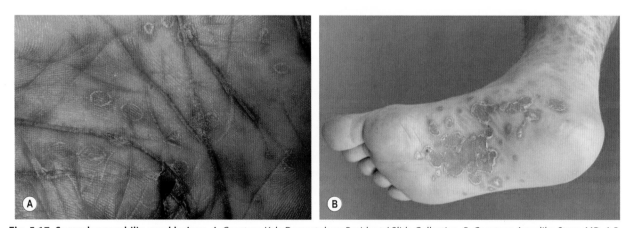

Fig. 5.17 Secondary syphilis, acral lesions. *A, Courtesy, Yale Dermatology Residents' Slide Collection. B, Courtesy, Angelika Stary, MD. A,B, From Bolognia JL, Schaffer JV, Duncan KO, Ko CJ. Dermatology Essentials, 1e. Philadelphia: Saunders, 2014, with permission.*

SMALL PLAQUE PARAPSORIASIS

Lesions <5 cm in diameter, exclusive of digitate dermatosis *(Fig. 5.18A)*

Digitate Dermatosis (a Type of Small Plaque Parapsoriasis)
Brown to pink thin plaques with subtle scale
Lesions arranged like "fingerprints" *(Fig. 5.18B)*

Histopathology:
Subtle spongiosis and scattered lymphocytes within the epidermis *(Fig. 5.18C)*

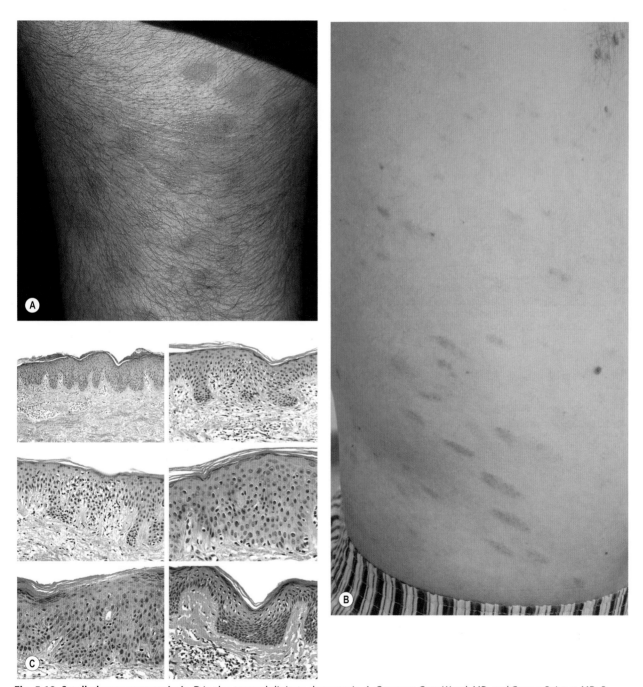

Fig. 5.18 Small plaque parapsoriasis. B is also termed digitate dermatosis. *A, Courtesy, Gary Wood, MD, and George Reizner, MD; B, Courtesy, Yale Dermatology Residents' Slide Collection. A, From Bolognia JL, Schaffer JV, Duncan KO, Ko CJ. Dermatology Essentials, 1e. Philadelphia: Saunders, 2014, with permission. C, From Belousova IE, Vanecek T, Samtsov AV, et al. A patient with clinicopathologic features of small plaque parapsoriasis presenting later with plaque-stage mycosis fungoides: report of a case and comparative retrospective study of 27 cases of "nonprogressive" small plaque parapsoriasis. J Am Acad Dermatol. 2008;59:474–82, © Elsevier.*

Scabies

Lesions of different morphology, including eczematous thin plaques and inflammatory papules *(see Fig. 16.6A)*

Pityriasis Rubra Pilaris

Classically erythroderma that descends from the head to the feet
Early lesions on the trunk can be discrete and scaly *(Fig. 5.19)*

Darier Disease (Keratosis Follicularis)

Autosomal dominant genodermatosis; *ATP2A2* mutations
Predilection for the scalp, face, chest, back (seborrheic areas) *(Fig. 5.20A)*; sometimes intertriginous
Crusted pink to brown papules that become confluent *(Fig. 5.20B,C)*
Acantholytic dyskeratosis capped by hyperkeratosis *(Fig. 5.20D)*

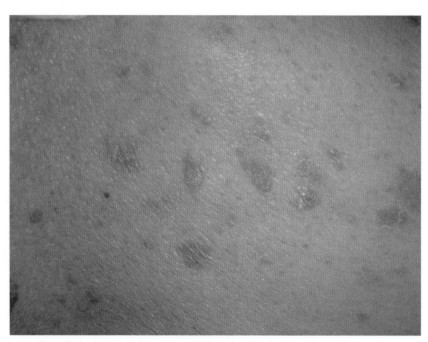

Fig. 5.19 Pityriasis rubra pilaris. Early papulosquamous lesions on the chest.

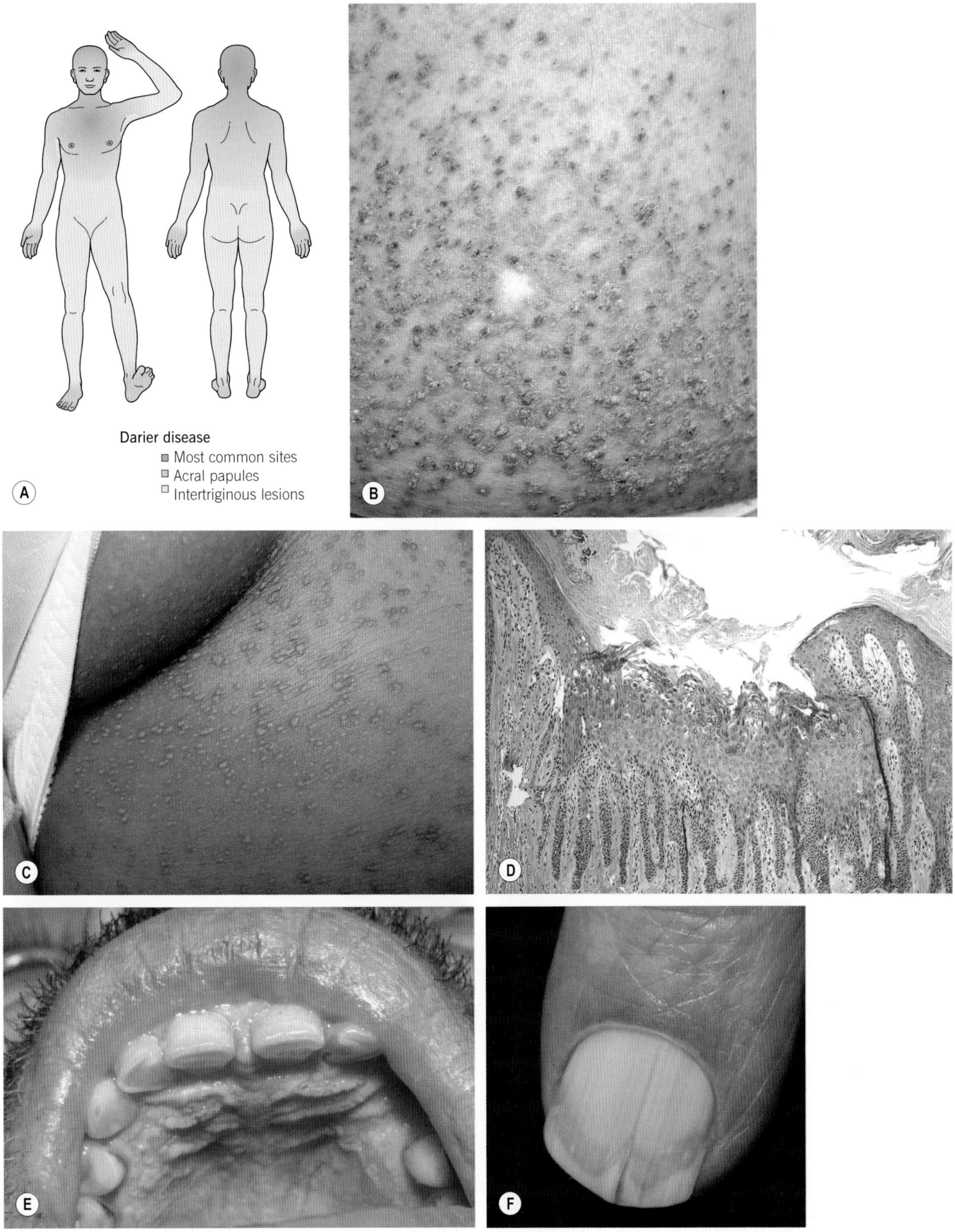

Fig. 5.20 Darier disease. A Typical distribution. **B–D** Typical lesions. **E** Oral lesions. **F** Nail changes can include white and red streaks (shown) and V-shaped notches. *B,F, Courtesy, Yale Dermatology Residents' Slide Collection. A, From Bolognia JL, Schaffer JV, Duncan KO, Ko CJ. Dermatology Essentials, 1e. Philadelphia: Saunders, 2014, with permission. E, Courtesy, Daniel Hohl, MD. E, From Bolognia JL, Jorizzo JL, Schaffer JV. Dermatology, 3e. London: Saunders, 2012, with permission.*

SMALL, SCALY LESIONS WITH ERYTHEMA

Key Differences (Fig. 5.21)

A. Guttate psoriasis – silvery scale over pink–red erythema

B. Pityriasis rosea – central or collarette scale over pink–red erythema

C. Lichen planus – linear, interconnecting scale (Wickham's striae) over violaceous, flat papules

D. Pityriasis lichenoides (chronica) – red–brown papules, some scaly

E. Digitate dermatosis – dull pink–brown elongated ovals

F. Syphilis – red–brown to violaceous papules

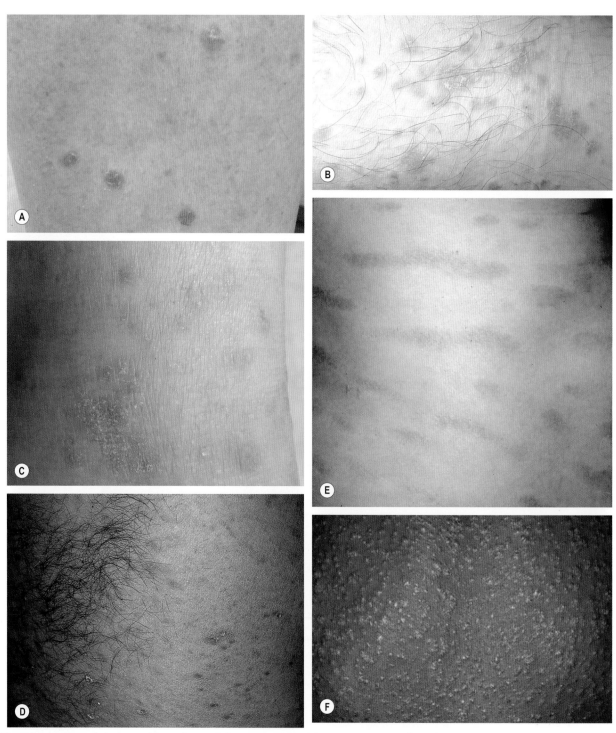

Fig. 5.21 Small, scaly lesions with erythema. A Guttate psoriasis. **B** Pityriasis rosea. **C** Lichen planus. **D** Pityriasis lichenoides (chronica). **E** Digitate dermatosis. **F** Syphilis. *D,F Courtesy, Yale Dermatology Residents' Slide Collection; B,E, From Schwarzenberger K, Werchniak AE, Ko C. General Dermatology. London: Saunders, 2009. D,F, From Bolognia JL, Jorizzo JL, Schaffer JV. Dermatology, 3e. London: Saunders, 2012, with permission.*

Spongiotic/Eczematous Processes 6

This chapter covers acute to subacute presentations of atopic dermatitis, seborrheic dermatitis, asteatotic eczema, stasis dermatitis, id reaction, nummular eczema, contact dermatitis and tinea.

Acute lesions – weeping or oozing +/– crusting over edematous pink papules or plaques *(see Fig. 1.32)*
Subacute lesions – scaly or crusted pink patches or plaques
Chronic – thickened plaques *(see Fig. 1.38 and Chapter 4)*

ATOPIC DERMATITIS

Infancy:
Distribution – favors face and extensor surfaces *(Figs 6.1, 6.2)*

Childhood:
Distribution – favors flexural surfaces *(see Fig. 4.18; Fig. 6.3)*

Adult:
(See Chapter 4)

Atopic Dermatitis Clues:
Keratosis pilaris, xerosis, ichthyosis, pityriasis alba – see Chapter 4

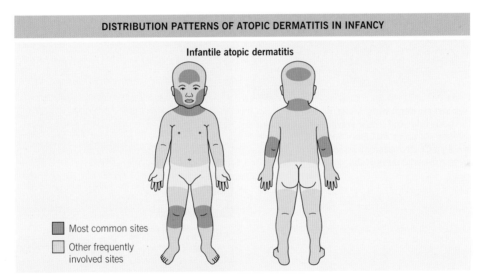

DISTRIBUTION PATTERNS OF ATOPIC DERMATITIS IN INFANCY

Infantile atopic dermatitis

■ Most common sites
□ Other frequently involved sites

Fig. 6.1 **Distribution patterns of atopic dermatitis in infancy.** *Courtesy, Julie V Schaffer, MD. From Bolognia JL, Schaffer JV, Duncan KO, Ko CJ. Dermatology Essentials, 1e. Philadelphia: Saunders, 2014, with permission.*

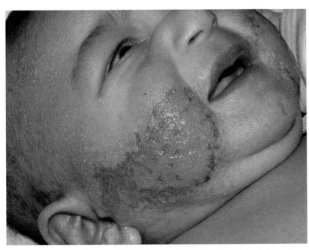

Fig. 6.2 **Atopic dermatitis, infancy.** Acute lesions involving the lower cheek. *Courtesy, Julie V Schaffer, MD. From Bolognia JL, Schaffer JV, Duncan KO, Ko CJ. Dermatology Essentials, 1e. Philadelphia: Saunders, 2014, with permission.*

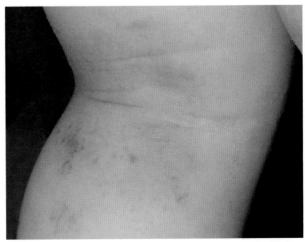

Fig. 6.3 **Atopic dermatitis, childhood.** Acute to subacute lesions in the popliteal fossa. *Courtesy, Julie V Schaffer, MD. From Bolognia JL, Schaffer JV, Duncan KO, Ko CJ. Dermatology Essentials, 1e. Philadelphia: Saunders, 2014, with permission.*

SEBORRHEIC DERMATITIS, INFANT

Moist, scaly plaques involving the folds *(see Fig. 2.14C; Fig. 6.4)*

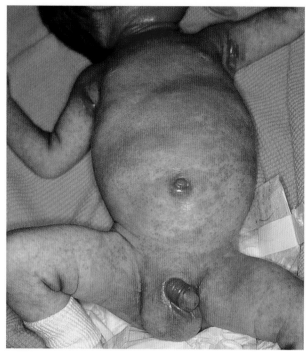

Fig. 6.4 **Infantile seborrheic dermatitis.** Moist, ill-defined plaques favoring the body folds but also involving other sites in this case. *Courtesy, Robert Hartman, MD. From Bolognia JL, Schaffer JV, Duncan KO, Ko CJ. Dermatology Essentials, 1e. Philadelphia: Saunders, 2014, with permission.*

SEBORRHEIC DERMATITIS, ADULT

Predilection for the scalp, posterior ears, central face, upper chest and back
Variably colored papules and plaques with flaking and/or greasy scale *(Fig. 6.5)*
Lesions may be annular *(see Fig. 2.9B)*

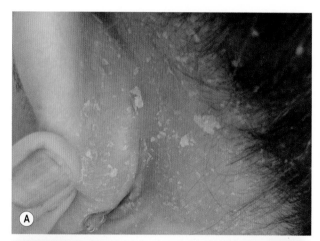

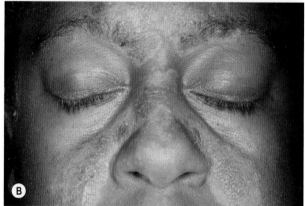

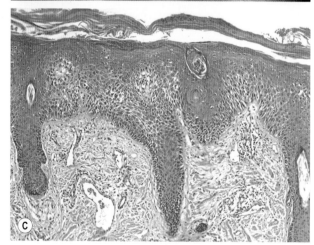

Fig. 6.5 **Seborrheic dermatitis, adult. A** Erythema and flaky white scale behind the ear. **B** Purplish papules and plaques in a typical distribution over the central face. **C** Parakeratosis adjacent to follicles with intercellular edema (spongiosis). *A, Courtesy, Norbert Reider, MD and Peter O Fritsch, MD; B, Courtesy, Jeffrey P Callen, MD. A,B, From Bolognia JL, Schaffer JV, Duncan KO, Ko CJ. Dermatology Essentials, 1e. Philadelphia: Saunders, 2014, with permission.*

ASTEATOTIC ECZEMA (XEROTIC ECZEMA, ECZEMA CRAQUELÉ)

Favors the lower extremities, flanks, and lateral upper back
In areas of dry skin, pruritus may be present
Superficial cracking of the skin *(Fig. 6.6)*

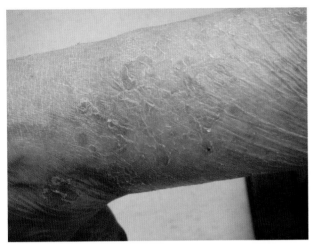

Fig. 6.6 Asteatotic eczema. *Courtesy, Kalman Watsky, MD.*

STASIS DERMATITIS

Predilection for the lower extremities, often bilateral
Associated lower extremity edema
+/– signs of venous hypertension – varicosities *(Fig. 6.7)*, petechiae, lipodermatosclerosis *(see Fig. 2.21)*, ulceration above medial malleolus *(Fig. 6.8;* see Chapter 17*)*, livedoid vasculopathy

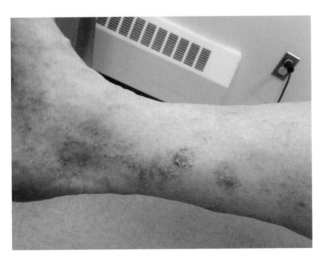

Fig. 6.7 Stasis dermatitis.

ID REACTION *(FIG. 6.8)*

Relatively widespread (may be generalized); predilection for extensor extremities
Associated with localized dermatitis (i.e. allergic contact dermatitis, stasis dermatitis, tinea)

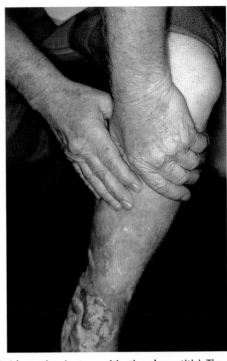

Fig. 6.8 Id reaction (autosensitization dermatitis). The extensor forearms are involved. The patient had allergic contact dermatitis to neomycin as well as stasis dermatitis. There is also a venous ulcer over the medial malleolus. *Courtesy, Jean L Bolognia, MD. From Bolognia JL, Schaffer JV, Duncan KO, Ko CJ. Dermatology Essentials, 1e. Philadelphia: Saunders, 2014, with permission.*

NUMMULAR ECZEMA *(FIG. 6.9)*

Classically on the arms and legs
Coin-shaped 2–3 cm plaques, classically weeping or oozing

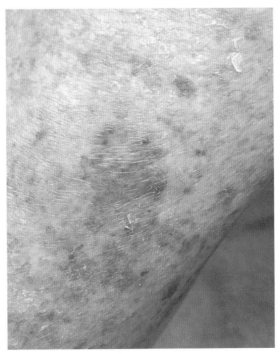

Fig. 6.9 Nummular eczema.

ALLERGIC CONTACT DERMATITIS *(FIGS 6.10, 6.11)*

Delayed-type hypersensitivity reaction in a previously sensitized person

Acute lesions more common than chronic lesions

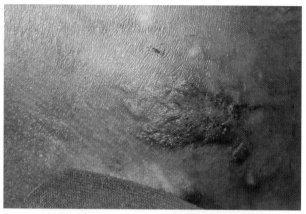

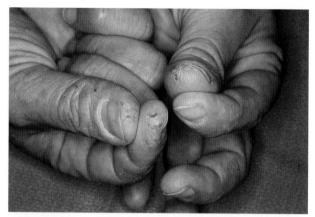

Fig. 6.10 Acute allergic contact dermatitis to chlorhexidine. *Courtesy, Yale Dermatology Residents' Slide Collection.*

Fig. 6.11 Chronic allergic contact dermatitis to glutaraldehyde in an optometrist. *Courtesy, Kalman Watsky, MD. From Bolognia JL, Schaffer JV, Duncan KO, Ko CJ. Dermatology Essentials, 1e. Philadelphia: Saunders, 2014, with permission.*

IRRITANT CONTACT DERMATITIS *(FIGS 6.12, 6.13)*

Due to a local toxic (non-immunologic) effect from a contactant

Chronic lesions more common than acute lesions

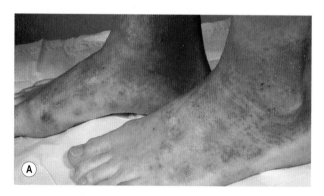

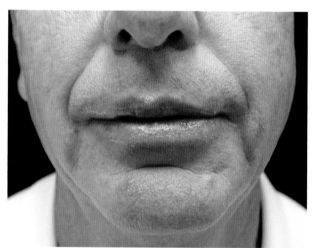

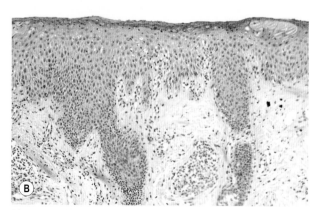

Fig. 6.13 Cheilitis and perioral involvement due to irritant contact dermatitis (lip licking). *Courtesy, Jeffrey P Callen, MD. From Bolognia JL, Schaffer JV, Duncan KO, Ko CJ. Dermatology Essentials, 1e. Philadelphia: Saunders, 2014, with permission.*

Fig. 6.12 Bilateral irritant contact dermatitis due to chronic wearing of occlusive footwear. *Courtesy, David Cohen, MD. From Bolognia JL, Schaffer JV, Duncan KO, Ko CJ. Dermatology Essentials, 1e. Philadelphia: Saunders, 2014, with permission.*

TINEA

Annular, scaly border (if present; KOH preparation can confirm the diagnosis) is a helpful clue *(Fig. 6.14A,B)*

BULLOUS PEMPHIGOID, ECZEMATOUS *(see Fig. 13.4C)*

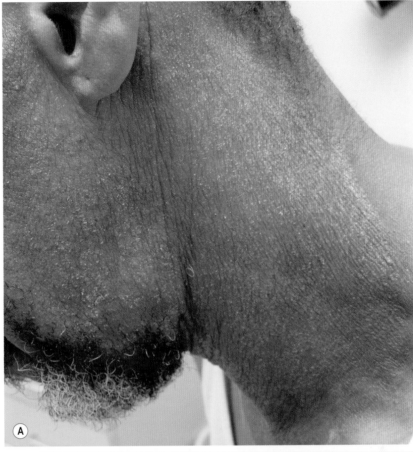

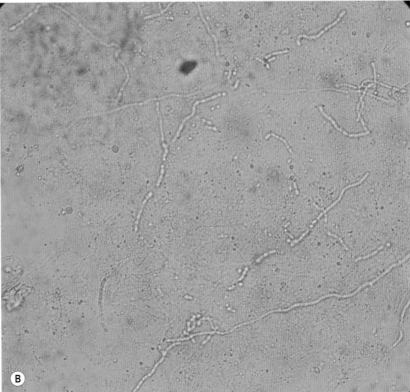

Fig. 6.14 Tinea corporis.

Epidermal Neutrophils | 7

Neutrophils in the epidermis often create pustules but sometimes lead to erythema and/or erosions. This chapter covers psoriasis, acute generalized exanthematous pustulosis, subcorneal pustular dermatosis, and IgA pemphigus.

EPIDERMAL NEUTROPHILS – PUSTULAR

Pustular Psoriasis, Generalized

Widespread *(Fig. 7.1)* erythema and sterile pustules, many coalescing into "lakes of pus" *(Fig. 7.2)*

Histopathology:
Abundant neutrophils (arrow) below the stratum corneum *(Fig. 7.3)*; may be indistinguishable from acute generalized exanthematous pustulosis and subcorneal pustular dermatosis

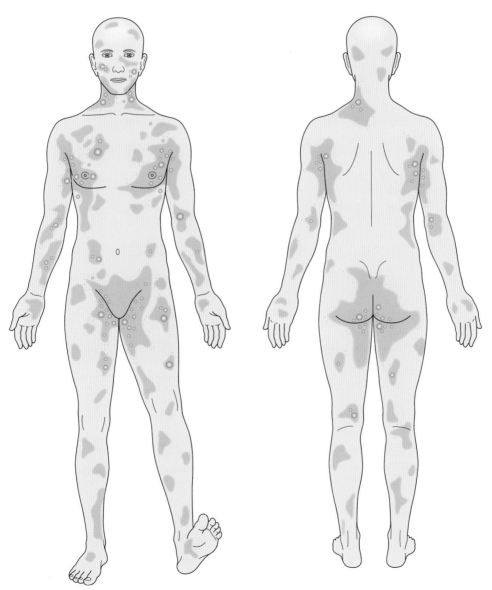

Fig. 7.1 Pustular psoriasis, generalized.

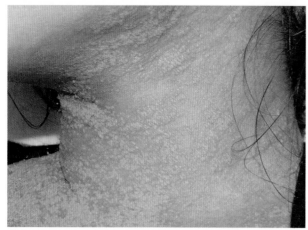

Fig. 7.2 Pustular psoriasis. *Courtesy, Julie V Schaffer, MD. From Bolognia JL, Schaffer JV, Duncan KO, Ko CJ. Dermatology Essentials, 1e. Philadelphia: Saunders, 2014, with permission.*

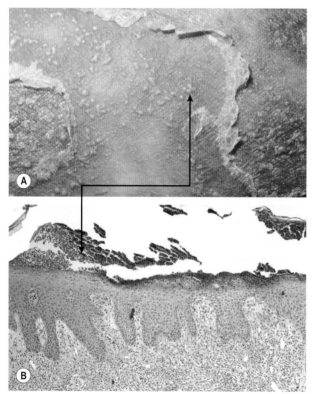

Fig. 7.3 Pustular psoriasis. Pustules correspond to subcorneal collections of neutrophils. *A, Courtesy, Kenneth Greer, MD. A, From Bolognia JL, Schaffer JV, Duncan KO, Ko CJ. Dermatology Essentials, 1e. Philadelphia: Saunders, 2014, with permission.*

Pustular Psoriasis, Variants

Localized – pustules limited to plaques of psoriasis *(Fig. 7.4)*
Annular – rings of erythema studded with peripheral pustules *(Fig. 7.5)*
Palmoplantar *(Fig. 7.6)*
Acrodermatitis continua of Hallopeau – distal digit with erythema/scale/pustules *(see Fig. 4.11B)*

Acute Generalized Exanthematous Pustulosis

Commonly induced by antibiotics (penicillins, macrolides)
Begins on the face/body folds and becomes generalized *(Fig. 7.7)*
Small, sterile pustules over edema and erythema *(Figs 7.8, 7.9)*

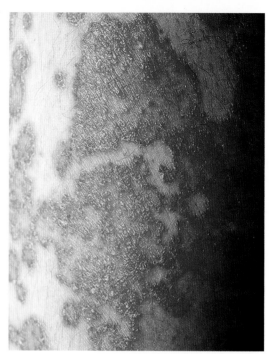

Fig. 7.4 Pustular psoriasis, localized. *Courtesy, Yale Dermatology Residents' Slide Collection. From Bolognia JL, Schaffer JV, Duncan KO, Ko CJ. Dermatology Essentials, 1e. Philadelphia: Saunders, 2014, with permission.*

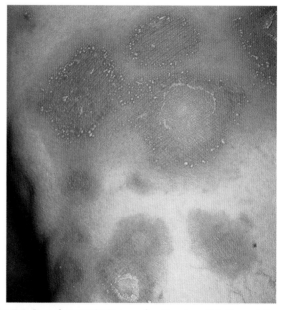

Fig. 7.5 Pustular psoriasis, annular. *Courtesy, Yale Dermatology Residents' Slide Collection. From Bolognia JL, Schaffer JV, Duncan KO, Ko CJ. Dermatology Essentials, 1e. Philadelphia: Saunders, 2014, with permission.*

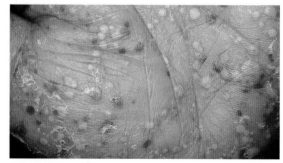

Fig. 7.6 Pustulosis of the palm. *Courtesy, Yale Dermatology Residents' Slide Collection. From Bolognia JL, Schaffer JV, Duncan KO, Ko CJ. Dermatology Essentials, 1e. Philadelphia: Saunders, 2014, with permission.*

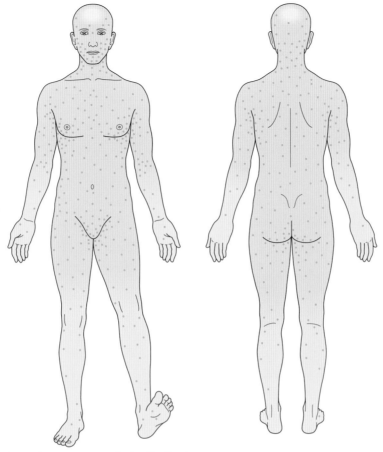

Fig. 7.7 Acute generalized exanthematous pustulosis, distribution.

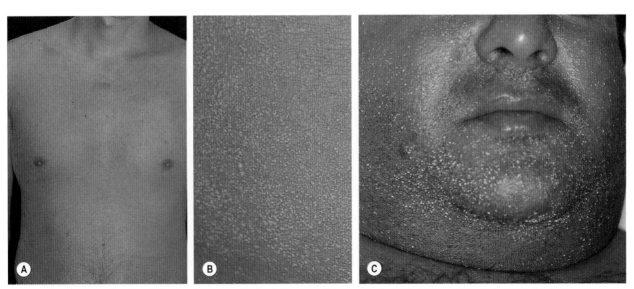

Fig. 7.8 Acute generalized exanthematous pustulosis. *C, Courtesy, Kalman Watsky, MD. A,B, From Min JA, Park HJ, Cho BK, Lee JY. Acute generalized exanthematous pustulosis induced by Rhus (lacquer). J Am Acad Dermatol. 2010;63:166–8, © Elsevier. C, From Bolognia JL, Jorizzo JL, Schaffer JV. Dermatology, 3e. London: Saunders, 2012, with permission.*

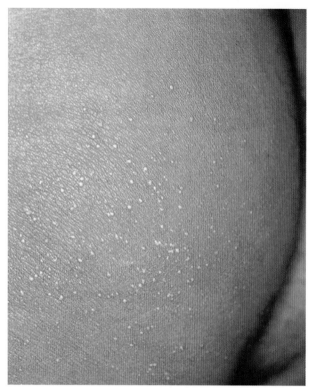

Fig. 7.9 Acute generalized exanthematous pustulosis. *Courtesy, Yale Dermatology Residents' Slide Collection. From Bolognia JL, Schaffer JV, Duncan KO, Ko CJ. Dermatology Essentials, 1e. Philadelphia: Saunders, 2014, with permission.*

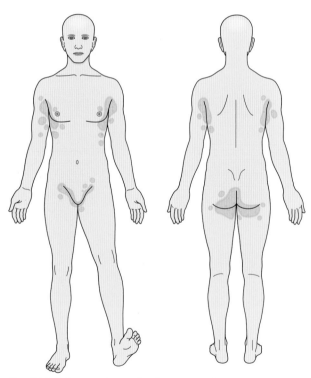

Fig. 7.10 Subcorneal pustular dermatosis, distribution.

Subcorneal Pustular Dermatosis (Sneddon-Wilkinson Disease)

Considered by some to be a variant of psoriasis
Tends to affect body folds *(Fig. 7.10)*
Annular lesions studded with pustules *(Fig. 7.11)*
Pustules may be "half and half" with clear fluid above pus *(Fig. 7.12)*

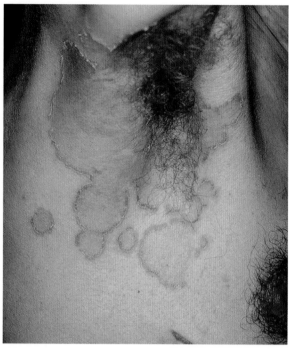

Fig. 7.11 Subcorneal pustular dermatosis. *Courtesy, Yale Dermatology Residents' Slide Collection. From Bolognia JL, Schaffer JV, Duncan KO, Ko CJ. Dermatology Essentials, 1e. Philadelphia: Saunders, 2014, with permission.*

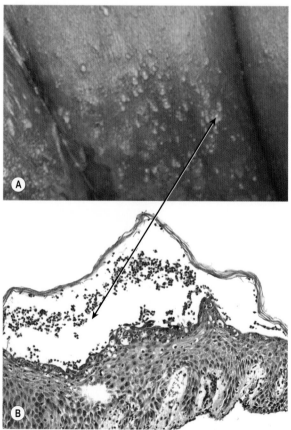

Fig. 7.12 Subcorneal pustular dermatosis. *Courtesy, Yale Dermatology Residents' Slide Collection.*

Other Causes of Pustules

Pustules can be seen in a variety of other settings. Sterile pustules are seen in acne *(Fig. 7.13)* and other acneiform processes as well as in neutrophil-rich processes like early pyoderma gangrenosum *(Fig. 7.14)* or acropustulosis of infancy *(Fig. 7.15)*. Scabies infestation may also present with pustules *(Fig. 7.16)*. Non-sterile pustules are due to various organisms *(Fig. 7.17*; green arrow)*; special stains and/or culture studies may be helpful.

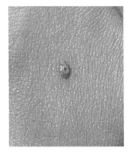

Fig. 7.14 Pyoderma gangrenosum, early papulopustule. *Courtesy, Yale Dermatology Residents' Slide Collection. From Bolognia JL, Schaffer JV, Duncan KO, Ko CJ. Dermatology Essentials, 1e. Philadelphia: Saunders, 2014, with permission.*

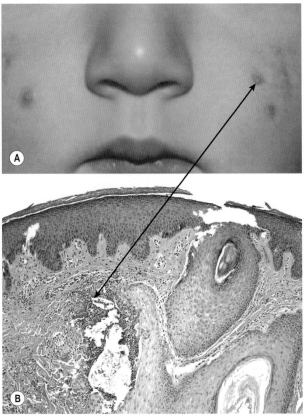

Fig. 7.13 Acne. *Courtesy, Kalman Watsky, MD. From Bolognia JL, Schaffer JV, Duncan KO, Ko CJ. Dermatology Essentials, 1e. Philadelphia: Saunders, 2014, with permission.*

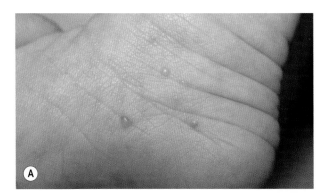

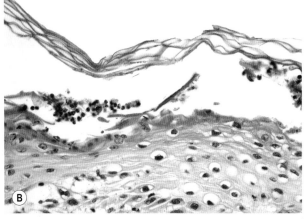

Fig. 7.15 Acropustulosis of infancy. Vesicles and pustules with absent burrows. *Courtesy, Deborah S Goddard, MD, Amy E Gilliam, MD, and Ilona J Frieden, MD. From Bolognia JL, Jorizzo JL, Schaffer JV. Dermatology, 3e. London: Saunders, 2012, with permission.*

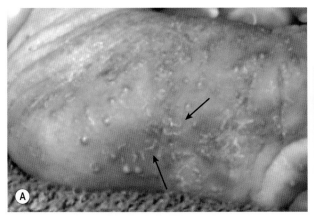

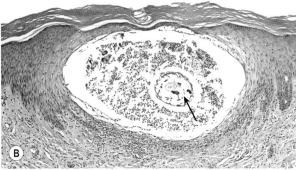

Fig. 7.16 Scabies infestation. A Multiple burrows (arrows) and small pustules. **B** A mite (arrow) is evident. *Courtesy, Anne Lucky, MD. From Schachner LA, Hansen RE. Pediatric Dermatology, 4e. London: Mosby, 2011.*

Fig. 7.17 Tinea corporis. Pustules within figurate plaques. Dermatophytes are evident (green arrow). *Courtesy, Yale Dermatology Residents' Slide Collection. From Bolognia JL, Schaffer JV, Duncan KO, Ko CJ. Dermatology Essentials, 1e. Philadelphia: Saunders, 2014, with permission.*

EPIDERMAL NEUTROPHILS – PUSTULAR OR NON-PUSTULAR

IgA Pemphigus

Two types, both with intercellular IgA deposition on immunofluorescence *(Fig. 7.18A)*

Typically affects the axillae/groin *(Fig. 7.19)*

Central crusts surrounded by flaccid vesicles or pustules *(Fig. 7.20)*

Two types:

1. subcorneal pustular dermatosis type (histologically indistinguishable from Sneddon–Wilkinson disease; *see Fig. 7.12B)*

2. intraepidermal neutrophilic type *(Fig. 7.18C)*

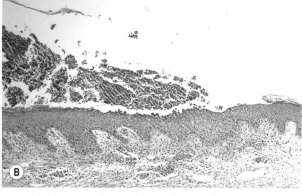

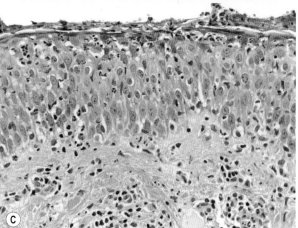

Fig. 7.18 IgA pemphigus. A Direct immunofluorescence – intercellular IgA deposition. **B** Subcorneal neutrophils in the subcorneal pustular dermatosis type. **C** Superficial erosion and intraepidermal neutrophils in the intraepidermal neutrophilic type. *C, Courtesy, Lorenzo Cerroni, MD. From Bolognia JL, Jorizzo JL, Schaffer JV. Dermatology, 3e. London: Saunders, 2012, with permission.*

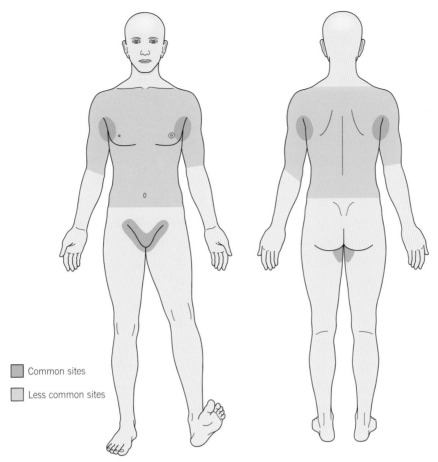

Fig. 7.19 IgA pemphigus, distribution.

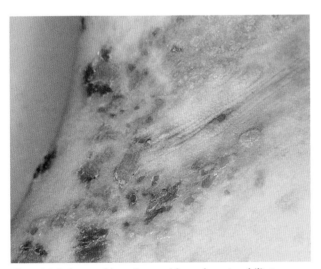

Fig. 7.20 IgA pemphigus, intraepidermal neutrophilic type.
Courtesy, Masayuki Amagai, MD. From Bolognia JL, Jorizzo JL, Schaffer JV. Dermatology, 3e. London: Saunders, 2012, with permission.

Rashes with Pustules

Key Differences (Fig. 7.21)

- Pustular psoriasis – lakes of pus (arrow)
- Acute generalized exanthematous pustulosis – edema may be present, small monomorphous pustules
- Subcorneal pustular dermatosis of Sneddon and Wilkinson – annular lesions with relatively normal center
- IgA pemphigus, subcorneal pustular dermatosis type – central crusts (arrows) surrounded by vesicles/pustules

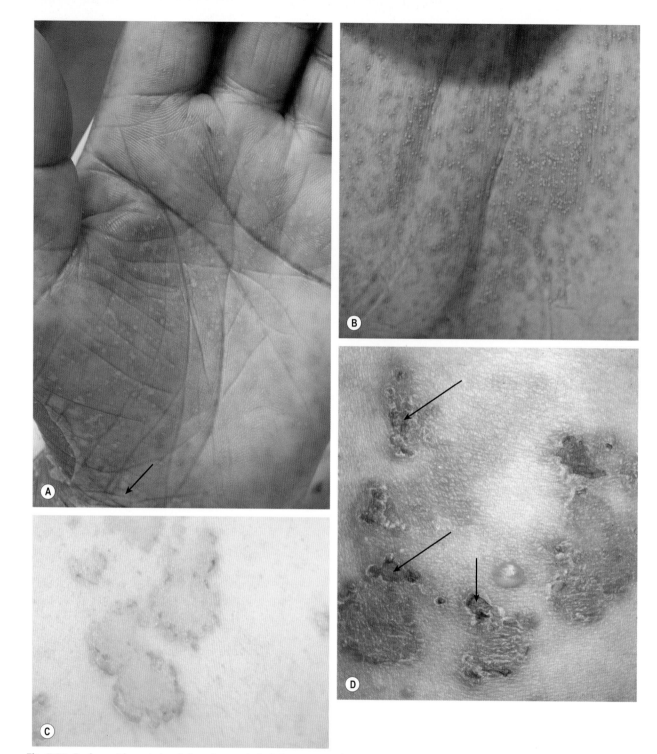

Fig. 7.21 Rashes with pustules. A Pustular psoriasis. **B** Acute generalized exanthematous pustulosis. **C** Subcorneal pustular dermatosis of Sneddon and Wilkinson. **D** IgA pemphigus, subcorneal pustular dermatosis type. *A, Courtesy, Yale Dermatology Residents' Slide Collection; B, Courtesy, Yale Dermatology Residents' Slide Collection; C, Courtesy, Dirk Elston, MD. D, Courtesy, Masayuki Amagai, MD. C, From Elston D. Clinical image collection. Dermatopathology, 2e. London: Saunders, 2014. D, From Bolognia JL, Jorizzo JL, Schaffer JV. Dermatology, 3e. London: Saunders, 2012, with permission.*

Epidermal Injury/Necrosis | 8

Epidermal injury/necrosis may be superficial, usually manifested as peeling or crusting of the skin *(Fig. 8.1A)*, or deeper secondary to dermal vascular injury, with early lesions presenting with a grayish hue to the skin *(Fig. 8.1C*; see Chapter 18).

The extent of epidermal injury can be important *(Fig. 8.2)*, and this chapter organizes diseases in that vein (extensive, extensive or limited, and often limited).

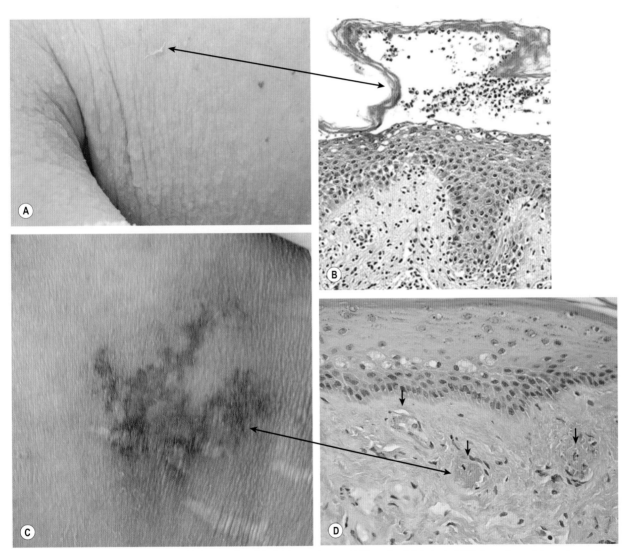

Fig. 8.1 Early epidermal necrosis. Staphylococcal scalded skin syndrome (**A,B**) and calciphylaxis (**C,D**; thrombosed dermal vessels above a deeper, calcified vessel). *A, Courtesy, Yale Dermatology Residents' Slide Collection. B, From Brinster NK, Liu V, McKee PH, Diwan H. Dermatopathology: High Yield Pathology. Philadelphia: Saunders, 2011. D, From Weenig RH. Pathogenesis of calciphylaxis: Hans Selye to nuclear factor kappa-B. J Am Acad Dermatol. 2008;58:458–71, © Elsevier.*

EXTENSIVE

Toxic Epidermal Necrolysis

Associated fever, lymphadenopathy, hepatitis
>30% of the body surface area *(Fig. 8.2)*
Mucosal erosions
Macular atypical targets
Bullae and erosions (arrow) over the skin *(Fig. 8.3)*

Histopathology:

Normal stratum corneum above epidermal necrosis, often with detachment of the epidermis from the dermis

Stevens–Johnson Syndrome

Covers <10% of the body surface area *(see Fig. 8.2)*
Similar lesions to toxic epidermal necrolysis, clinically and histologically *(Fig. 8.4)*

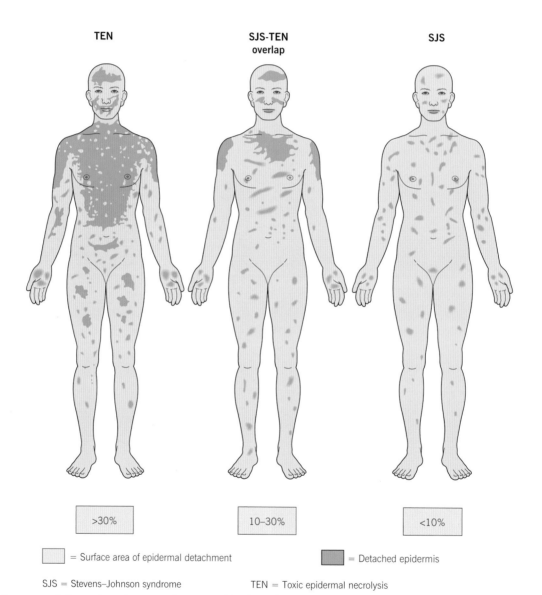

TEN

SJS-TEN
overlap

SJS

>30%

10–30%

<10%

= Surface area of epidermal detachment

= Detached epidermis

SJS = Stevens–Johnson syndrome

TEN = Toxic epidermal necrolysis

Fig. 8.2 Spectrum of disease based upon surface area of epidermal detachment. *Adapted from Bastuji-Garin S, Rzany B, Stern RS, et al. Clinical classification of cases of toxic epidermal necrolysis, Stevens-Johnson syndrome, and erythema multiforme. Arch Dermatol. 1993;129:92–6. From Bolognia JL, Schaffer JV, Duncan KO, Ko CJ. Dermatology Essentials, 1e. Philadelphia: Saunders, 2014, with permission.*

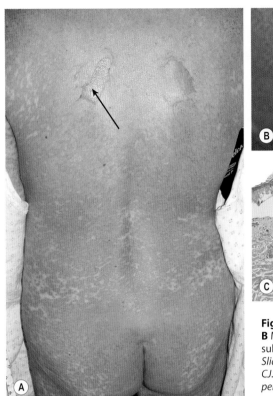

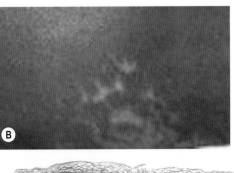

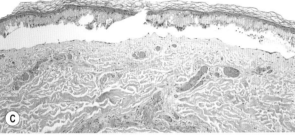

Fig. 8.3 Toxic epidermal necrolysis. A Sloughing of skin. **B** Macular atypical targets. **C** Epidermal necrosis with subepidermal cleft. *A, B, Courtesy, Yale Dermatology Residents' Slide Collection. B, From Bolognia JL, Schaffer JV, Duncan KO, Ko CJ. Dermatology Essentials, 1e. Philadelphia: Saunders, 2014, with permission.*

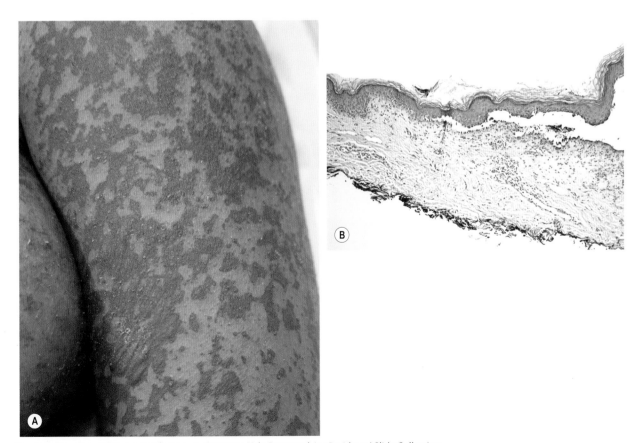

Fig. 8.4 Stevens–Johnson syndrome. *A, Courtesy, Yale Dermatology Residents' Slide Collection.*

EXTENSIVE OR LIMITED

Sunburn (Phototoxicity)

Acute erythema *(Fig. 8.5)*
Later stages – sloughing of skin

Thermal Burn

Body surface area affected can be estimated using a "rule of nines" *(Fig. 8.6A)*
Acute erythema; in more severe cases, sloughing, erosion, and/or ulceration *(Fig. 8.6B–D)*

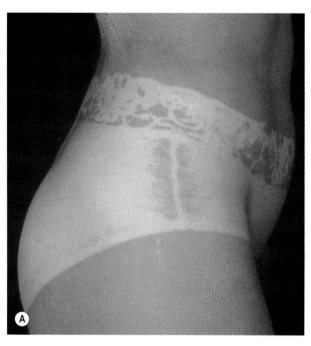

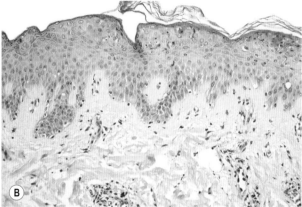

Fig. 8.5 Sunburn. A Twenty-four hours after an accidental 10-fold overdose of UVB prescribed as phototherapy. **B** Scattered necrotic keratinocytes in the epidermis. *With permission, Department of Dermatology, University of Würzburg, Germany. A, From Bolognia JL, Jorizzo JL, Schaffer JV. Dermatology, 3e. London: Saunders, 2012, with permission. B, From Brinster NK, Liu V, McKee PH, Diwan H. Dermatopathology: High Yield Pathology. Philadelphia: Saunders, 2011.*

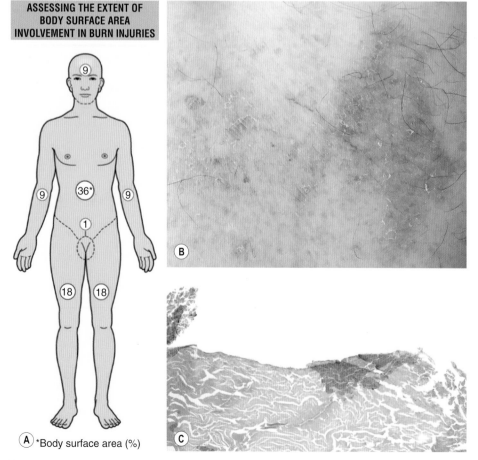

ASSESSING THE EXTENT OF BODY SURFACE AREA INVOLVEMENT IN BURN INJURIES

9
9 36* 9
1
18 18

A *Body surface area (%)

Fig. 8.6 Thermal burn. A Assessing the extent of body surface area involvement: rule of nines. **B** Erythema, erosion, and scale secondary to a burn from spilling hot tea. **C** The epidermis is completely absent in this burn. *A, Courtesy, Karynne O Duncan, MD. A, From Bolognia JL, Schaffer JV, Duncan KO, Ko CJ. Dermatology Essentials, 1e. Philadelphia: Saunders, 2014, with permission.*

Erythema Multiforme

Favors acral sites

Classic lesion – target with central deep red erythema surrounded by a halo of lighter color and an outer red rim *(Fig. 8.7A)*

Papular atypical targets (only 2 zones; *Fig. 8.7B*)

Histopathology:

Normal stratum corneum (blue arrow) above interface change (green arrow) with sparse lymphocytic inflammation *(Fig. 8.7C)*

A. Erythema multiforme – papular atypical targets with 2 zones of color – central deep pink to red and lighter rim

B. Urticaria multiforme – center of lesions is normal skin

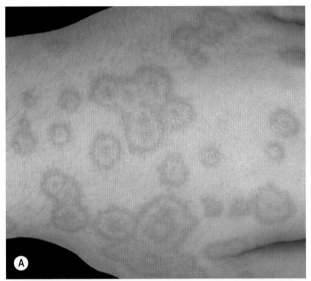

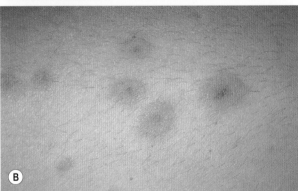

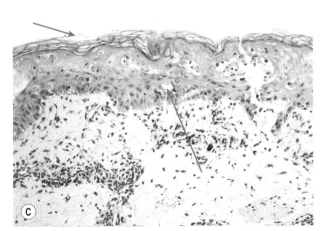

Fig. 8.7 Erythema multiforme. A Classic lesion. **B** Papular atypical targets. **C** Apoptotic keratinocytes. *A,B, Courtesy, Yale Dermatology Residents' Slide Collection. A,B, From Bolognia JL, Schaffer JV, Duncan KO, Ko CJ. Dermatology Essentials, 1e. Philadelphia: Saunders, 2014, with permission.*

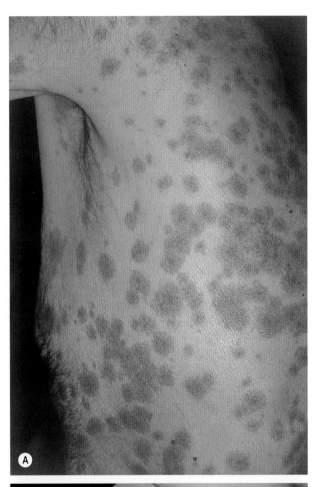

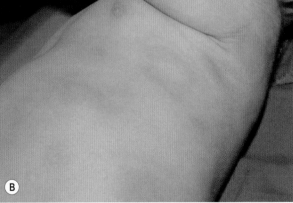

Fig. 8.8 Lesions with 2 zones of color. A Erythema multiforme. **B** Urticaria multiforme. *A, Courtesy, Yale Dermatology Residents' Slide Collection. B, Courtesy, Julie V Schaffer, MD. A,B, From Bolognia JL, Schaffer JV, Duncan KO, Ko CJ. Dermatology Essentials, 1e. Philadelphia: Saunders, 2014, with permission.*

Paraneoplastic Pemphigus

Characteristic hemorrhagic crusts over the vermilion lips *(Fig. 8.9)*

Lesions as in erythema multiforme or pemphigus vulgaris (flaccid blisters; *see Fig. 13.1*)

Histopathology:

For erythema multiforme-like lesions – interface change *(Fig. 8.9B)*; vesicular lesions – acantholysis *(Fig. 8.9C)*

Direct immunofluorescence – linear IgG and C3 at the dermal–epidermal junction and intercellular IgG and C3 *(Fig. 8.9D)*

Lupus Erythematosus

In particular, subacute lupus erythematosus

Papulosquamous lesions *(Fig. 8.10A)*, sometimes annular, over the trunk and proximal upper extremities

Histopathology:

Interface change with scattered apoptotic cells (arrow; *Fig. 8.10B)*

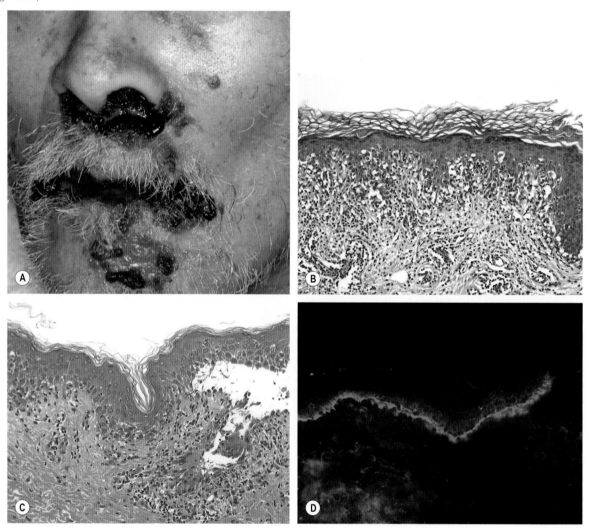

Fig. 8.9 Paraneoplastic pemphigus. *A,C, Courtesy, Masayuki Amagai, MD. D, Courtesy, Matthew Fleming, MD. A,C, From Bolognia JL, Jorizzo JL, Schaffer JV. Dermatology, 3e. London: Saunders, 2012, with permission. D, From Weidner N, Cote RJ, Suster S, Weiss LM. Modern Surgical Pathology, 2e. Philadelphia: Saunders, 2009.*

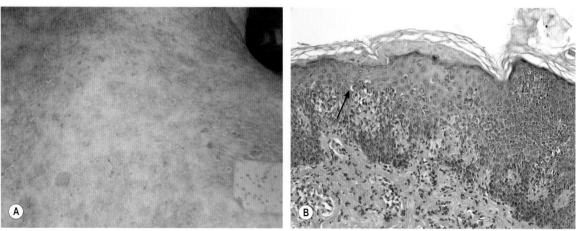

Fig. 8.10 Subacute lupus erythematosus.

Fixed Drug Eruption *(Fig. 8.11)*

Common inciting drugs include naproxen, allopurinol, antibiotics

Oval to round lesion(s), erythematous to violaceous, bullae may form

May resolve with hyperpigmentation *(Fig. 8.11E)*

Histopathology:

Early lesions with interface change and superficial and deep mixed inflammation *(Fig. 8.11B)*; later lesions with pigment incontinence and variable inflammation *(Fig. 8.11F)*

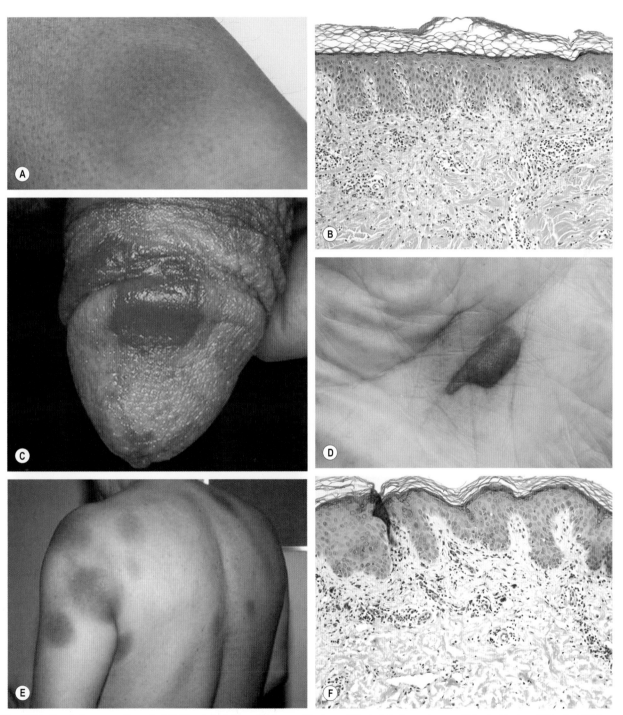

Fig. 8.11 Fixed drug eruption. A–C,E Characteristic oval to round lesions. **B** Early interface change. **C** Eroded lesion. **D** Central blister with detachment of the epidermis. **E** Oval areas of postinflammatory hyperpigmentation. **F** Pigment incontinence. *A,D Courtesy, Yale Dermatology Residents' Slide Collection; C, Courtesy, Kalman Watsky, MD; E, Courtesy, Mary Stone, MD. C,E, From Bolognia JL, Schaffer JV, Duncan KO, Ko CJ. Dermatology Essentials, 1e. Philadelphia: Saunders, 2014, with permission.*

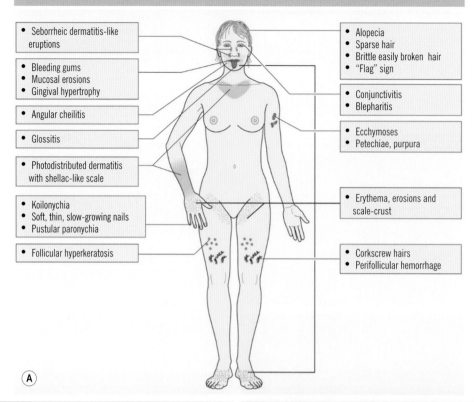

- Seborrheic dermatitis-like eruptions

- Bleeding gums
- Mucosal erosions
- Gingival hypertrophy

- Angular cheilitis

- Glossitis

- Photodistributed dermatitis with shellac-like scale

- Koilonychia
- Soft, thin, slow-growing nails
- Pustular paronychia

- Follicular hyperkeratosis

- Alopecia
- Sparse hair
- Brittle easily broken hair
- "Flag" sign

- Conjunctivitis
- Blepharitis

- Ecchymoses
- Petechiae, purpura

- Erythema, erosions and scale-crust

- Corkscrew hairs
- Perifollicular hemorrhage

Ⓐ

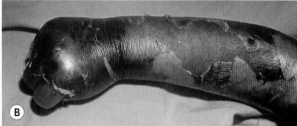

Ⓑ

Fig. 8.12 Nutritional deficiency. A Mucocutaneous clues that suggest a possible nutritional disorder. **B** Kwashiorkor. Edema and superficial epidermal necrosis with an "enamel paint" appearance. **C** Marasmus. Emaciation, hyperpigmentation, and superficial necrosis of the skin. *A, Courtesy, Karynne O Duncan, MD; B,C Courtesy, Ramón Ruiz-Maldonado, MD. A, From Bolognia JL, Schaffer JV, Duncan KO, Ko CJ. Dermatology Essentials, 1e. Philadelphia: Saunders, 2014, with permission. B,C, From Bolognia JL, Jorizzo JL, Schaffer JV. Dermatology, 3e. London: Saunders, 2012, with permission.*

Nutritional Deficiency

Particular nutritional deficiencies have classic associated findings (e.g. vitamin C deficiency and bleeding gums; *Fig. 8.12A*); importantly, patients can be deficient in more than one nutrient. Several different deficiencies can produce erythema and superficial scale corresponding to superficial epidermal necrosis (*Fig. 8.12B,C*); most of these present in periorificial, intertriginous, and acral areas (e.g. zinc, biotin, or essential fatty acid deficiency) except for pellagra, which favors sun-exposed sites.

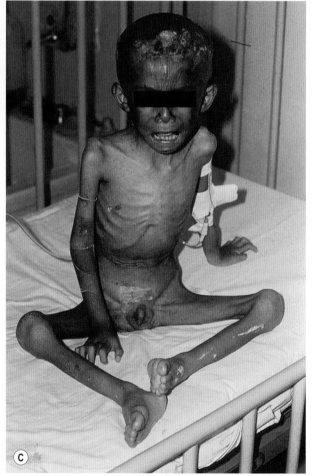

Ⓒ

Niacin/Nicotinic Acid (Vitamin B₃) Deficiency (Pellagra; see Chapter 3)

Classic triad – diarrhea, dementia, dermatitis
Favors sun-exposed sites and perianal areas
Erythema with subsequent hyperpigmentation, desquamation *(Fig. 8.13A, see asterisk)*, crusting

Clinical clues – Casal's necklace (broad area of involvement around the neck)

Histopathology:
Confluent parakeratosis and/or upper epidermal necrosis *(Fig. 8.13B, see asterisk)*

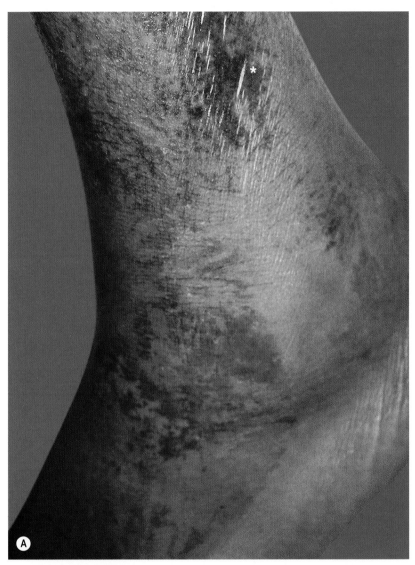

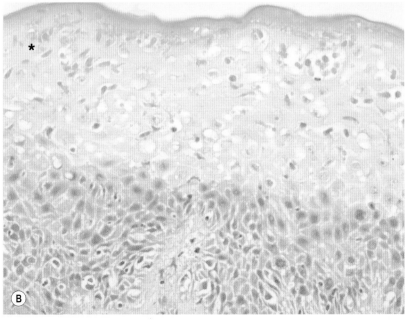

Fig. 8.13 Pellagra. *A, Courtesy, Yale Dermatology Residents' Slide Collection. A, From Bolognia JL, Jorizzo JL, Schaffer JV. Dermatology, 3e. London: Saunders, 2012, with permission. B, From Weidner N, Cote RJ, Suster S, Weiss LM. Modern Surgical Pathology, 2e. Philadelphia: Saunders, 2009.*

Zinc Deficiency (Acquired or Genetic, the Latter Is Termed Acrodermatitis Enteropathica)

Classic triad – diarrhea, dermatitis, alopecia
Favors periorificial, intertriginous, and acral sites
(Fig. 8.14A–D)

Erythema, erosions, crusting, and superficial desquamation
Clinical clue – pustular paronychia

Histopathology:
Parakeratosis and/or superficial necrosis of the epidermis
(Fig. 8.14E)

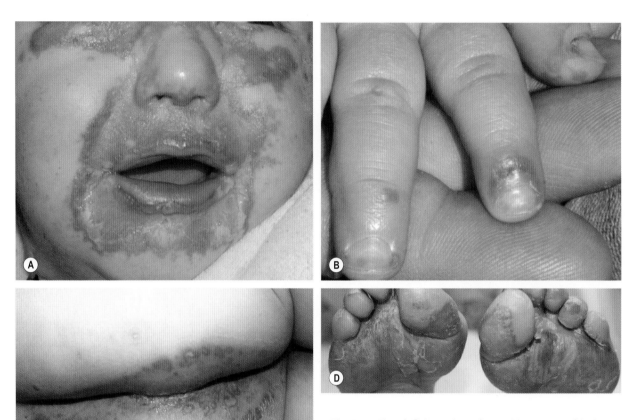

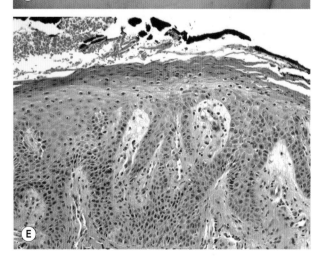

Fig. 8.14 Zinc deficiency (acrodermatitis enteropathica). *A,B, Courtesy Julie V Schaffer, MD. C, Courtesy, Jason Lott, MD; D, Courtesy, Yale Dermatology Residents' Slide Collection. A,B, From Bolognia JL, Jorizzo JL, Schaffer JV. Dermatology, 3e. London: Saunders, 2012, with permission.*

Necrolytic Acral Erythema

Associated with hepatitis C infection
Acral sites *(Fig. 8.15A)*

Histopathology:
Superficial necrosis of the epidermis *(Fig. 8.15B)*

Necrolytic Migratory Erythema *(Fig. 8.16)*

Associated with a glucagon-secreting pancreatic tumor
Angular cheilitis and eroded plaques with a predilection
for intertriginous sites (especially the groin)

Histopathology:
Superficial necrosis of the epidermis similar to necrolytic
acral erythema

Calciphylaxis *(see Figs. 8.1C and 18.4B)*

Warfarin-Induced Skin Necrosis
(see Fig. 18.4G)

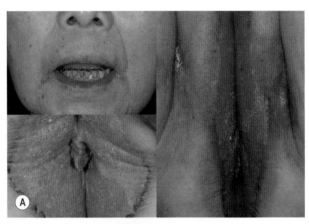

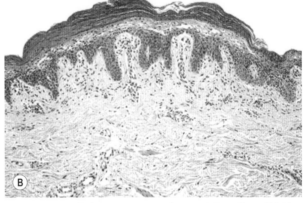

Fig. 8.16 Necrolytic migratory erythema. *A, From Tseng HC, Liu CT, Ho JC, Lin SH. Necrolytic migratory erythema and glucagonoma rising from pancreatic head. Pancreatology. 2013;13:455–7, © 2013 IAP and EPC. B, From Brinster NK, Liu V, McKee PH, Diwan H. Dermatopathology: High Yield Pathology. Philadelphia: Saunders, 2011.*

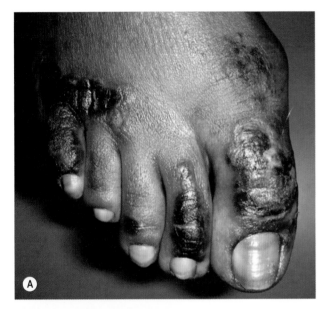

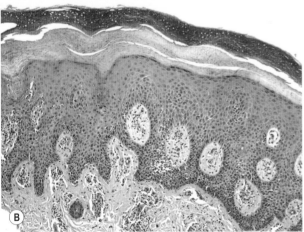

Fig. 8.15 Necrolytic acral erythema. *A, Courtesy, Jeffrey P Callen, MD. A, From Bolognia JL, Jorizzo JL, Schaffer JV. Dermatology, 3e. London: Saunders, 2012, with permission.*

OFTEN LIMITED

Spider Bite

Some species of spiders will bite humans and cause
epidermal and dermal necrosis (e.g. the brown recluse
spider, *Loxosceles reclusa*)
Initial erythema may become dusky and eventuate in
bullae and/or necrosis *(Fig. 8.17)*

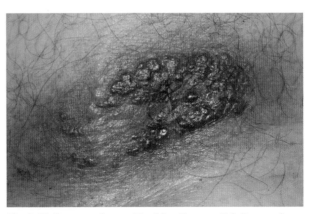

Fig. 8.17 Brown recluse spider bite. *Courtesy, Yale Dermatology Residents' Slide Collection.*

Follicular Processes | 9

Follicular processes have lesions that are either pierced by a hair shaft or are distributed in a pattern corresponding to hair follicles. This chapter covers acne, rosacea, folliculitis, keratosis pilaris, pityriasis rubra pilaris, discoid lupus erythematosus, lichen planopilaris, follicular mucinosis, scurvy, vitamin A deficiency, and trichodysplasia spinulosa.

ACNE

Typically affects the face, chest, and back
Lesions include comedones, papules, pustules, and nodules *(Figs 9.1, 9.2)*

Sequelae include scarring and postinflammatory pigmentary changes *(see Fig. 9.2)*

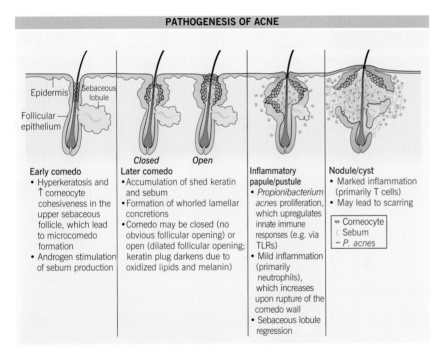

PATHOGENESIS OF ACNE

Early comedo
- Hyperkeratosis and ↑ corneocyte cohesiveness in the upper sebaceous follicle, which lead to microcomedo formation
- Androgen stimulation of sebum production

Later comedo
- Accumulation of shed keratin and sebum
- Formation of whorled lamellar concretions
- Comedo may be closed (no obvious follicular opening) or open (dilated follicular opening; keratin plug darkens due to oxidized lipids and melanin)

Inflammatory papule/pustule
- *Propionibacterium acnes* proliferation, which upregulates innate immune responses (e.g. via TLRs)
- Mild inflammation (primarily neutrophils), which increases upon rupture of the comedo wall
- Sebaceous lobule regression

Nodule/cyst
- Marked inflammation (primarily T cells)
- May lead to scarring

▽ Corneocyte
ℓ Sebum
– *P. acnes*

Epidermis
Sebaceous lobule
Follicular epithelium
Closed *Open*

Fig. 9.1 Pathogenesis of acne. *From Bolognia JL, Schaffer JV, Duncan KO, Ko CJ. Dermatology Essentials, 1e. Philadelphia: Saunders, 2014, with permission.*

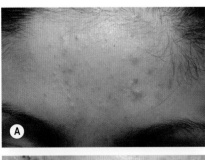

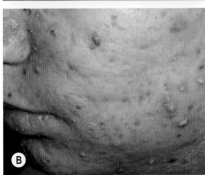

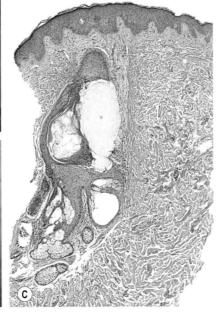

Fig. 9.2 Acne. A Open and closed comedones and several inflammatory papules. **B** Papulopustules and scarring. **C** Follicular rupture and inflammation. *A, Courtesy Kalman Watsky, MD; B, Courtesy, Andrew Zaenglein, MD and Diane Thiboutot, MD. A,B, From Bolognia JL, Schaffer JV, Duncan KO, Ko CJ. Dermatology Essentials, 1e. Philadelphia: Saunders, 2014, with permission.*

ROSACEA

Most commonly affects the face *(Fig. 9.3)*; rarely scalp, chest
Papulopustular form and granulomatous variant are folliculo-centric

Histopathology:
Perifollicular and perivascular lymphocytes
+/– histiocytes
Dilated vessels

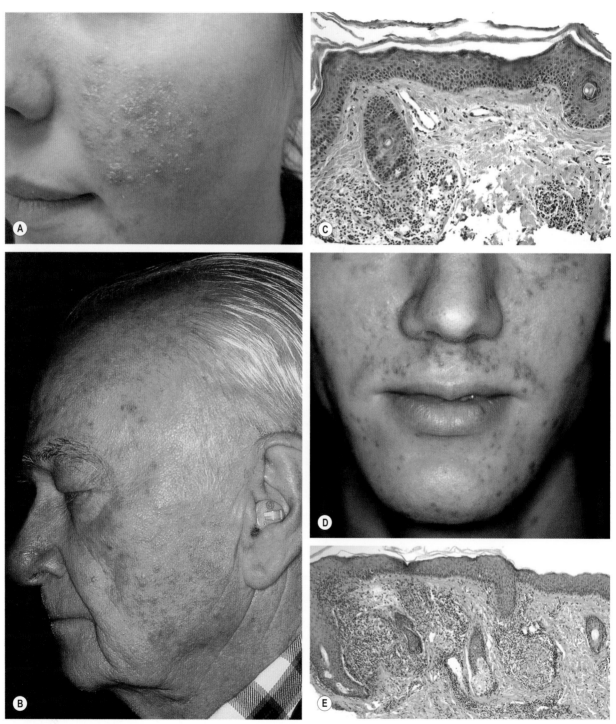

Fig. 9.3 Rosacea. A–C Papulopustular form. Lymphocytes surround follicles. **D,E** Granulomatous rosacea (perifollicular granulomas). *A, Courtesy, Kalman Watsky, MD; B,D, Courtesy, Yale Dermatology Residents' Slide Collection. B,D, From From Bolognia JB, Jorizzo JL, Rapini RP. Dermatology, 2e. London: Saunders, 2008, with permission.*

FOLLICULITIS

Folliculitis is inflammation of hair follicles and can be superficial or deep, infectious *(Fig. 9.4)* or non-infectious *(Figs 9.5, 9.6)*

Papules and/or pustules, sometimes crusted, affect various sites

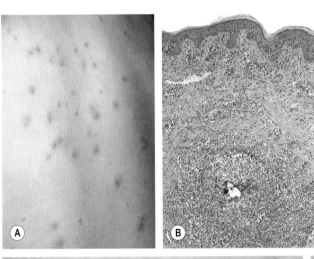

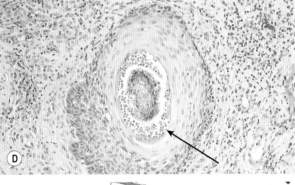

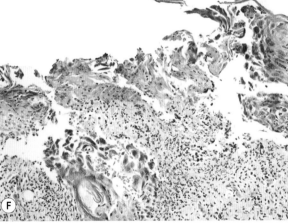

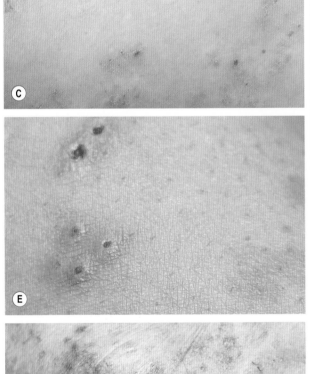

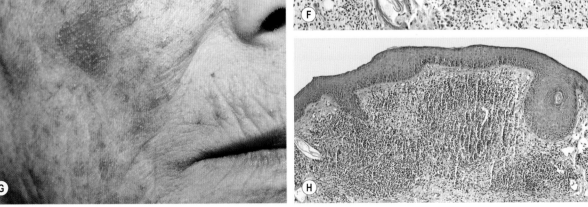

Fig. 9.4 Infectious folliculitis. A,B Bacterial (*Staphylococcus aureus*) folliculitis. Clumps of bacteria are present in an inflamed follicle. **C,D** Fungal folliculitis. Around the hair shaft, there are hyphae cut in cross-section (arrow). In addition to erythematous papules, there are plaques with annular scale. **E,F** Viral (herpes simplex virus) folliculitis. There is acantholysis with multinucleate cells. **G,H** *Demodex* folliculitis. *Demodex* mites are located in the dermis with surrounding inflammation. *A, Courtesy, Julie V Schaffer, MD; E, Courtesy, Yale Dermatology Residents' Slide Collection; G, Courtesy, Kalman Watsky, MD. A, From Bolognia JL, Schaffer JV, Duncan KO, Ko CJ. Dermatology Essentials, 1e. Philadelphia: Saunders, 2014, with permission.*

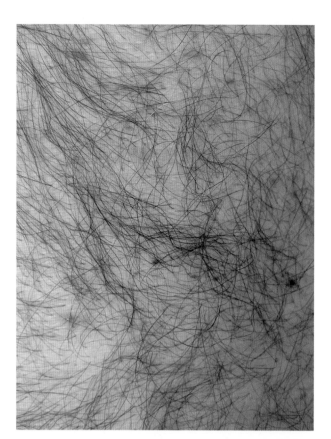

Fig. 9.5 Sterile (culture-negative) folliculitis. Note the pustule pierced by a hair shaft.

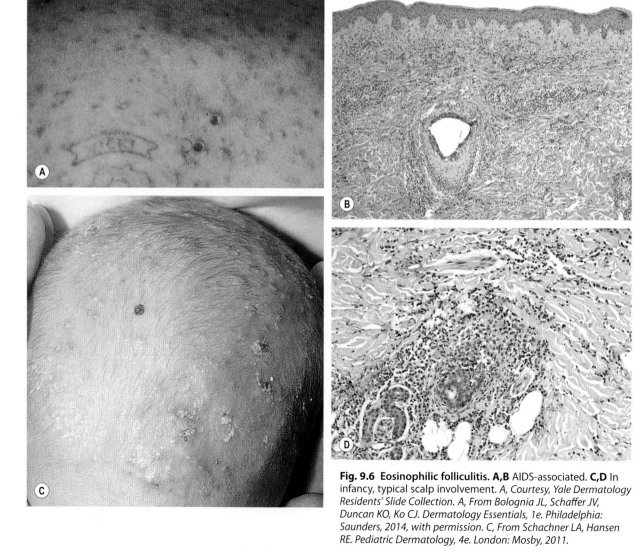

Fig. 9.6 Eosinophilic folliculitis. A,B AIDS-associated. **C,D** In infancy, typical scalp involvement. *A, Courtesy, Yale Dermatology Residents' Slide Collection. A, From Bolognia JL, Schaffer JV, Duncan KO, Ko CJ. Dermatology Essentials, 1e. Philadelphia: Saunders, 2014, with permission. C, From Schachner LA, Hansen RE. Pediatric Dermatology, 4e. London: Mosby, 2011.*

KERATOSIS PILARIS

Favors the upper arms *(Fig. 9.7)* and thighs, as well as the lateral cheeks in children
Keratotic follicular papules, +/– erythema

Histopathology:
Keratin-plugged hair follicle, sometimes with surrounding inflammation

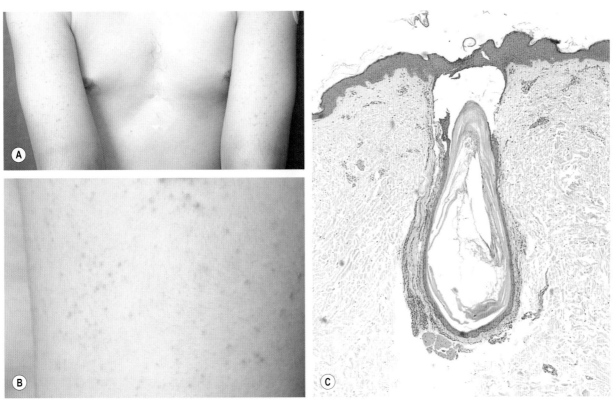

Fig. 9.7 Keratosis pilaris. *A,B, Courtesy, Kathleen Suozzi, MD.*

PITYRIASIS RUBRA PILARIS (see also Chapter 4)

Nutmeg grater-like follicular papules *(Fig. 9.8)*

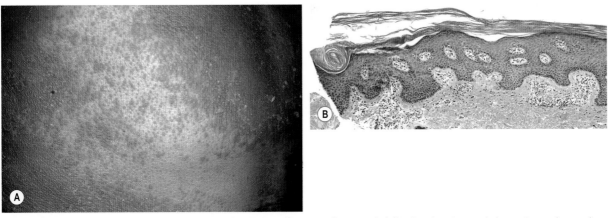

Fig. 9.8 Pityriasis rubra pilaris. A,B Follicular papules and confluent erythema with follicular plugging and alternating ortho- and parakeratosis. *A, Courtesy, Yale Dermatology Residents' Slide Collection. A, From Bolognia JL, Schaffer JV, Duncan KO, Ko CJ. Dermatology Essentials, 1e. Philadelphia: Saunders, 2014, with permission.*

DISCOID LUPUS ERYTHEMATOSUS

Follicular plugging, often easily appreciated in the conchal bowl *(Fig. 9.9)*
Associated scarring, dyspigmentation, and/or atrophy

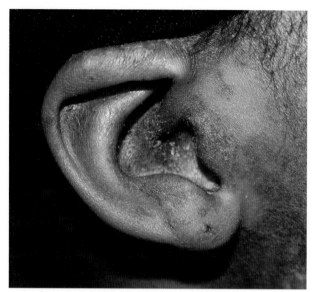

Fig. 9.9 Discoid lupus erythematosus. *Courtesy, Yale Dermatology Residents' Slide Collection.*

LICHEN PLANOPILARIS

Scalp with areas of hair loss *(Fig. 9.10)* sometimes with plugged, erythematous follicles
Skin, mucosa, or nails may show signs of lichen planus

Histopathology:
Lymphocytes surrounding the upper part of the follicle with destruction of the follicular epithelium

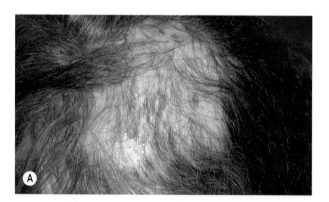

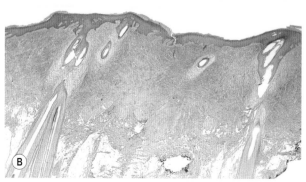

Fig. 9.10 Lichen planopilaris.

FOLLICULAR MUCINOSIS

Grouped follicular papules with alopecia *(Fig. 9.11; see also Fig. 2.7A)*
Violet–brown plaques may be present

Histopathology:
Mucin within follicles creating white–blue space between keratinocytes

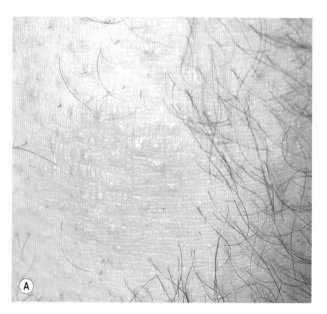

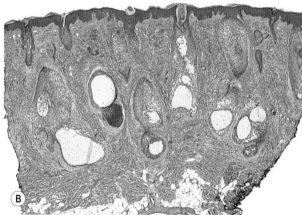

Fig. 9.11 Follicular mucinosis.

SCURVY

Perifollicular hemorrhage and corkscrew hairs *(Fig. 9.12)*
Other clues – gingival bleeding, purpura

Histopathology:
Plugged follicles surrounded by inflammation and erythrocytes

VITAMIN A DEFICIENCY

Phrynoderma (clusters of hyperkeratotic follicular papules) over extensor surfaces *(Fig. 9.13)*
Xerosis
Night blindness

Histopathology:
Plugged follicle

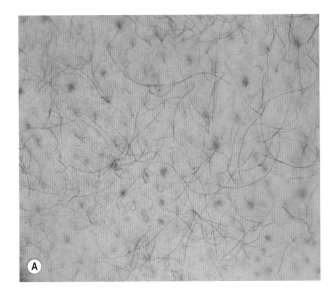

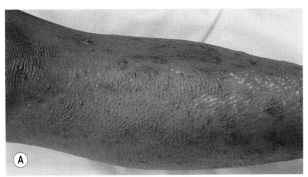

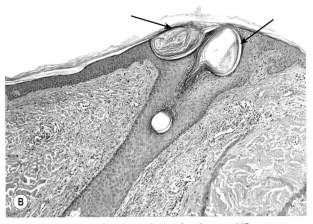

Fig. 9.12 Scurvy. *A, Courtesy, Christopher Stamey, MD.*

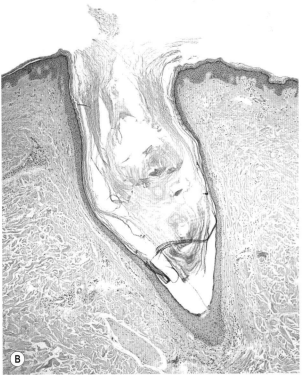

Fig. 9.13 Phrynoderma. *A, Courtesy, Chad M Hivnor, MD. A, From Bolognia JL, Schaffer JV, Duncan KO, Ko CJ. Dermatology Essentials, 1e. Philadelphia: Saunders, 2014, with permission.*

TRICHODYSPLASIA SPINULOSA

Follicular papules *(Fig. 9.14)*, sometimes with prominent protruding spines

Histopathology:
Expanded follicles with abnormal outer root sheath and absent hair shaft; viral intracytoplasmic bodies may be evident.

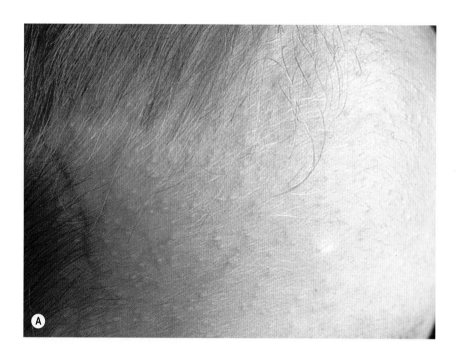

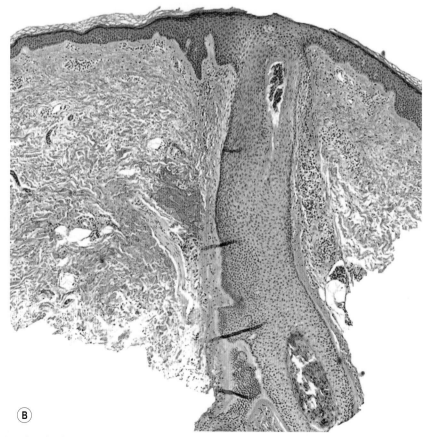

Fig. 9.14 Viral-associated trichodysplasia. Follicular papules on the forehead (**A**). Dilated follicles with abnormal parakeratosis (**B**).
A, Courtesy, Danielle Tashakori, PA.

Small Papules Secondary to a Dermal Process

10

The focus of this chapter is on dermal processes with minimal surface epidermal change, in particular histiocytic/granulomatous disorders that produce multiple small papules on the skin. Entities in this chapter include lichen nitidus, histiocytoses, sarcoidosis, granuloma annulare, eruptive xanthoma, urticaria pigmentosa, and lichen myxedematosus. Not covered in this chapter are dermal tumors/cysts (e.g. cherry angiomas, *see Fig. 20.8A,B*; neurofibromas, *see Fig. 20.11A,B*; steatocystomas, *see Fig. 21.6A,B*; vellus hair cysts, *see Fig. 21.7A,B*) and epidermal tumors/processes, which can also produce multiple papules (e.g. warts, *see Fig. 19.16A,B*; molluscum, *see Fig. 19.17A,B*; multiple facial papules, *see Fig. 2.1*).

LICHEN NITIDUS

Shiny, tiny (~1 mm) papules *(Fig. 10.1)*

Histopathology:
Epidermal rete demarcating a lymphohistiocytic infiltrate in the superficial dermis

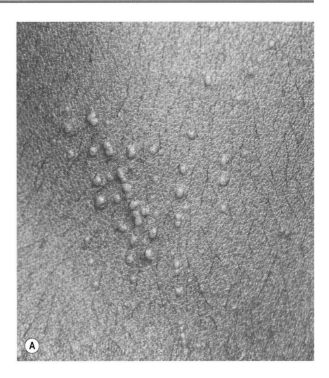

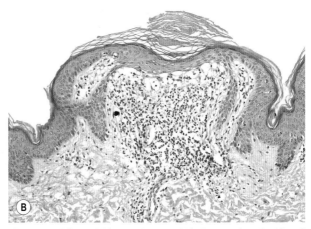

Fig. 10.1 Lichen nitidus. *A, Courtesy, Yale Dermatology Residents' Slide Collection.*

HISTIOCYTOSES

There are classic presentations of different histiocytoses (*Fig. 10.2, Table 10.1*), and the typical lesion is a dermal red–brown to pink papule for non-Langerhans cell histiocytoses. Such papules may also be seen in Langerhans cell histiocytosis (LCH), but the more common LCH lesion is an eroded and purpuric papule or plaque. In practice, there is significant overlap between various histiocytoses; the clinical distribution, other clinical lesions, and/or histopathologic features may be helpful in categorization.

Table 10.1 Classic features of selected histiocytoses

Histiocytosis	Classic clinical features	Classic histopathologic features
Langerhans cell histiocytosis (*Fig. 10.3A–C*)	• Eroded, purpuric papules/plaques in intertriginous zones • Ulcerations • Pink to red–brown dermal-based papules without surface change	• Dermal Langerhans cells (Langerin+, CD1a+ [*Fig. 10.3B,C*], S-100+) • Eosinophils may be present
Generalized eruptive histiocytoma (*Fig. 10.3D,E*)	• Favors the face and trunk • Red–brown papules	• Dermal histiocytic infiltrate (CD68+), often without obvious giant cells
Indeterminate cell histiocytosis	• Favors the trunk and proximal extremities • Red–brown papules	• Dermal histiocytic infiltrate (S-100+, CD68+, CD1a–, Langerin–)
Multicentric reticulohistiocytosis (*Fig. 10.3F,G*)	• Favors acral sites • Pink to red–brown papules	• Two-toned giant cells
Rosai–Dorfman disease (*Fig. 10.3H–K*)	• Red–brown papules or plaque(s)/nodule(s) • Massive, painless bilateral cervical lymphadenopathy is characteristic	• Emperipolesis • S100+ multinucleate cells (*Fig. 10.3J–K*) • CD68+

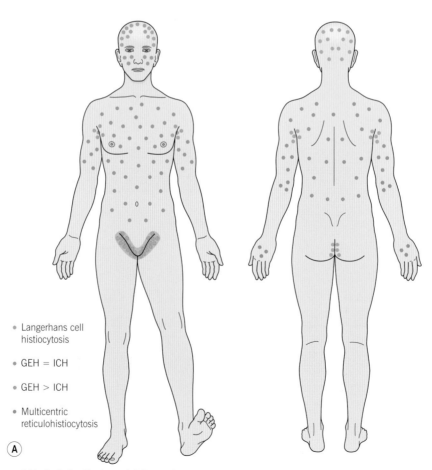

- Langerhans cell histiocytosis
- GEH = ICH
- GEH > ICH
- Multicentric reticulohistiocytosis

(A)

Fig. 10.2 Histiocytoses. A Typical distribution of different histiocytoses. GEH, generalized eruptive histiocytosis; ICH, indeterminate cell histiocytosis.

Continued

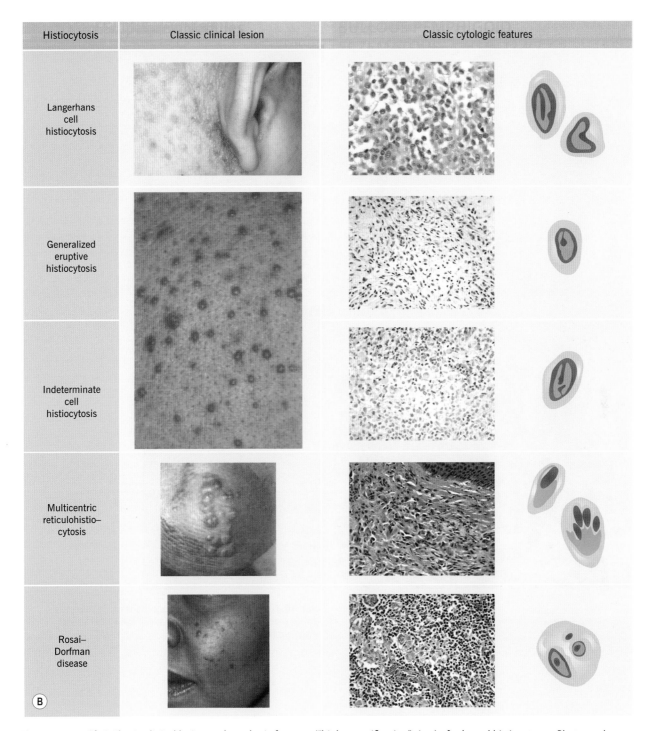

Histiocytosis	Classic clinical lesion	Classic cytologic features
Langerhans cell histiocytosis		
Generalized eruptive histiocytosis		
Indeterminate cell histiocytosis		
Multicentric reticulohistiocytosis		
Rosai– Dorfman disease		

Fig. 10.2, cont'd B Classic clinical lesion and cytologic features ("high magnification" view) of selected histiocytoses. *Photographs courtesy, Irwin Braverman, MD; Ingo Haase, MD, and Iliana Tantcheva-Poor, MD; Jean L Bolognia, MD and Yale Dermatology Residents' Slide Collection. From Bolognia JL, Jorizzo JL, Schaffer JV. Dermatology, 3e. London: Saunders, 2012, with permission.*

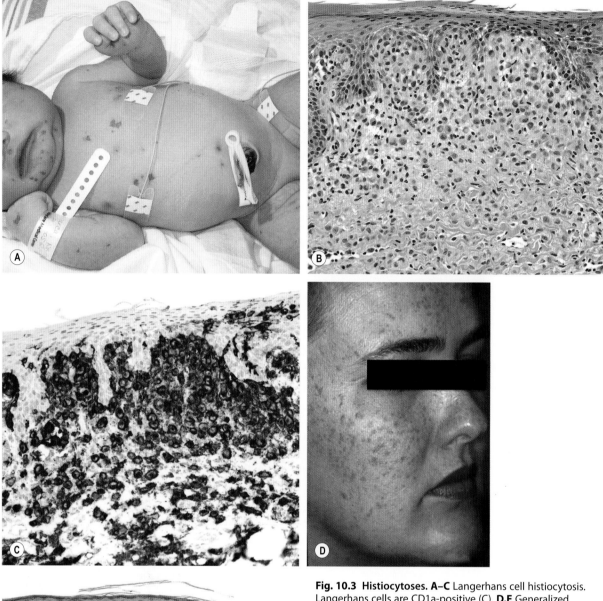

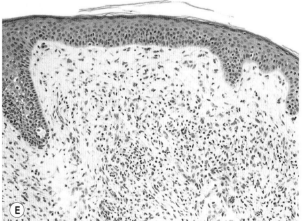

Fig. 10.3 Histiocytoses. A–C Langerhans cell histiocytosis. Langerhans cells are CD1a-positive (C). **D,E** Generalized eruptive histiocytoma.

Continued

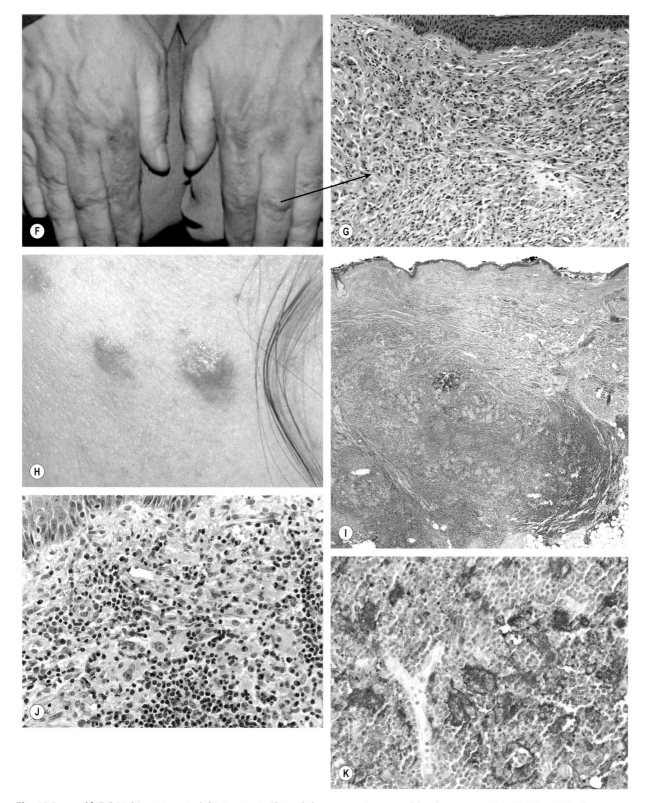

Fig. 10.3, cont'd F,G Multicentric reticulohistiocytosis. This subtle presentation resembles dermatomyositis. **H–K** Rosai–Dorfman disease. *A, Courtesy, Deborah S Goddard, MD, Amy E Gilliam, MD, and Ilona J Frieden, MD; D,H Courtesy, Jennifer M McNiff, MD. F, Courtesy, Kalman Watsky, MD. A,E, From Bolognia JL, Schaffer JV, Duncan KO, Ko CJ. Dermatology Essentials, 1e. Philadelphia: Saunders, 2014, with permission.*

SARCOIDOSIS

May affect the skin only or be multisystemic *(Fig. 10.4A)*
Any cutaneous site may be affected
Classically multiple red–brown to pink papules, sometimes forming annular arrangements *(Fig. 10.4B)*

Sarcoidosis can be a mimic of many other diseases *(Fig. 10.4D,E)*

Histopathology:
Naked dermal granulomas *(Fig. 10.4C)*

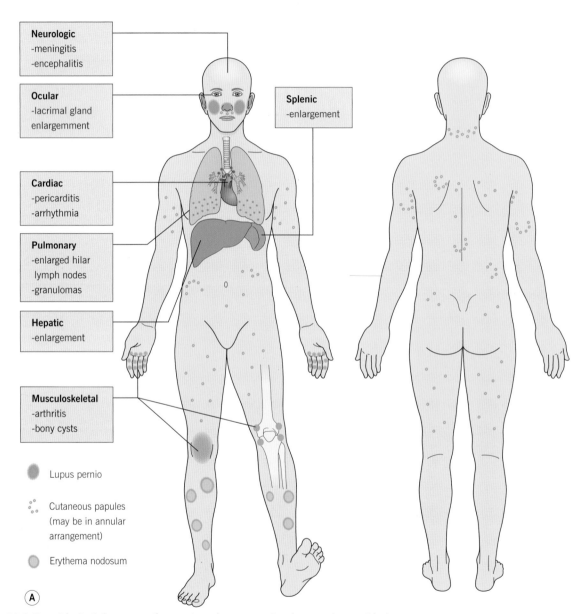

Neurologic
-meningitis
-encephalitis

Ocular
-lacrimal gland enlargemment

Splenic
-enlargement

Cardiac
-pericarditis
-arrhythmia

Pulmonary
-enlarged hilar lymph nodes
-granulomas

Hepatic
-enlargement

Musculoskeletal
-arthritis
-bony cysts

Lupus pernio

Cutaneous papules (may be in annular arrangement)

Erythema nodosum

(A)

Fig. 10.4 Sarcoidosis. A Spectrum of systemic and cutaneous involvement in sarcoidosis.

Continued

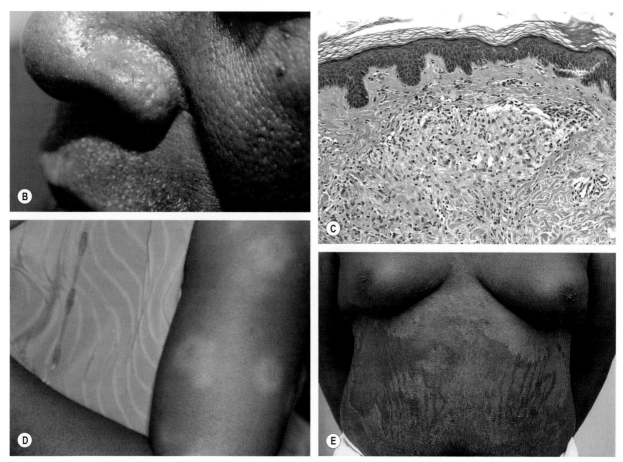

Fig. 10.4, cont'd B,C Sarcoidosis, classic papules with granuloma formation in the dermis. **D** Hypopigmented variant. **E** Ichthyosiform variant. *B, Courtesy, Yale Dermatology Residents' Slide Collection; D, Courtesy, Louis A Fragola, Jr, MD; E, Courtesy, Jean L Bolognia, MD. D,E, From Bolognia JL, Schaffer JV, Duncan KO, Ko CJ. Dermatology Essentials, 1e. Philadelphia: Saunders, 2014, with permission.*

GRANULOMA ANNULARE

Typically acral, but may be generalized *(Fig. 10.5A)*
Pink papules that may form annular arrangements

Histopathology:
Dermal mucin surrounded by palisades of histiocytes *(Fig. 10.5B)*

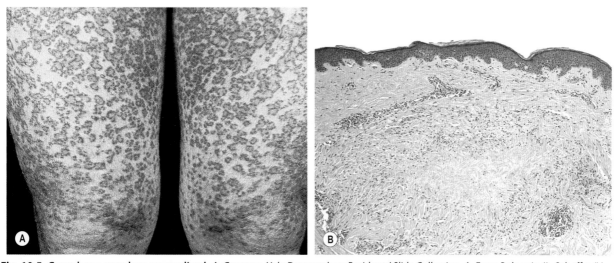

Fig. 10.5 Granuloma annulare, generalized. *A, Courtesy, Yale Dermatology Residents' Slide Collection. A, From Bolognia JL, Schaffer JV, Duncan KO, Ko CJ. Dermatology Essentials, 1e. Philadelphia: Saunders, 2014, with permission.*

ERUPTIVE XANTHOMA

Typically affects the buttocks/thighs *(Fig. 10.6A)*
In the setting of uncontrolled diabetes mellitus, and/or elevated lipids (i.e. hypertriglyceridemia)
Yellow–pink papules *(Fig. 10.6B)*

Histopathology:
Intracellular and extracellular lipid *(Fig. 10.6C)*

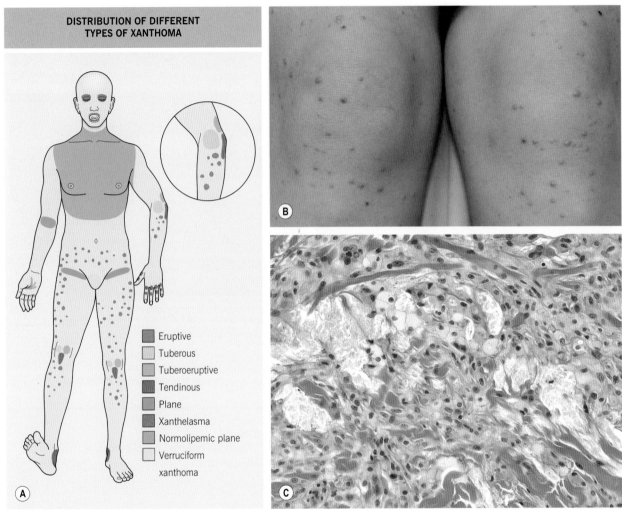

DISTRIBUTION OF DIFFERENT TYPES OF XANTHOMA

- Eruptive
- Tuberous
- Tuberoeruptive
- Tendinous
- Plane
- Xanthelasma
- Normolipemic plane
- Verruciform xanthoma

Fig. 10.6 Xanthoma. A Typical distribution of different types of xanthoma. **B,C** Eruptive xanthoma. *B,C, Courtesy, Yale Dermatology Residents' Slide Collection. A, From Bolognia JL, Schaffer JV, Duncan KO, Ko CJ. Dermatology Essentials, 1e. Philadelphia: Saunders, 2014, with permission.*

URTICARIA PIGMENTOSA

Favors the trunk *(Fig. 10.7A,C)*
Red–brown papules that may urticate with stroking
(Darier's sign)

Histopathology:
Dermal mast cells *(Fig. 10.7B,D,E)*

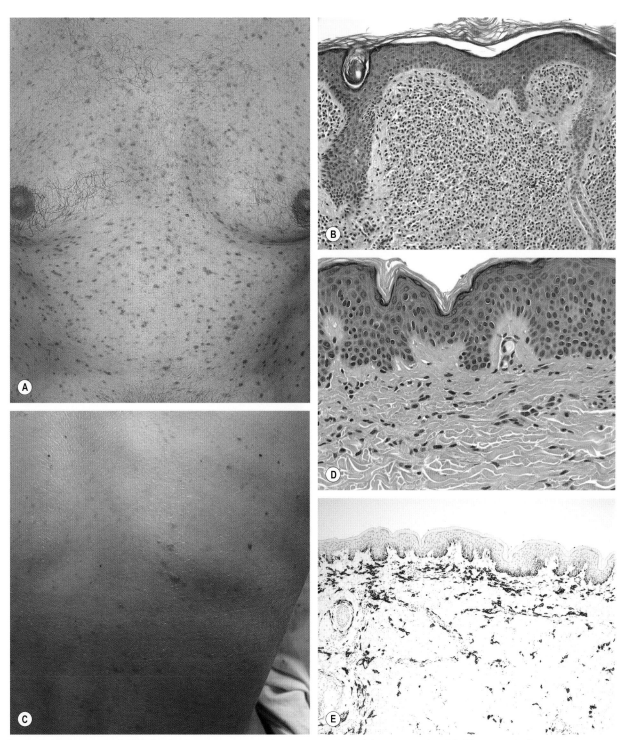

Fig. 10.7 Mastocytosis. A,B Urticaria pigmentosa presenting as numerous red–brown papules. **C,D** Mastocytosis that appears more urticarial clinically with a subtler infiltrate histopathologically. **E** Mastocytosis – CD117 staining is positive. *A, Courtesy, Michael Tharp, MD; C, Courtesy, Yale Dermatology Residents' Slide Collection; D,E, Courtesy, Nemanja Rodic, MD, PhD. A, From Bolognia JL, Schaffer JV, Duncan KO, Ko CJ. Dermatology Essentials, 1e. Philadelphia: Saunders, 2014, with permission.*

LICHEN MYXEDEMATOSUS *(Fig. 10.8)*

1–2 mm flesh-colored papules, sometimes in linear or clustered arrays

Histopathology:
Spindle cells, often with increased stromal mucin

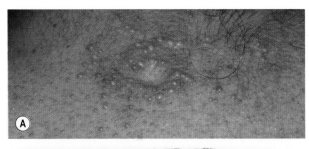

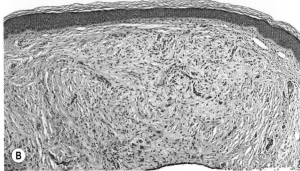

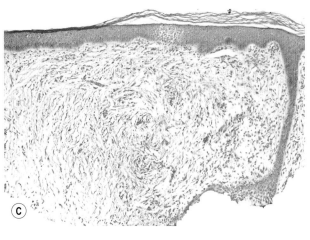

Fig. 10.8 Lichen myxedematosus. *A, Courtesy, Kalman Watsky, MD.*

STEATOCYSTOMAS

Often on the trunk when multiple *(see Fig. 21.6A)*
May discharge an oily substance
Skin-colored papulonodules

Histopathology:
Cyst wall lined by epithelium with a bright pink serrated surface *(see Fig. 21.6B)*

MILIA

White papules
If the surface is punctured, white material (keratin) can be extruded

Histopathology:
Cystic space lined by epithelium resembling the normal epidermis

VELLUS HAIR CYSTS

Variably colored small papules *(see Fig. 21.7A)*

Histopathology:
Cystic space containing keratin and vellus hairs *(see Fig. 21.7B)*

ACNE VULGARIS AND ACNE ROSACEA (see Chapter 9)

Dermal Inflammation | 11

Neutrophilic infiltrates may have a characteristic acute, non-treated appearance that is red and "hot" due to inflammation *(see Fig. 1.47)*. Mixed inflammatory infiltrates (lymphocytes and histiocytes with neutrophils or eosinophils) are in general a lighter pink–red.

Granulomatous disorders often produce monomorphous papules with a red–brown to violaceous color (see Chapter 10 and *Fig. 2.7G*). This chapter covers neutrophilic, mixed, and lymphocytic infiltrates.

NEUTROPHILIC ("HOT")

Sweet Syndrome

Any site, but predilection for facial and acral locations Edematous/pseudovesicular to crusted papules and plaques, sometimes targetoid *(Fig. 11.1A,B)*

Histopathology:
Dense dermal infiltrate of neutrophils, sometimes with papillary dermal edema *(Fig. 11.1C)*

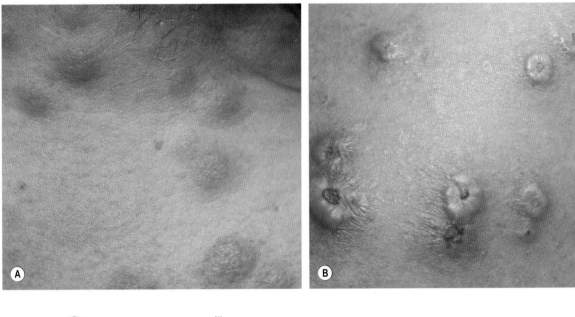

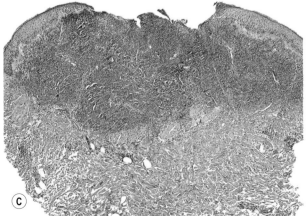

Fig. 11.1 Sweet syndrome. *A,B, Courtesy, Yale Dermatology Residents' Slide Collection.*

Pyoderma Gangrenosum *(Fig. 11.2)*

Any site, but commonly on the legs
Early lesion is an inflamed pustule *(see Fig. 7.14)*
Well-developed lesions often ulcerated with a violet–gray undermined border

Histopathology:
Inflamed lesions have a dense dermal infiltrate of neutrophils

Erythema Elevatum Diutinum, Acute Stage *(Fig. 11.3)*

Symmetric, often acral (extensor surfaces of elbows/hands), red–violet to pink–brown papules and plaques

Histopathology:
Infiltrate of neutrophils with vascular damage
Late stage becomes clinically indurated and histologically fibrotic *(see Fig. 22.16)*

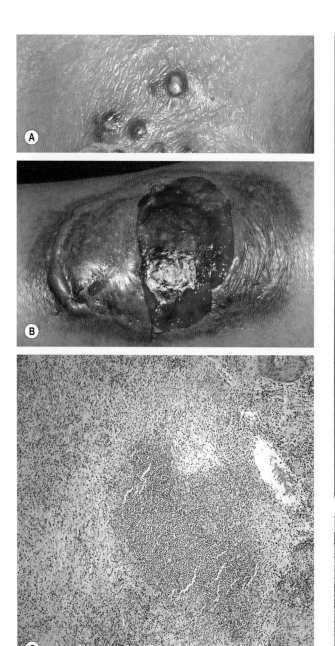

Fig. 11.2 Pyoderma gangrenosum. *A,B, Courtesy, Yale Dermatology Residents' Slide Collection.*

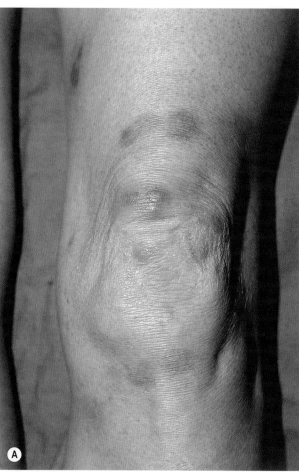

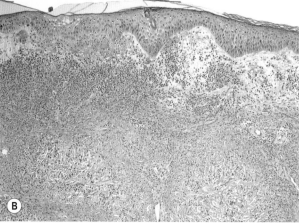

Fig. 11.3 Erythema elevatum diutinum. *A, Courtesy, Kenneth Greer, MD. A, From Bolognia JL, Jorizzo JL, Schaffer JV. Dermatology, 3e. London: Saunders, 2012, with permission.*

Cellulitis *(Fig. 11.4)*

Any site, but commonly affects the lower legs
Warm, tender, bright red plaque
Often associated fever and elevated white cell count

Histopathology:
Interstitial infiltrate of neutrophils

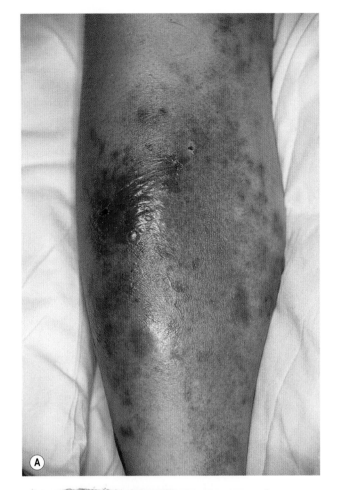

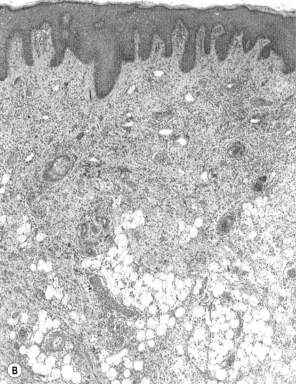

Fig. 11.4 Cellulitis (group A streptococci). *A, Courtesy, Yale Dermatology Residents' Slide Collection. A, From Bolognia JL, Jorizzo JL, Schaffer JV. Dermatology, 3e. London: Saunders, 2012, with permission. B, From Guarner J. Skin and soft tissue infections. In: Procop GW, Pritt BS (eds). Pathology of Infectious Diseases. London: Saunders, 2015.*

MIXED WITH NEUTROPHILS AND EOSINOPHILS OR PREDOMINANT EOSINOPHILS (PINK–RED)

Wells' Syndrome *(Eosinophilic Cellulitis; Fig. 11.5)*

Pink edematous plaques that may resemble cellulitis

Histopathology:
Interstitial infiltrate of eosinophils and neutrophils, often with flame figures (collagen encrusted with granular red–purple material)

Arthropod Bite Reaction *(Fig. 11.6)*

Various arthropods can assault or bite humans
Lesions are pink–red papules, sometimes crusted or vesicular

Histopathology:
Superficial and deep perivascular and interstitial mixed infiltrate

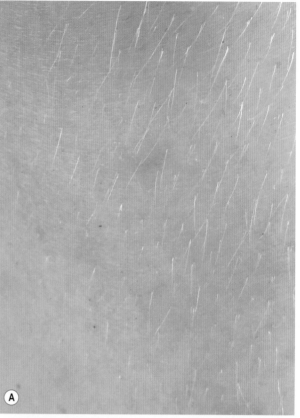

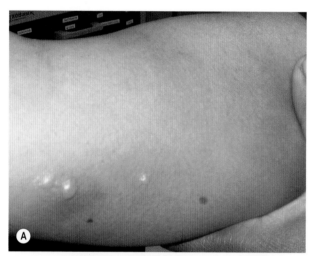

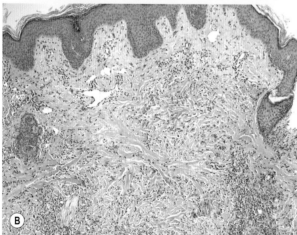

Fig. 11.5 Wells' syndrome. *A, Courtesy, Yale Dermatology Residents' Slide Collection.*

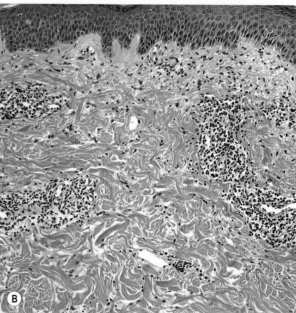

Fig. 11.6 Arthropod bite reaction.

Palisaded Neutrophilic and Granulomatous Disorder (Fig. 11.7)

Associated with connective tissue disorders such as rheumatoid arthritis, lupus erythematosus, and granulomatosis with polyangiitis
Erythematous papules, sometimes with central "punched out" ulceration
Favors the elbows and extensor digits

Histopathology:
Neutrophilic infiltrates with vasculitis and/or palisading granulomas

Granuloma Faciale (Fig. 11.8; see Fig. 2.7E)

Typically on the face but may affect other sites
Red–brown papule or plaque, often with prominent follicular openings

Histopathology:
Mixed infiltrate below a grenz zone (rim of spared papillary dermis)

Fixed Drug Eruption

(see Chapter 8)

Urticaria (see Fig. 1.47I,J)

Transient, edematous pink papules/plaques

Histopathology:
Mostly perivascular neutrophils, lymphocytes, and/or eosinophils

Urticarial Bullous Pemphigoid

(see Chapter 13)

Eosinophilic Folliculitis

(see Chapter 9)

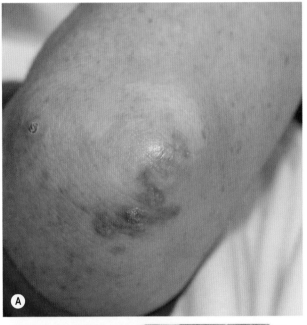

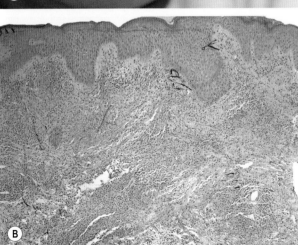

Fig. 11.7 Palisaded neutrophilic and granulomatous disorder.

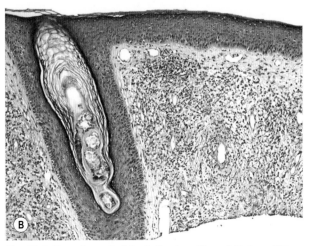

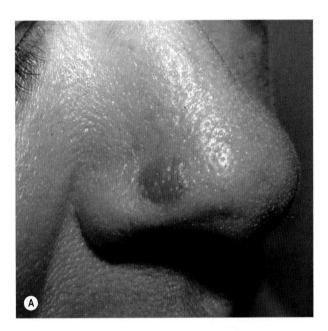

Fig. 11.8 Granuloma faciale. *A, Courtesy, Cloyce L Stetson, MD; B, Courtesy, Anjela Galan, MD. A, From Bolognia JL, Schaffer JV, Duncan KO, Ko CJ. Dermatology Essentials, 1e. Philadelphia: Saunders, 2014, with permission.*

Polymorphic Eruption of Pregnancy (Pruritic Urticarial Papules and Plaques of Pregnancy) *(Fig. 11.9)*

Abdomen and upper thighs, sparing the umbilicus
Pink to pink–brown (the latter in darker skin types) papules and plaques; can be urticarial, targetoid, vesicular, or eczematous

Histopathology:
Perivascular lymphocytic infiltrate, +/– eosinophils; epidermal changes may be present depending on the type of lesion biopsied

Lyme Disease *(Fig. 11.10)*

Classic lesion is targetoid with darker center and 1–2 cm wide pink rim
Lesions may be multiple

Histopathology:
Non-specific perivascular inflammation

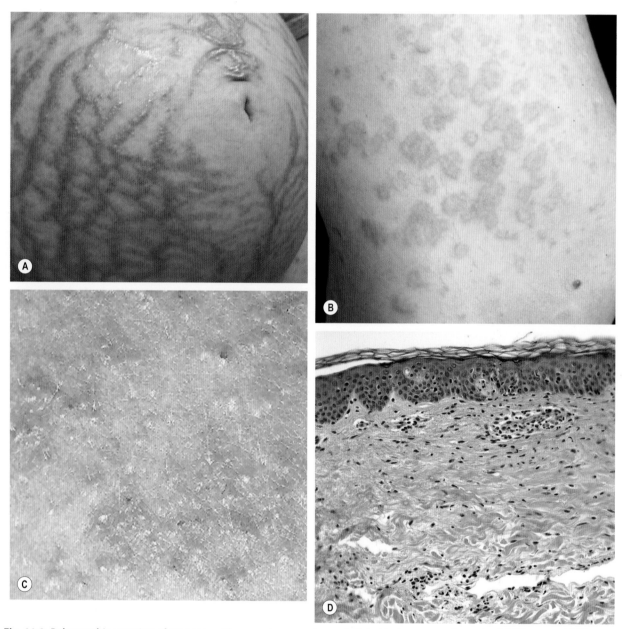

Fig. 11.9 Polymorphic eruption of pregnancy. There can be a spectrum of clinical lesions – macular, urticarial (**A**), targetoid (**B**), vesicular, and eczematous (**C**). *A, Courtesy, Yale Dermatology Residents' Slide Collection; B,C, Courtesy, Christina M Ambros-Rudolph, MD. B,C, From Bolognia JL, Schaffer JV, Duncan KO, Ko CJ. Dermatology Essentials, 1e. Philadelphia: Saunders, 2014, with permission.*

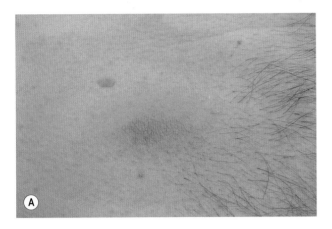

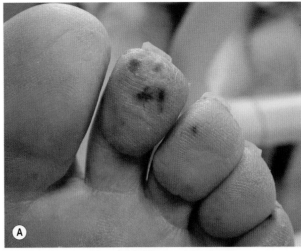

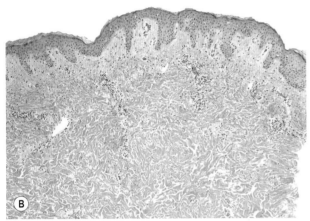

Fig. 11.10 Lyme disease. *A, Courtesy, Yale Dermatology Residents' Slide Collection.*

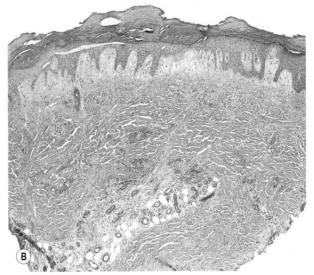

Fig. 11.11 Perniosis. *A, Courtesy, Jean L Bolognia, MD. A, From Bolognia JL, Jorizzo JL, Schaffer JV. Dermatology, 3e. London: Saunders, 2012, with permission.*

Perniosis *(Fig. 11.11)*

Pink to purple macules and/or papules, sometimes with petechiae, typically on the digits (acral sites)

Histopathology:
Superficial and deep perivascular lymphocytic inflammation, often with papillary dermal edema

Lupus Tumidus

Typically affects the face/upper trunk *(see Fig. 2.7B)*
Edematous, pink papules and plaques *(Fig. 11.12A)*

Histopathology:
Perivascular lymphocytic inflammation, classically with increased dermal mucin *(Fig. 11.12C)*

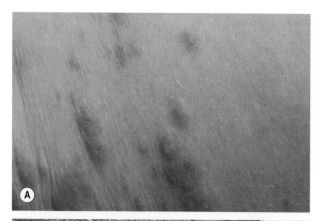

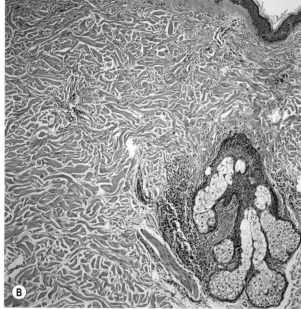

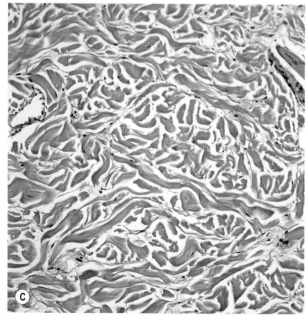

Fig. 11.12 Lupus tumidus. Increased mucin is shown in (**C**). *A, Courtesy, Yale Dermatology Residents' Slide Collection.*

Lymphocytic Infiltrate of Jessner

Typically affects the upper trunk or face *(Fig. 11.13; see Fig. 2.7C)*

Juicy pink papules or plaques, sometimes annular

Histopathology:

Perivascular lymphocytic inflammation, classically without increased dermal mucin

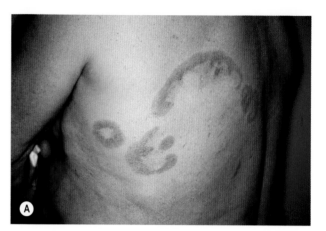

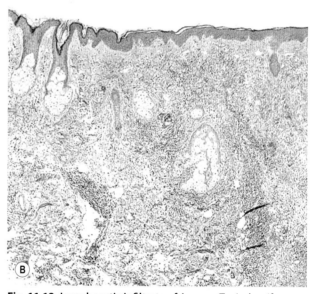

Fig. 11.13 Lymphocytic infiltrate of Jessner. Typical arciform plaques on the back. *A, From Rémy-Leroux V, Léonard F, Lambert D, et al. Comparison of histopathologic-clinical characteristics of Jessner's lymphocytic infiltration of the skin and lupus erythematosus tumidus: Multicenter study of 46 cases. J Am Acad Dermatol. 2008;58:217–23, © Elsevier.*

Sclerosing Disorders | 12

Induration, or hardening, of the skin can be a manifestation of systemic disease (e.g. systemic sclerosis) or limited to the skin (e.g. morphea), and generalized or localized (e.g. extragenital lichen sclerosus). Typically, these diseases favor certain sites *(Fig. 12.1)*. Sclerosis involving the subcutis often shows rippling of the skin (e.g. eosinophilic fasciitis; *see Fig. 12.1)*. Patients with chronic graft-versus-host disease can have skin findings that resemble any of the sclerosing disorders *(Fig. 12.2, bolded text)*. Induration of the skin can be due to exogenous substances (i.e. gadolinium – nephrogenic systemic fibrosis). This chapter covers systemic sclerosis, scleromyxedema, scleredema, eosinophilic fasciitis, linear melorheostotic scleroderma, morphea, and lichen sclerosus.

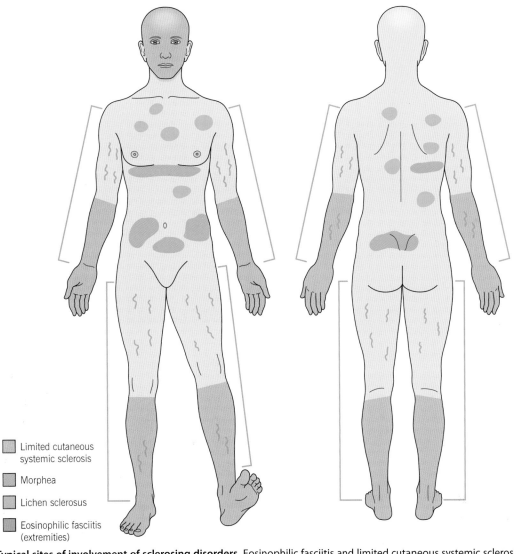

Limited cutaneous systemic sclerosis

Morphea

Lichen sclerosus

Eosinophilic fasciitis (extremities)

Fig. 12.1 Typical sites of involvement of sclerosing disorders. Eosinophilic fasciitis and limited cutaneous systemic sclerosis both involve the extremities, but the deeper involvement of the former is evidenced by rippling of the skin. Morphea and extragenital lichen sclerosus tend to affect the trunk.

MANIFESTATIONS OF CHRONIC GRAFT-VERSUS-HOST DISEASE

Keratoconjunctivitis sicca, blepharitis

Photosensitive eruption, resembling lupus erythematosus or dermatomyositis

Lichen sclerosus-like

Impaired sweating

Eczema craquelé-like

Lichen planus-like

Nail dystrophy

Morphea-like

Fasciitis/subcutaneous sclerosis

Ulceration

Angiomatous papule

Alopecia (often scarring)

Oral involvement

Poikiloderma

Keratosis pilaris-like

Leopard-like hyperpigmentation

Xerosis

Vitiligo-like leukoderma

Genital involvement

Psoriasiform

Ichthyosiform

Eczematous with plantar hyperkeratosis

(A)

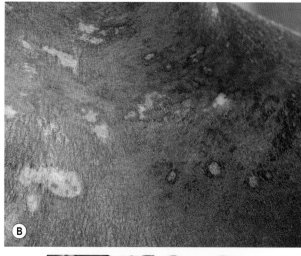

(B)

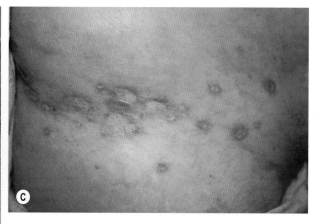

(C)

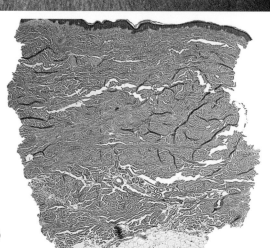

(D)

Fig. 12.2 Graft-versus-host disease. A–C Graft-versus-host disease, chronic. **B** Lichen sclerosus-like changes. **C,D** Morphea-like changes. There are superficial ulcerations. Biopsy findings are those of morphea, with sclerosis of the dermis. *B,C, Courtesy, Yale Dermatology Residents' Slide Collection. A, From Bolognia JL, Schaffer JV, Duncan KO, Ko CJ. Dermatology Essentials, 1e. Philadelphia: Saunders, 2014, with permission.*

SYSTEMIC SCLEROSIS (SCLERODERMA)

Three main types of systemic sclerosis *(Fig. 12.3)*

Systemic Sclerosis – Clues

Leukoderma – retention of perifollicular pigment, producing a "salt and pepper" appearance *(Fig. 12.4; see Fig. 2.26)*

Acral signs – in particular, the hands can show many features suggestive of systemic sclerosis *(Fig. 12.5)*
Telangiectasias – often on the face, borders are squared off *(Fig. 12.6)*

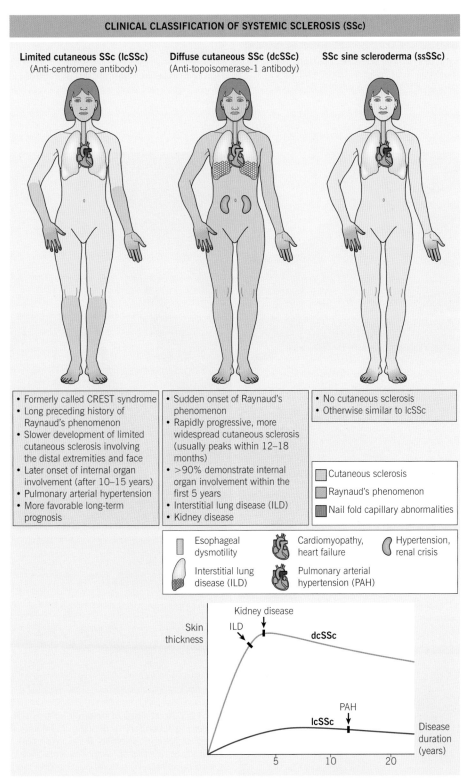

Fig. 12.3 Clinical classification of systemic sclerosis. *Courtesy, Karynne O Duncan, MD. From Bolognia JL, Schaffer JV, Duncan KO, Ko CJ. Dermatology Essentials, 1e. Philadelphia: Saunders, 2014, with permission.*

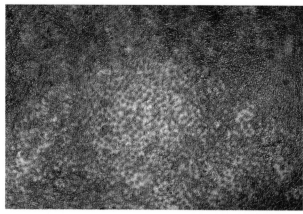

Fig. 12.4 Leukoderma of systemic sclerosis. *Courtesy, M Kari Connolly, MD. From Bolognia JL, Schaffer JV, Duncan KO, Ko CJ. Dermatology Essentials, 1e. Philadelphia: Saunders, 2014, with permission.*

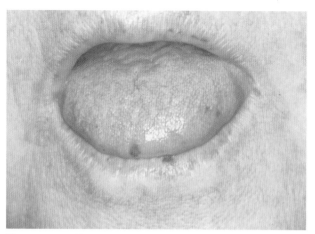

Fig. 12.6 Mat-like telangiectasias. *Courtesy, Irwin Braverman, MD.*

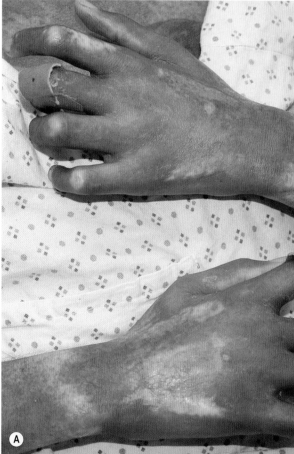

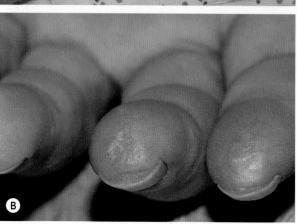

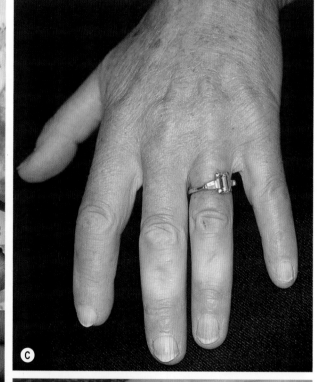

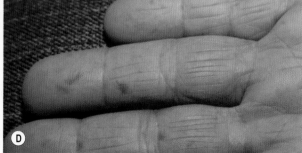

Fig. 12.5 Acral signs of systemic sclerosis. A Sclerodactyly. **B** Scarring secondary to digital pulp infarcts. **C** Edematous phase of systemic sclerosis. **D** Calcinosis cutis. Telangiectasias. *A, Courtesy, Yale Dermatology Residents' Slide Collection; B,D, Courtesy, Kalman Watsky, MD; C, Courtesy, Jean L Bolognia, MD. B,C, From Bolognia JL, Schaffer JV, Duncan KO, Ko CJ. Dermatology Essentials, 1e. Philadelphia: Saunders, 2014, with permission.*

SCLEROMYXEDEMA

Involves the hands and forearms, head (especially glabellar region), upper trunk, and thighs
Linear arrays of small papules *(Fig. 12.7)*

Histopathology:
Increased fibroblasts and mucin

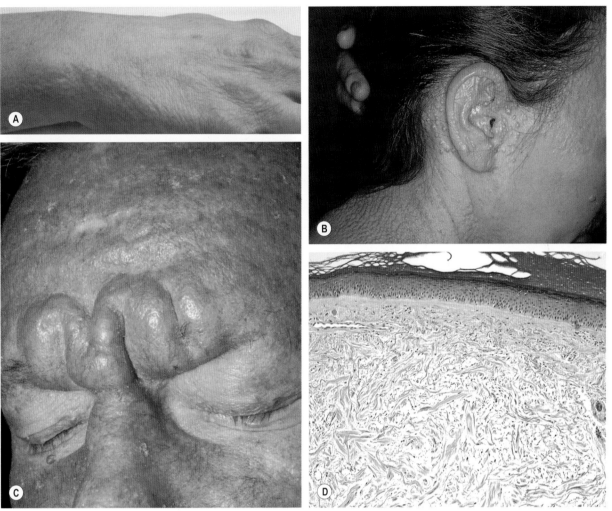

Fig. 12.7 Scleromyxedema. *A,B, Courtesy, Yale Dermatology Residents' Slide Collection; C, Courtesy, Joyce Rico, MD. B,C, From Bolognia JL, Schaffer JV, Duncan KO, Ko CJ. Dermatology Essentials, 1e. Philadelphia: Saunders, 2014, with permission.*

SCLEREDEMA

Typically involves the posterior neck and upper back
Less commonly involves the upper extremities and face
Induration +/– erythema *(Fig. 12.8)*

Histopathology:
Increased space between collagen bundles +/– increased mucin

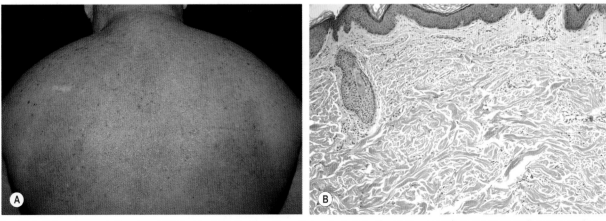

Fig. 12.8 Scleredema. *A, Courtesy, USC Residents' Collection. From Bolognia JL, Schaffer JV, Duncan KO, Ko CJ. Dermatology Essentials, 1e. Philadelphia: Saunders, 2014, with permission.*

EOSINOPHILIC FASCIITIS

Involves the extremities +/– the trunk
Induration often preceded by an edematous phase
Skin surface often rippled *(Fig. 12.9)*

Histopathology:
Thickening and inflammation of the fascia +/– dermal involvement

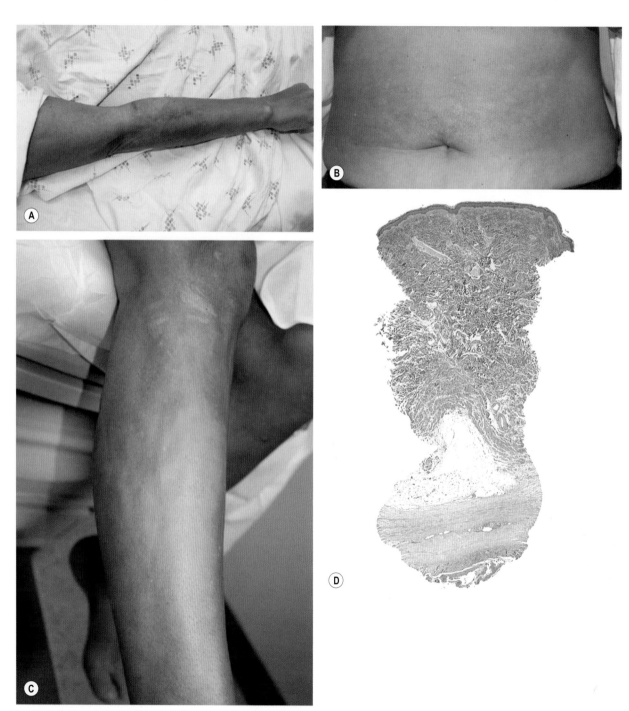

Fig. 12.9 Eosinophilic fasciitis. *A–C, Courtesy, Yale Dermatology Residents' Slide Collection.*

LINEAR MELORHEOSTOTIC SCLERODERMA

Often unilateral
Favors the extremities
Induration of the skin, rippling may be present
(Fig. 12.10)
Involvement of bone (melorheostosis) may be associated

Histopathology:
Adipocytes interspersed between thickened collagen bundles

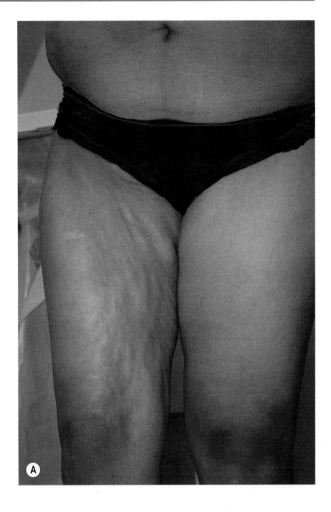

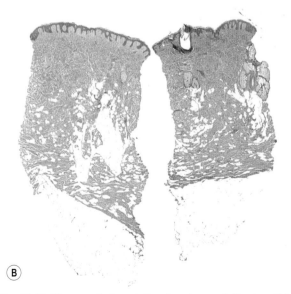

Fig. 12.10 Linear melorheostotic scleroderma. *A, Courtesy, Yale Dermatology Residents' Slide Collection.*

MORPHEA (CIRCUMSCRIBED, PLAQUE)

Favors pressure sites of the trunk (i.e. hips, waist, bra-line in women)
Discrete, indurated plaques, may be hyperpigmented (*Fig. 12.11*)

Histopathology:
Thickened collagen with decreased space (fenestrations) between collagen bundles, loss of fat around eccrine glands

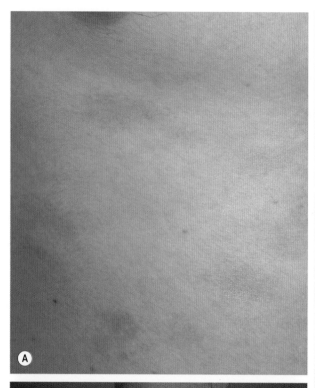

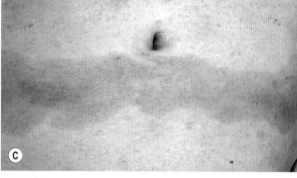

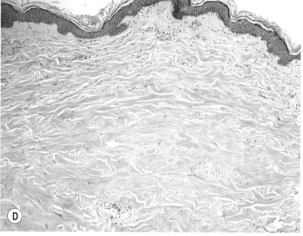

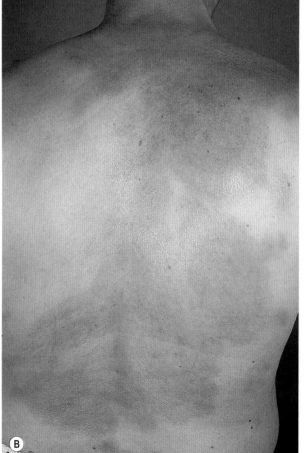

Fig. 12.11 Morphea, patch/plaque type. A Inflammatory stage. **B** Hyperpigmented plaques with erythematous borders. **C** Late stage with hyperpigmentation in a characteristic configuration. **D** Thickened collagen bundles. *A, Courtesy, Yale Dermatology Residents' Slide Collection and Kamran Ghoreschi, MD. B, Courtesy, NYU Residents' Slide Collection. B, From Bolognia JL, Schaffer JV, Duncan KO, Ko CJ. Dermatology Essentials, 1e. Philadelphia: Saunders, 2014, with permission.*

MORPHEA, LINEAR

Commonly in children
Favors the head or extremities; on the extremities,
a rippled appearance suggests deep involvement
(Fig. 12.12)

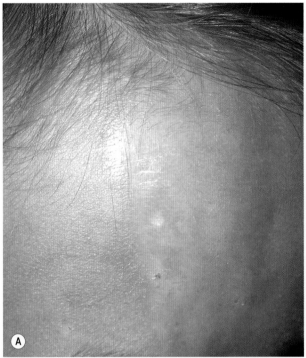

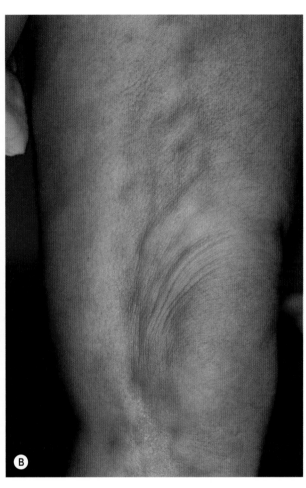

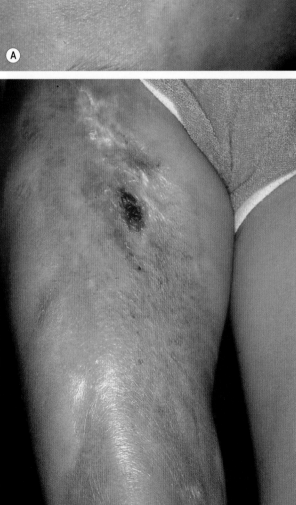

Fig. 12.12 Linear morphea. *A–C, Courtesy, Yale Dermatology Residents' Slide Collection. B,C, From Bolognia JL, Schaffer JV, Duncan KO, Ko CJ. Dermatology Essentials, 1e. Philadelphia: Saunders, 2014, with permission.*

LICHEN SCLEROSUS, EXTRAGENITAL

Predilection for the trunk *(see Fig. 2.16A,B for vulvar lichen sclerosus)*
Atrophic, wrinkled, white macules and patches *(Fig. 12.13)*

Histopathology:
Vacuolar change, dermal hyalinization, and underlying lymphocytes

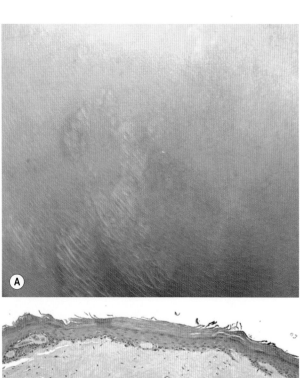

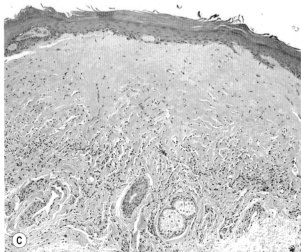

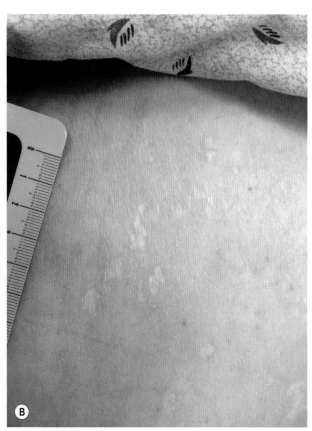

Fig. 12.13 Lichen sclerosus.

Vesiculobullous, Numerous Lesions | 13

Many different factors are clues to the diagnosis of blistering disorders. Some diseases have particular sites of predilection (*Table 13.1*). The morphology and arrangement of the individual lesions are important (i.e. tense vs flaccid, erythematous vs non-erythematous base [*Fig. 13.1*], clustered [*Fig. 13.2*]). The location of the split is also a key factor to consider (*Table 13.2*). For many blistering disorders, there are particular direct immunofluorescence patterns (*Table 13.3*) as well as characteristic circulating antibodies (*Table 13.4*).

This chapter focuses on bullous pemphigoid, pemphigoid gestationis, cicatricial pemphigoid, epidermolysis bullosa acquisita, porphyria cutanea tarda, linear IgA disease, dermatitis herpetiformis, bullous lupus erythematosus, bullous lichen planus, pemphigus, herpes, and coxsackie virus infection.

Table 13.1 Blistering disorders – characteristic distribution

Blistering disorder	Site(s)
Bullous pemphigoid Pemphigus vulgaris Pemphigus foliaceus Linear IgA disease	Trunk and extremities
Pemphigoid gestationis	Abdomen
Cicatricial pemphigoid (Brunsting–Perry variant)	Scalp
Epidermolysis bullosa acquisita* Porphyria cutanea tarda Hand-foot-and-mouth disease	Acral
Dermatitis herpetiformis	Elbows/knees Buttocks Scalp
Pemphigus vegetans	Body folds

*May also be generalized

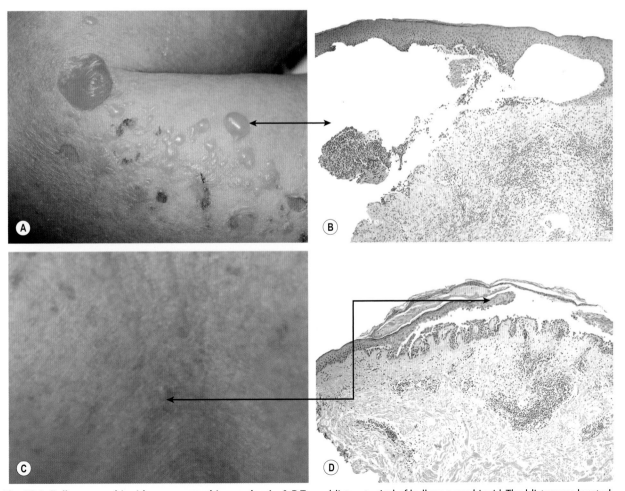

Fig. 13.1 Bullous pemphigoid versus pemphigus vulgaris. A,B Tense blisters typical of bullous pemphigoid. The blisters are located within pink, urticarial plaques. **C,D** Flaccid blisters typical of pemphigus vulgaris. The base of the blister is non-erythematous. *A, Courtesy, Yale Dermatology Residents' Slide Collection.*

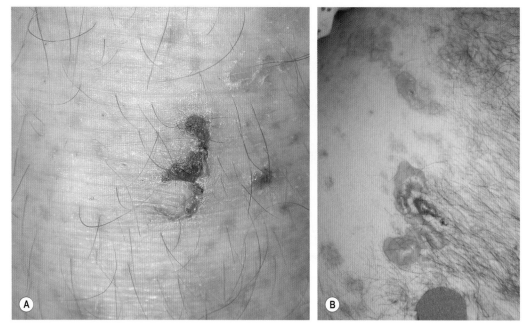

Fig. 13.2 Clustered vesicles/bullae. A Dermatitis herpetiformis. Clustered small vesicles ("herpetiform") and erosions. **B** Linear IgA disease. Clusters of larger vesicles/bullae in annular arrangements. *Courtesy, Yale Dermatology Residents' Slide Collection.*

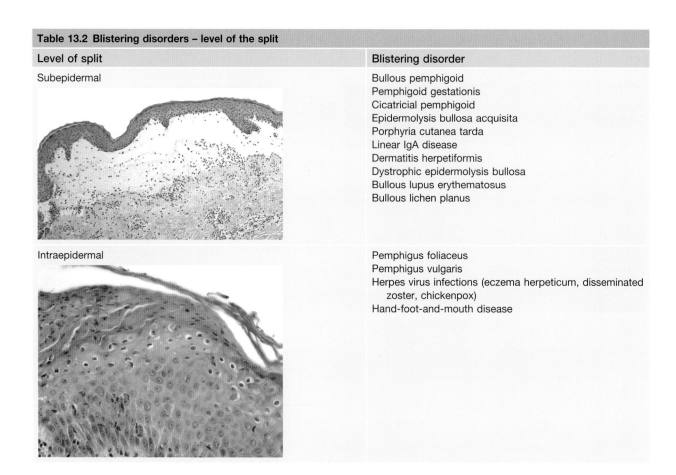

Table 13.2 Blistering disorders – level of the split	
Level of split	**Blistering disorder**
Subepidermal	Bullous pemphigoid
	Pemphigoid gestationis
	Cicatricial pemphigoid
	Epidermolysis bullosa acquisita
	Porphyria cutanea tarda
	Linear IgA disease
	Dermatitis herpetiformis
	Dystrophic epidermolysis bullosa
	Bullous lupus erythematosus
	Bullous lichen planus
Intraepidermal	Pemphigus foliaceus
	Pemphigus vulgaris
	Herpes virus infections (eczema herpeticum, disseminated zoster, chickenpox)
	Hand-foot-and-mouth disease

Table 13.3 Blistering disorders – usual direct immunofluorescence patterns

Direct immunofluorescence pattern	Blistering disorder
Linear C3 and IgG at the dermal–epidermal junction 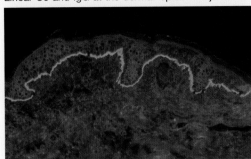	Bullous pemphigoid Pemphigoid gestationis Cicatricial pemphigoid Epidermolysis bullosa acquisita Bullous lupus erythematosus*
Intercellular IgG and C3 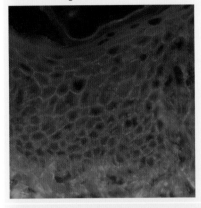	Pemphigus vulgaris Pemphigus foliaceus
Linear IgA at the dermal–epidermal junction 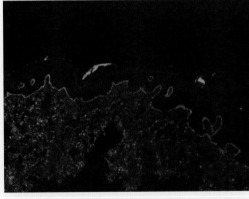	Linear IgA disease Cicatricial pemphigoid
Granular IgA in the papillary dermis 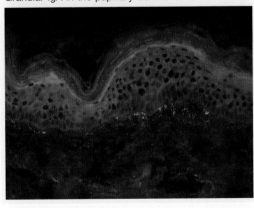	Dermatitis herpetiformis

*Often has IgA and IgM as well

Table 13.4 Blistering disorders – antibody profiles

Blistering disorder	Antibodies directed against
Bullous pemphigoid	BPAg1, BPAg2
Pemphigus vulgaris	Desmoglein 3
Pemphigus foliaceus	Desmoglein 1
Dermatitis herpetiformis	Epidermal transglutaminase
Linear IgA	BPAg2
Cicatricial pemphigoid	BPAg2
Pemphigoid gestationis	BPAg2
Epidermolysis bullosa acquisita	Type VII collagen
Bullous lupus erythematosus	

BULLOUS PEMPHIGOID

Generalized or localized tense blisters *(Fig. 13.3A)*
Blister base erythematous or skin-colored

Histopathology:
Subepidermal split with numerous eosinophils
(Fig. 13.3B)

Direct Immunofluorescence:
Linear C3 and IgG

Salt-Split Skin:
Localization of immunoreactants to the blister roof, base, or both

Bullous Pemphigoid, Variants *(Fig. 13.4)*

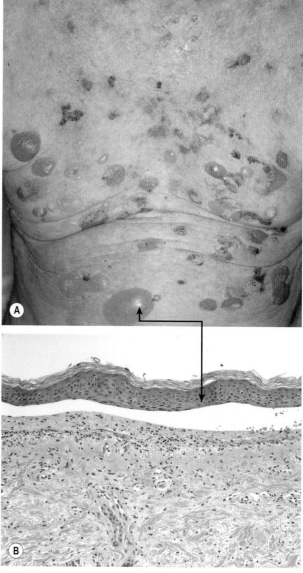

Fig. 13.3 Bullous pemphigoid. *A, Courtesy, Yale Dermatology Residents' Slide Collection. A, From Bolognia JL, Jorizzo JL, Schaffer JV. Dermatology, 3e. London: Saunders, 2012, with permission.*

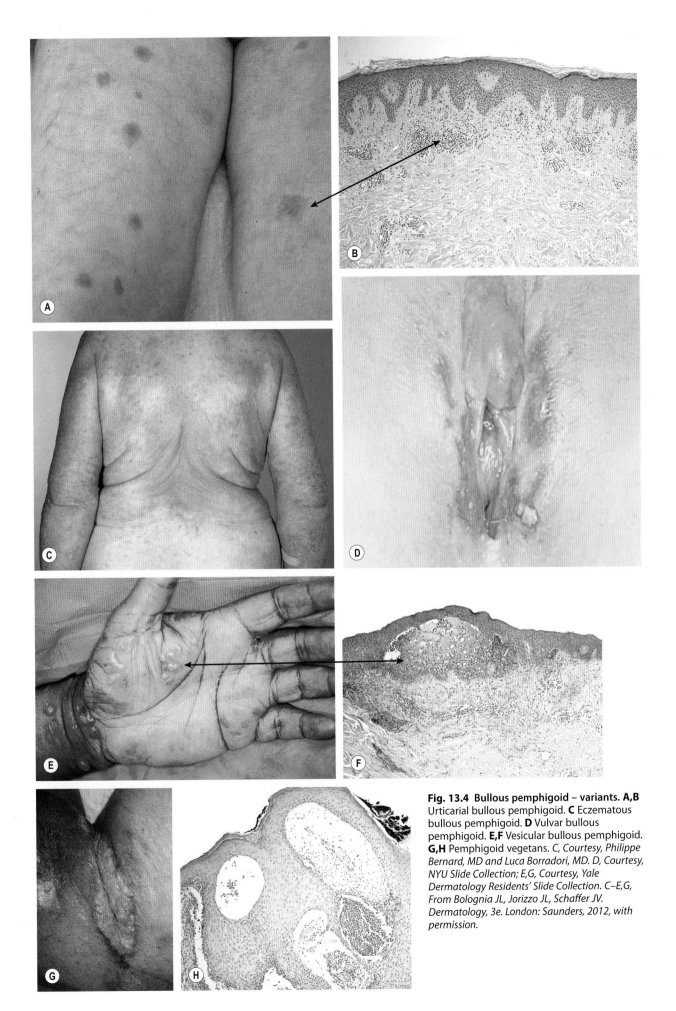

Fig. 13.4 Bullous pemphigoid – variants. A,B Urticarial bullous pemphigoid. **C** Eczematous bullous pemphigoid. **D** Vulvar bullous pemphigoid. **E,F** Vesicular bullous pemphigoid. **G,H** Pemphigoid vegetans. *C, Courtesy, Philippe Bernard, MD and Luca Borradori, MD. D, Courtesy, NYU Slide Collection; E,G, Courtesy, Yale Dermatology Residents' Slide Collection. C–E,G, From Bolognia JL, Jorizzo JL, Schaffer JV. Dermatology, 3e. London: Saunders, 2012, with permission.*

PEMPHIGOID GESTATIONIS

Affects pregnant women
Tense blisters, initially on the abdomen *(Fig. 13.5)*
Histopathology and direct immunofluorescence like
bullous pemphigoid

Biopsy of an urticarial lesion may only show mixed
perivascular inflammation *(Fig. 13.5B)*, and direct
immunofluorescence studies are helpful *(Fig. 13.5C
– linear C3 at the dermal-epidermal junction).*

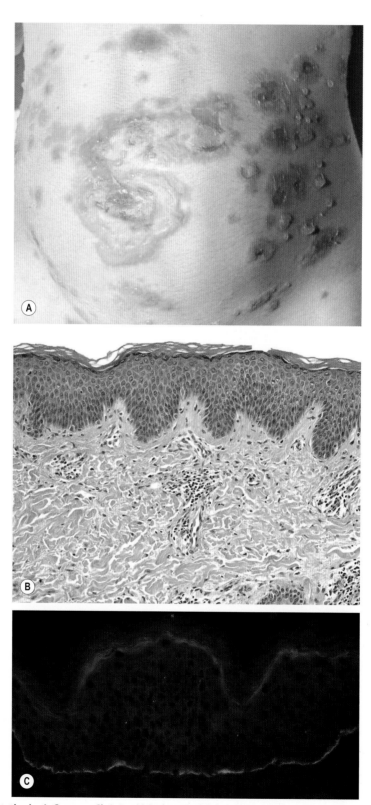

Fig. 13.5 Pemphigoid gestationis. *A, Courtesy, Christina M Ambros-Rudolph, MD. From Bolognia JL, Jorizzo JL, Schaffer JV. Dermatology, 3e. London: Saunders, 2012, with permission.*

CICATRICIAL PEMPHIGOID

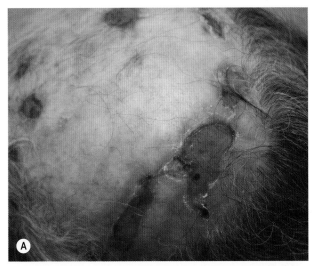

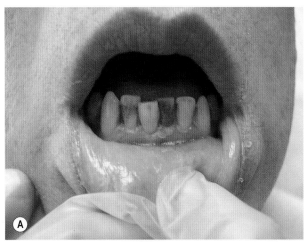

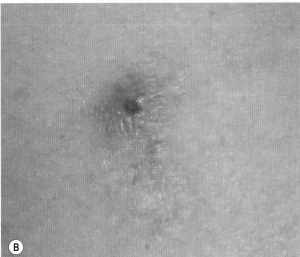

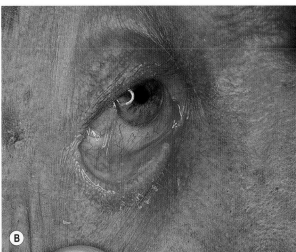

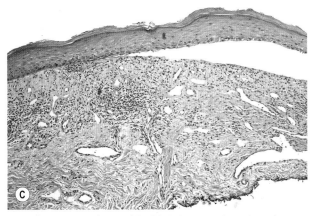

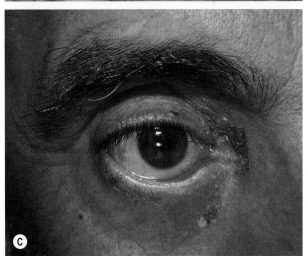

Fig. 13.6 Cicatricial pemphigoid. A Scarring alopecia and resolving lesions on the scalp. **B** Recurrent lesion at the site of a scar from a prior lesion. **C** Dermal scarring is a clue.

Fig. 13.7 Cicatricial pemphigoid. A Desquamative gingivitis. **B,C** Ocular lesions. *B, Courtesy, Yale Dermatology Residents' Slide Collection; C, Courtesy, Louis A Fragola, MD. B,C, From Bolognia JL, Jorizzo JL, Schaffer JV. Dermatology, 3e. London: Saunders, 2012, with permission.*

Brunsting–Perry variant – blisters localized to the scalp *(Fig. 13.6A)*

Blisters may reform in scars from previous blisters *(Fig. 13.6B)*

Desquamative gingivitis, ocular lesions *(Fig. 13.7)*

Histopathology (dermal scarring may be a clue) and direct immunofluorescence may resemble bullous pemphigoid

EPIDERMOLYSIS BULLOSA ACQUISITA

Classically localized to areas of frequent trauma (hands/elbows; *Fig. 13.8*)
May be generalized

Histopathology:
Subepidermal split with variable inflammation

Direct Immunofluorescence:
Linear C3 and IgG, sometimes with IgM and/or IgA

Salt-Split Skin:
Localization of immunoreactants to the blister base

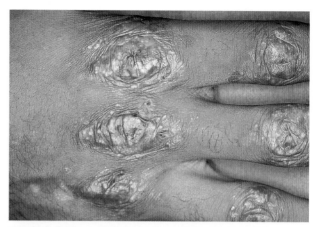

Fig. 13.8 Epidermolysis bullosa acquisita. *Courtesy, Yale Dermatology Residents' Slide Collection. From Bolognia JL, Jorizzo JL, Schaffer JV. Dermatology, 3e. London: Saunders, 2012, with permission.*

PORPHYRIA CUTANEA TARDA

Tense blisters or crusted lesions on dorsal hands *(Fig. 13.9A)*
Hypertrichosis of lateral face

Histopathology:
Non-inflamed subepidermal split with thickened basement membrane *(Fig. 13.9B)*

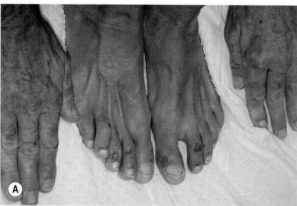

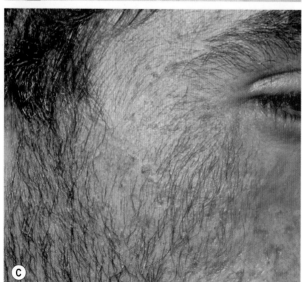

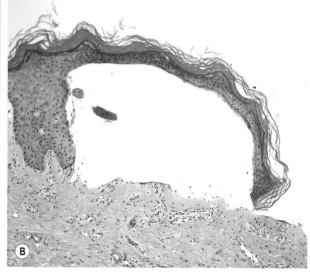

Fig. 13.9 Porphyria cutanea tarda. A Erosions on dorsal hands/feet. **B** Subepidermal split with minimal inflammation. **C** Hypertrichosis. *A, Yale Dermatology Residents' Slide Collection; C, Courtesy, Kurt Stenn, MD. C, From Bolognia JL, Jorizzo JL, Schaffer JV. Dermatology, 3e. London: Saunders, 2012, with permission.*

LINEAR IgA DISEASE

Predilection for body folds but may be generalized
Clusters of tense vesicles or bullae *(Fig. 13.10A,B)*

Histopathology:
Subepidermal split with neutrophils *(Fig. 13.10C)*

Direct Immunofluorescence:
Linear IgA

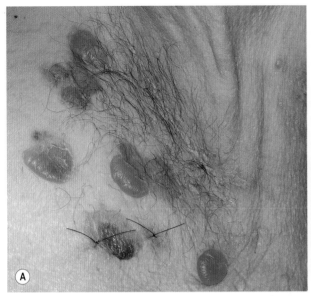

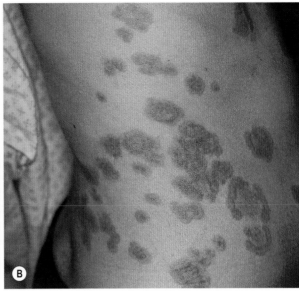

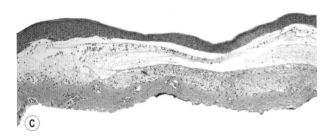

Fig. 13.10 Linear IgA disease. *A, Courtesy, Yale Dermatology Residents' Slide Collection. B, Courtesy, John J Zone, MD. B, From Bolognia JL, Jorizzo JL, Schaffer JV. Dermatology, 3e. London: Saunders, 2012, with permission.*

DERMATITIS HERPETIFORMIS

Favors the elbows/knees, scalp, lower back
Excoriated vesicles *(Fig. 13.11A)*

Histopathology:
Neutrophils in dermal papillae +/– subepidermal split
(Fig. 13.11B)

Direct Immunofluorescence:
Granular (rarely fibrillar) IgA in the dermal papillae

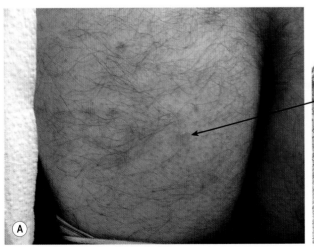

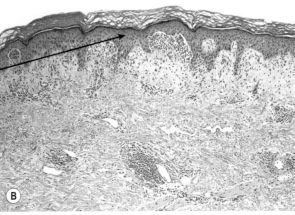

Fig. 13.11 Dermatitis herpetiformis.

BULLOUS LUPUS ERYTHEMATOSUS

Bullae in a patient with underlying systemic lupus erythematosus *(Fig. 13.12A)*

Histopathology:
Subepidermal split with neutrophils *(Fig. 13.12B)*

Direct Immunofluorescence:
Linear IgG, IgM, IgA; intranuclear labeling of antinuclear antibodies may be seen *(Fig. 13.12C)*

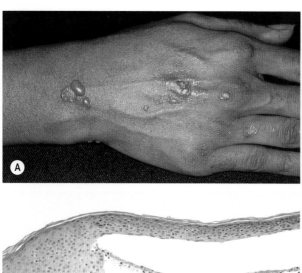

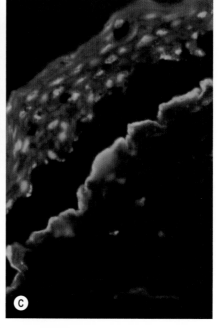

Fig. 13.12 Bullous lupus erythematosus. *A, Courtesy, Yale Dermatology Residents' Slide Collection. A, From Bolognia JL, Jorizzo JL, Schaffer JV. Dermatology, 3e. London: Saunders, 2012, with permission. C, From Patterson JW. Practical Skin Pathology: A Diagnostic Approach. Philadelphia: Saunders, 2013.*

BULLOUS LICHEN PLANUS

Violaceous papule/plaque that blisters *(Fig. 13.13A)*

Histopathology:
Subepidermal cleft with lymphocytes, pigment incontinence *(Fig. 13.13B)*

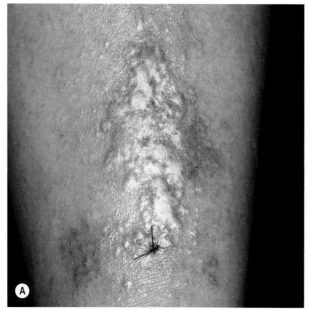

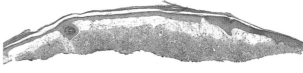

Fig. 13.13 Bullous lichen planus. *A, Courtesy, Yale Dermatology Residents' Slide Collection. A, From Bolognia JL, Jorizzo JL, Schaffer JV. Dermatology, 3e. London: Saunders, 2012, with permission.*

PEMPHIGUS VULGARIS

Often generalized, may be localized
Flaccid bullae and erosions *(Fig. 13.14)*

Histopathology:
Suprabasilar acantholysis (see *Fig. 13.1D*)

Direct Immunofluorescence:
Intercellular IgG and C3 (see *Table 13.3*)

PEMPHIGUS VARIANTS

IgA Pemphigus
(see Chapter 7)

Pemphigus Vegetans
Favors body folds
Thick, eroded plaques *(Fig. 13.15A)*

Histopathology:
Acanthosis with eosinophilic abscesses *(Fig. 13.15B)*
Acantholysis may not be evident

Pemphigus Foliaceus
(see Chapter 4)

Paraneoplastic Pemphigus
(see Chapter 8)

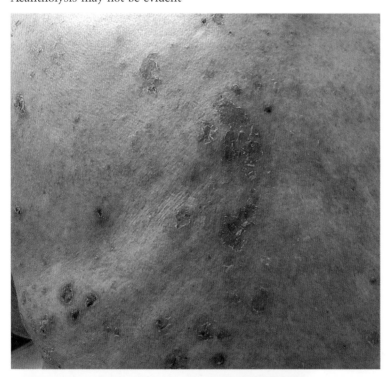

Fig. 13.14 Pemphigus vulgaris.

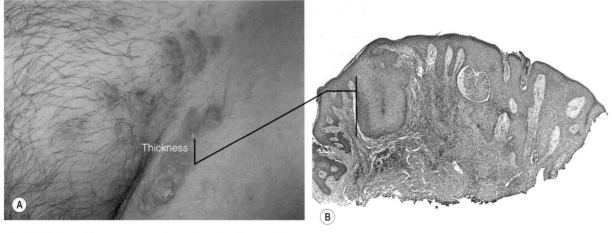

Thickness

Fig. 13.15 Pemphigus vegetans. *A, Courtesy, Ann Strong, MD.*

HERPES VIRUS INFECTIONS (ECZEMA HERPETICUM, DISSEMINATED ZOSTER, CHICKENPOX)

Eczema Herpeticum

Background of atopic dermatitis
Punched out 3–5 mm monomorphous ulcerations
(Fig. 13.16A)

Disseminated Zoster

Individual lesions similar to chickenpox or eczema herpeticum *(Fig. 13.16B)*

Histopathology:
Acantholysis, epidermal necrosis, multinucleate cells

Varicella (Chickenpox)

2–4 mm papule on an erythematous base *(Fig. 13.16C)*

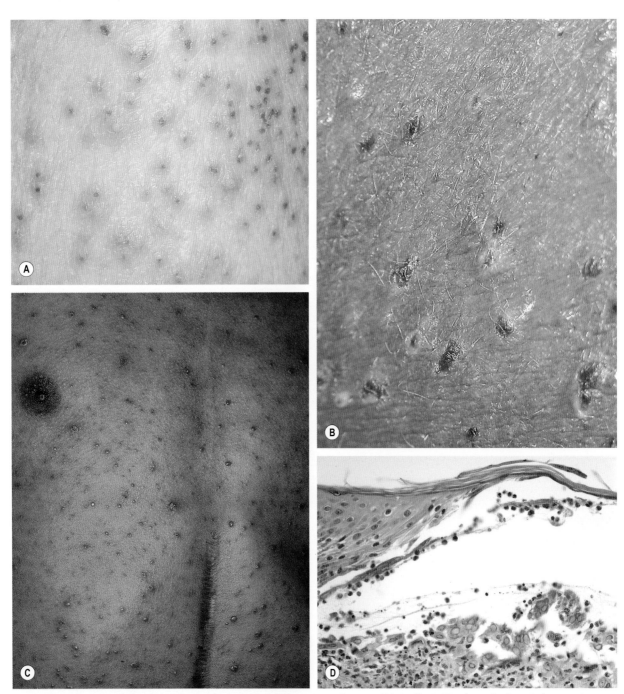

Fig. 13.16 Herpes virus infection. A Eczema herpeticum. **B** Disseminated zoster. **C** Varicella. **D** Histologic findings in herpes virus infections. Acantholytic cells and multinucleate cells with rimming of chromatin. *A,B, Courtesy, Yale Dermatology Residents' Slide Collection; C, Courtesy, Robert Hartman, MD. C, From Bolognia JL, Jorizzo JL, Schaffer JV. Dermatology, 3e. London: Saunders, 2012, with permission.*

HAND-FOOT-AND-MOUTH DISEASE

Due to enteroviruses, particularly coxsackie virus
Typical acral distribution (hands, feet, intraoral)
Atypical variants can involve the skin more extensively
(Fig. 13.17A) and/or affect sites of atopic dermatitis
(eczema coxsackium; *Fig. 13.17B)*
Oval vesicles, may be crusted or eroded

Histopathology:
Superficial necrotic keratinocytes (arrow), papillary
dermal edema, lymphocytic infiltrate *(Fig. 13.17C)*

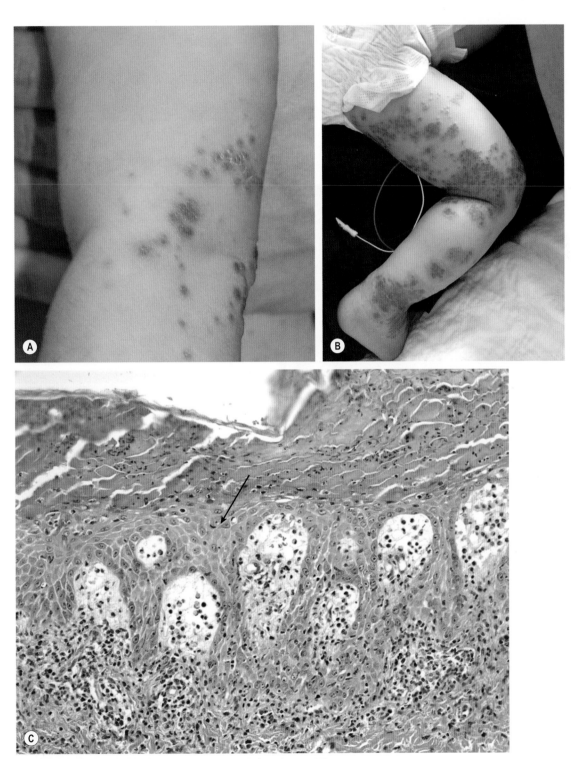

Fig. 13.17 Hand-foot-and-mouth disease. *A,B, Courtesy, Robert Stavert, MD.*

ADDITIONAL DIRECT IMMUNOFLUORESCENCE IMAGES *(Figs 13.18–13.20)*

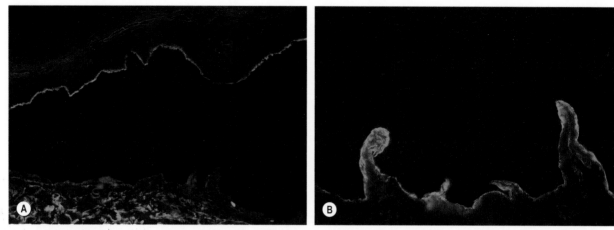

Fig. 13.18 Salt-split skin patterns. A Deposition of immunoreactant on the base of the roof, a typical pattern of bullous pemphigoid. **B** Deposition of immunoreactant on the floor (dermis), a typical pattern of epidermolysis bullosa acquisita that can also be associated with bullous pemphigoid.

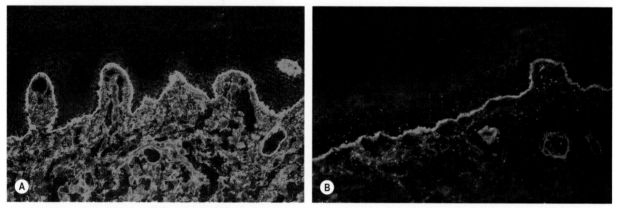

Fig. 13.19 Serrated patterns on direct immunofluorescence testing. A n-serrated (bullous pemphigoid). **B** u-serrated (epidermolysis bullosa acquisita or bullous lupus erythematosus).

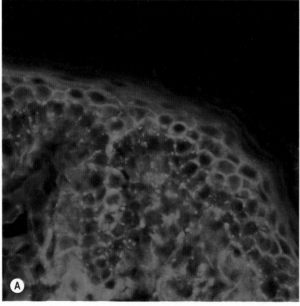

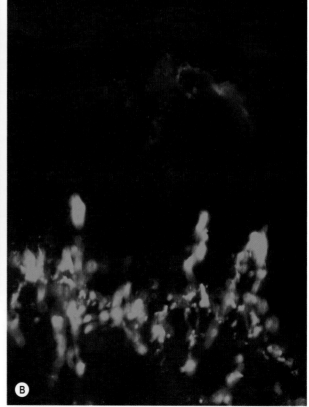

Fig. 13.20 Less common patterns on direct immunofluorescence testing. A Punctate intercellular pattern of IgG deposition in pemphigus. **B** Fibrillar IgA deposition in the papillary dermis in dermatitis herpetiformis.

Blistering, Localized | 14

In addition to morphology, body site affected, and clues from history, the microscopic findings (i.e. subcorneal, intraepidermal, or subepidermal split) in localized blistering conditions can aid in the correct diagnosis *(Fig. 14.1)*.

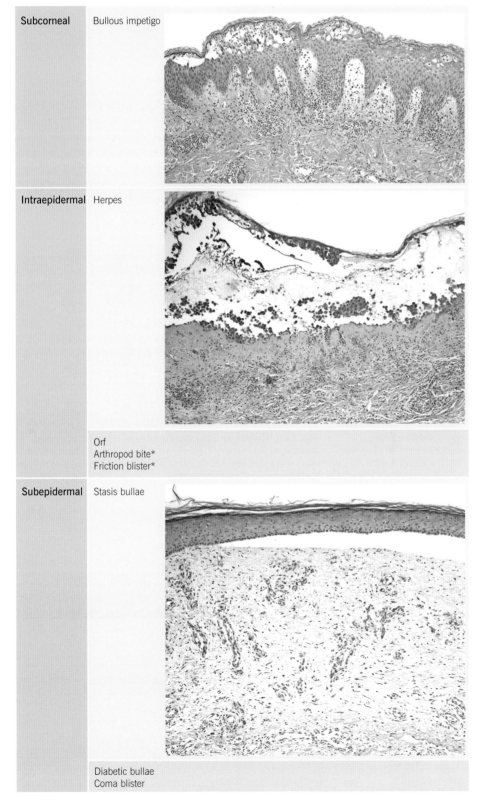

Subcorneal	Bullous impetigo
Intraepidermal	Herpes
	Orf Arthropod bite* Friction blister*
Subepidermal	Stasis bullae
	Diabetic bullae Coma blister

Fig. 14.1 Microscopy of selected localized blistering conditions. *Can also be subepidermal.

DISORDERS WITH A CHARACTERISTIC MORPHOLOGY

Bullous impetigo *(Fig. 14.2)* – somewhat tense vesicles/bullae or superficial erosions with collarettes of scale
Herpes virus infection *(Fig. 14.3)* – clustered vesicles and crusts (borders of coalescing lesions may be scalloped),

often on an erythematous base; older lesions may be eroded/ulcerated
Leukocytoclastic vasculitis *(Fig. 14.4)* – palpable purpura, sometimes with focal blisters

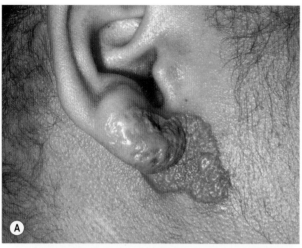

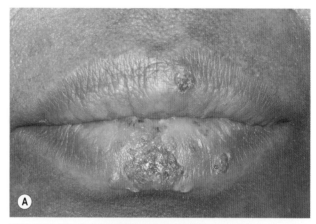

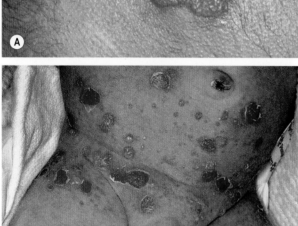

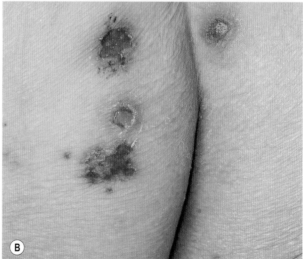

Fig. 14.2 Bullous impetigo. *A,B, Courtesy, Yale Dermatology Residents' Slide Collection. B, From Bolognia JL, Jorizzo JL, Schaffer JV. Dermatology, 3e. London: Saunders, 2012, with permission.*

Fig. 14.3 Herpes simplex virus infection. Note the scalloped borders to the coalescing lesions. Older lesions can be punched-out ulcerations (**B**). *A,B, Courtesy, Yale Dermatology Residents' Slide Collection.*

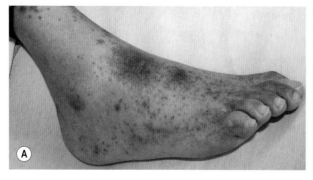

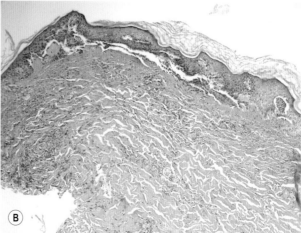

Fig. 14.4 Leukocytoclastic vasculitis. Purpuric red–purple papules are focally surmounted by bullae. *A, Courtesy, William Damsky, MD.*

DISORDERS THAT ARE OFTEN ACRAL

Orf *(Fig. 14.5)* – generally on the hand; varying morphology depending on stage

Diabetic bullae *(Fig. 14.6)* – predilection for the legs; often tense, non-inflamed blisters; patient with history of diabetes mellitus

Stasis bullae – predilection for the legs; other signs of venous insufficiency (i.e. venulectasia, brown discoloration secondary to hemosiderin deposition)

Localized epidermolysis bullosa *(Fig. 14.7)* – favors the feet or other areas prone to trauma

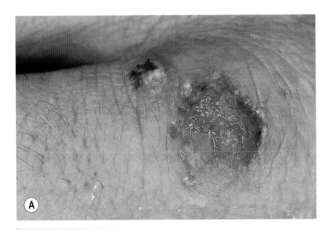

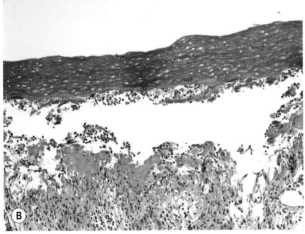

Fig. 14.5 Orf. Reticular degeneration is shown in **B**. *A, Courtesy, Anthony Mancini, MD. From Bolognia JL, Jorizzo JL, Schaffer JV. Dermatology, 3e. London: Saunders, 2012, with permission.*

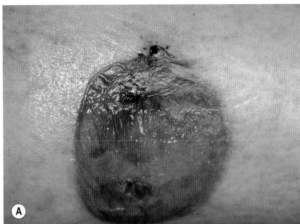

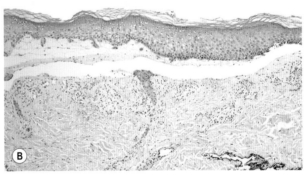

Fig. 14.6 Diabetic bullae, non-inflamed subepidermal split.

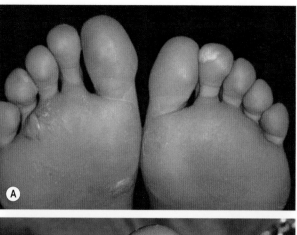

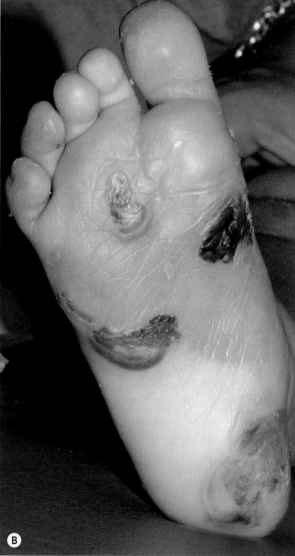

Fig. 14.7 Localized epidermolysis bullosa. *A, Courtesy, Yale Dermatology Residents' Slide Collection; B, Courtesy, Julie V Schaffer, MD. A,B, From Bolognia JL, Jorizzo JL, Schaffer JV. Dermatology, 3e. London: Saunders, 2012, with permission.*

TYPICAL HISTORY

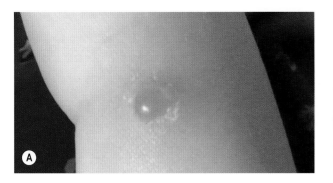

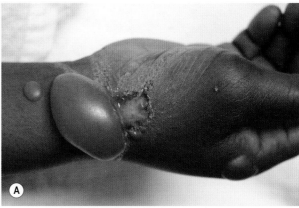

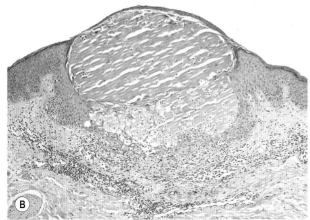

Fig. 14.8 Bullous arthropod bites. Intraepidermal serum and mixed inflammation (**B**). *A, Courtesy, Yale Dermatology Residents' Slide Collection.*

Bullous arthropod bite *(Fig. 14.8)* – history of outdoor activity and contact with arthropods
Friction – history of friction
Coma *(Fig. 14.9)* – history of pressure on the affected area during a coma

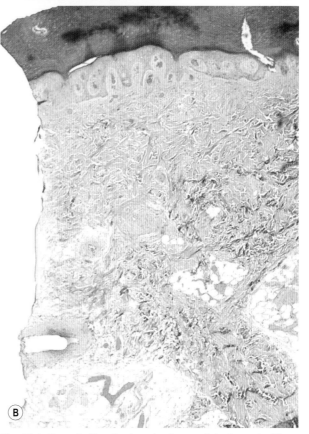

Fig. 14.9 Coma bullae. Eccrine gland necrosis is shown in (**B**). *A, Courtesy, Yale Dermatology Residents' Slide Collection.*

Vesicles and Papulopustules in Infants | 15

Vesicular and papular disorders in infants often have a characteristic distribution (i.e. head, body folds, acral).

HEAD

Neonatal Cephalic Pustulosis *(Fig. 15.1)*

Papulopustules on the face of infants from about 2–3 weeks of age to 2–3 months of age
Absent comedones

Benign Cephalic Histiocytosis *(Fig. 15.2)*

Typically on the face or neck
Small (<5 mm) brown–red papules
Spontaneous resolution over time (months to years)

Histopathology:
Histiocytes (CD1a-negative) within the dermis

Eosinophilic Folliculitis

(see Chapter 9)

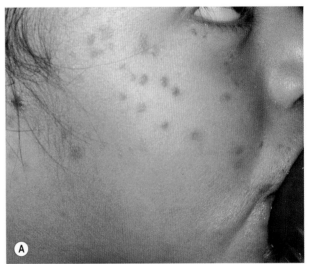

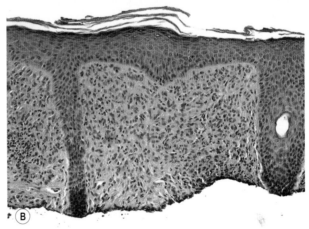

Fig. 15.2 Benign cephalic histiocytosis. *A, Courtesy, Yale Dermatology Residents' Slide Collection. A, From Bolognia JL, Schaffer JV, Duncan KO, Ko CJ. Dermatology Essentials, 1e. Philadelphia: Saunders, 2014, with permission.*

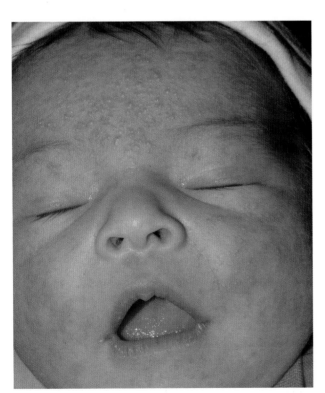

Fig. 15.1 Neonatal cephalic pustulosis. *Courtesy, Julie V Schaffer, MD. From Bolognia JL, Schaffer JV, Duncan KO, Ko CJ. Dermatology Essentials, 1e. Philadelphia: Saunders, 2014, with permission.*

BODY FOLDS

Langerhans Cell Histiocytosis *(Fig. 15.3)*

Favors the scalp and body folds
Pink to red–brown papules, often with petechiae,
sometimes eroded/ulcerated

Histopathology:
Histiocytes with reniform (kidney-shaped) nuclei that are
langerin-, CD1a-, S100-positive

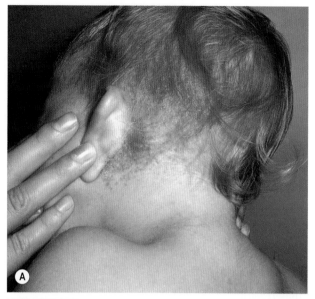

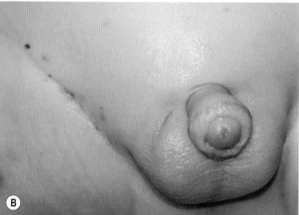

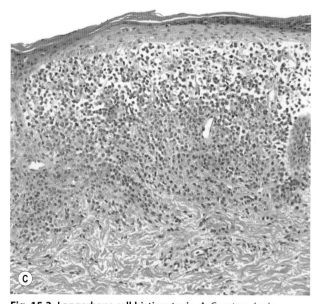

Fig. 15.3 Langerhans cell histiocytosis. *A, Courtesy, Irwin Braverman, MD; B, Courtesy, Jonathan Leventhal, MD.*

Acropustulosis of Infancy *(Fig. 15.4)*

Cyclical, typical age is 3 to 6 months up to 2–3 years of age
Pruritic vesicles

Histopathology:
Intraepidermal pustules

Scabies *(Fig. 15.5, See Fig. 7.16A,B)*

Can present like acropustulosis of infancy

Histopathology:
Evidence of scabies (mite – arrow) infestation on scraping or biopsy

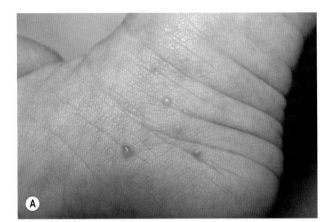

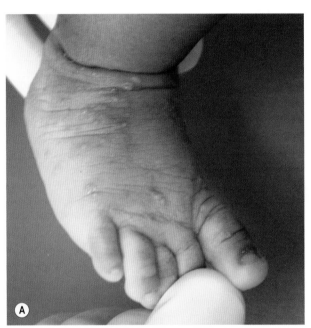

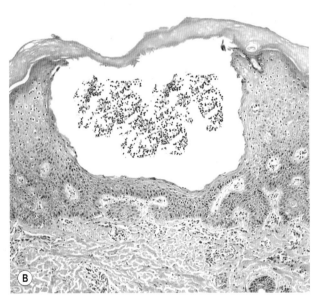

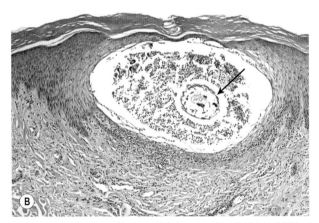

Fig. 15.4 Acropustulosis of infancy. *A, Courtesy, Deborah S Goddard, MD, Amy E Gilliam, MD, and Ilona J Frieden, MD. A, From Bolognia JL, Schaffer JV, Duncan KO, Ko CJ. Dermatology Essentials, 1e. Philadelphia: Saunders, 2014, with permission.*

Fig. 15.5 Scabies. *A, Courtesy, Yale Dermatology Residents' Slide Collection.*

OTHER DISORDERS

Erythema Toxicum Neonatorum *(Fig. 15.6)*

Typically develops day 1 or 2 of life and resolves within a week

Progresses from the face to the body

Erythematous papules and vesicles and pustules that may be surrounded by a pink flare

Histopathology:
Eosinophilic pustules within the epidermis

Transient Neonatal Pustular Melanosis *(Fig. 15.7)*

Favors the face, neck, back, shins

Superficial small vesiculopustules that rupture and leave collarettes of scale, eventuating in brown macules

Histopathology:
Neutrophils below the stratum corneum

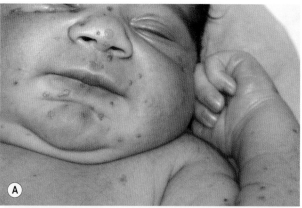

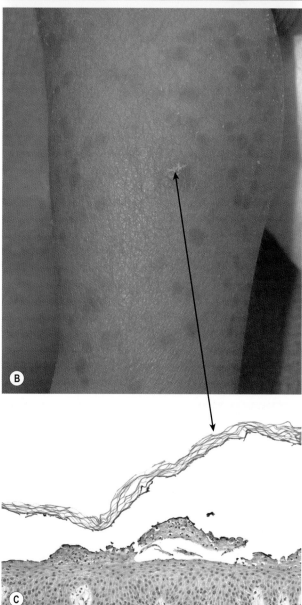

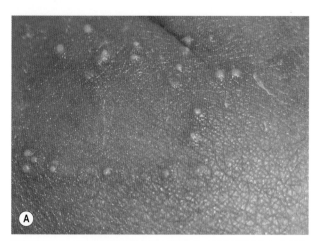

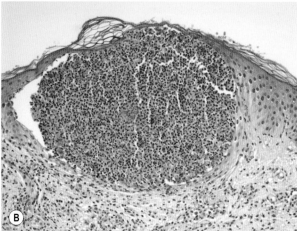

Fig. 15.6 Erythema toxicum neonatorum. *A, Courtesy, Yale Dermatology Residents' Slide Collection. B, From Patterson JW. Practical Skin Pathology: A Diagnostic Approach. Philadelphia: Saunders, 2013.*

Fig. 15.7 Transient neonatal pustular melanosis. *A,B, Courtesy, Yale Dermatology Residents' Slide Collection. B, From Bolognia JL, Schaffer JV, Duncan KO, Ko CJ. Dermatology Essentials, 1e. Philadelphia: Saunders, 2014, with permission.*

Miliaria Crystallina *(Fig. 15.8)*

Often secondary to increased perspiration
Favors the face, trunk, and arms
Clear, short-lived vesicles, non-inflamed

Miliaria Rubra *(Fig. 15.9)*

Favors occluded areas like the neck, trunk
Red papules

Histopathology:
Spongiosis and inflammation of the eccrine duct where
it enters the epidermis

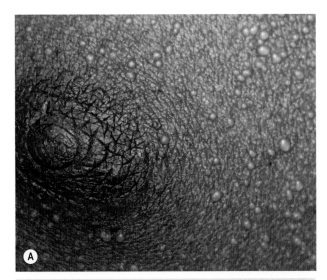

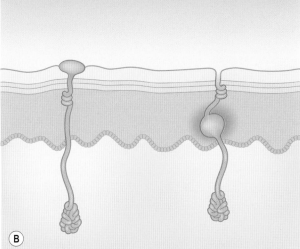

Fig. 15.8 Miliaria crystallina. A Miliaria crystallina. **B** Miliaria crystallina affects the surface of the acrosyringium; miliaria rubra affects the acrosyringium as it crosses the stratum spinosum. *A, Courtesy, Yale Dermatology Residents' Slide Collection. B, From Weston WL, Lane AT, Morelli JG. Color Textbook of Pediatric Dermatology, 4e. St Louis: Mosby, 2007.*

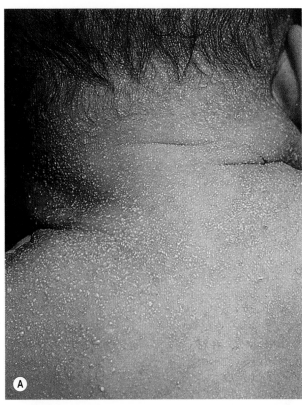

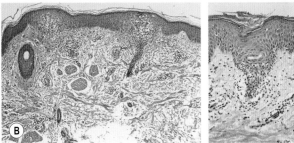

Fig. 15.9 Miliaria rubra. *A, Courtesy, Lawrence Eichenfeld, MD. A, From Bolognia JL, Schaffer JV, Duncan KO, Ko CJ. Dermatology Essentials, 1e. Philadelphia: Saunders, 2014, with permission. B, From Patterson JW. Weedon's Skin Pathology, 4e. London: Churchill Livingstone, 2015.*

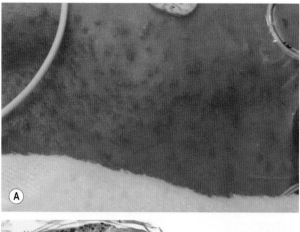

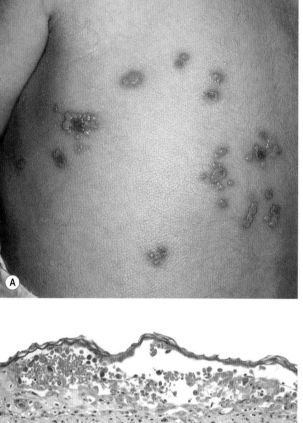

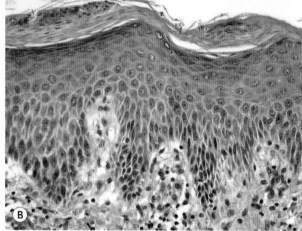

Fig. 15.10 Candidiasis. *A, Courtesy, Yale Dermatology Residents' Slide Collection.*

Candidiasis *(Fig. 15.10)*

Acquired *in utero*
Often evident at birth
Erythematous papules and/or pustules with fine scale; in premature infants, diffuse erythema and erosions

Histopathology:
Yeast and pseudohyphae in the stratum corneum

Herpes Virus Infection *(Fig. 15.11)*

Grouped vesicles on an erythematous base, scalloped borders

Histopathology:
Acantholysis, multinucleate cells

Epidermolysis Bullosa

Inherited skin disorders

Histopathology:
Blistering within or below the epidermis *(Fig. 15.12)*

Incontinentia Pigmenti *(Table 15.1; see Fig. 1.28A)*

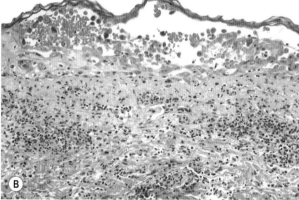

Fig. 15.11 Herpes simplex virus infection. *A, Courtesy, Yale Dermatology Residents' Slide Collection. A, From Bolognia JL, Schaffer JV, Duncan KO, Ko CJ. Dermatology Essentials, 1e. Philadelphia: Saunders, 2014, with permission.*

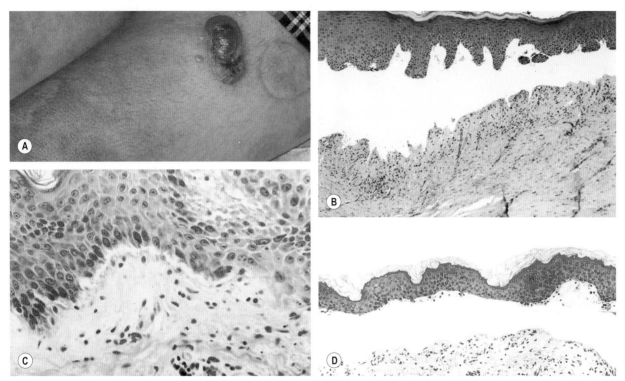

Fig. 15.12 Epidermolysis bullosa. A Dystrophic epidermolysis bullosa. Blistering and scarring at sites of previous blisters. Location of the split in dystrophic epidermolysis bullosa (in the papillary dermis, with scarring, **B**). The split is higher in epidermolysis bullosa simplex (within the basal cell, **C**), and junctional epidermolysis bullosa (below the basal cell, **D**). *A, Courtesy, Yale Dermatology Residents' Slide Collection. B–D, From Patterson JW. Practical Skin Pathology: A Diagnostic Approach. Philadelphia: Saunders, 2013.*

Table 15.1 Four stages of incontinentia pigmenti *(see Fig. 1.28)*

Stage	Typical age of presentation	Typical resolution
1 – Vesicular *(see Fig. 3.12G,H)*	Rarely congenital Birth to 2–3 weeks	In weeks to months
2 – Verrucous	2–6 weeks	In weeks to months
3 – Hyperpigmented	2–6 months	Fades during childhood
4 – Hypopigmented	Puberty	None

Helminths/Arthropods | 16

This chapter covers pediculosis, scabies, *Demodex* folliculitis, strongyloidiasis, tungiasis, cutaneous larva migrans, myiasis, tick bites, and filariasis.

PEDICULOSIS

Lice of different species primarily affect the head (*Pediculus humanus capitis*), clothing (*Pediculus humanus corporis*), and pubic hair/eyelashes (*Pthirus pubis*) (Figs 16.1–16.4).

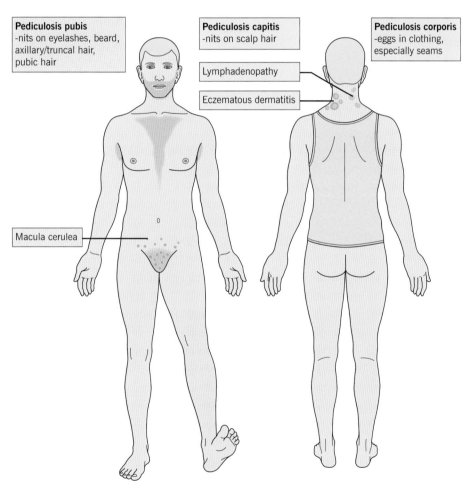

Pediculosis pubis
-nits on eyelashes, beard, axillary/truncal hair, pubic hair

Pediculosis capitis
-nits on scalp hair

Pediculosis corporis
-eggs in clothing, especially seams

Lymphadenopathy

Eczematous dermatitis

Macula cerulea

Fig. 16.1 Pediculosis, sites affected.

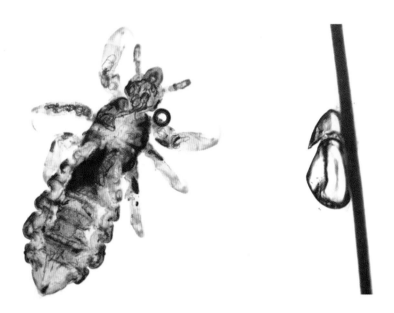

Fig. 16.2 Head louse (*Pediculus humanus capitis*) and an empty egg casing (the operculum is at the top) attached to a hair shaft.

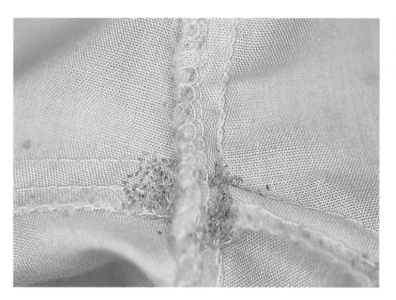

Fig. 16.3 Body lice eggs in the seams of clothing. *Courtesy, Yale Dermatology Residents' Slide Collection. From Bolognia JL, Jorizzo JL, Schaffer JV. Dermatology, 3e. London: Saunders, 2012, with permission.*

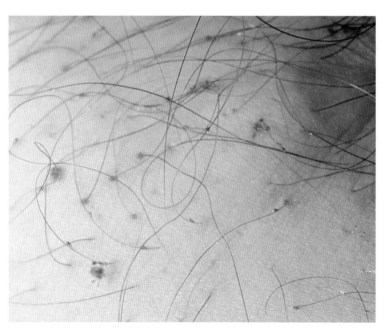

Fig. 16.4 Crab lice and eggs on pubic hair. *Courtesy, Louis A Fragola, MD. From Bolognia JL, Jorizzo JL, Schaffer JV. Dermatology, 3e. London: Saunders, 2012, with permission.*

SCABIES

Infestation with *Sarcoptes scabiei* var. *hominis*
Various skin manifestations *(Figs 16.5–16.8)*

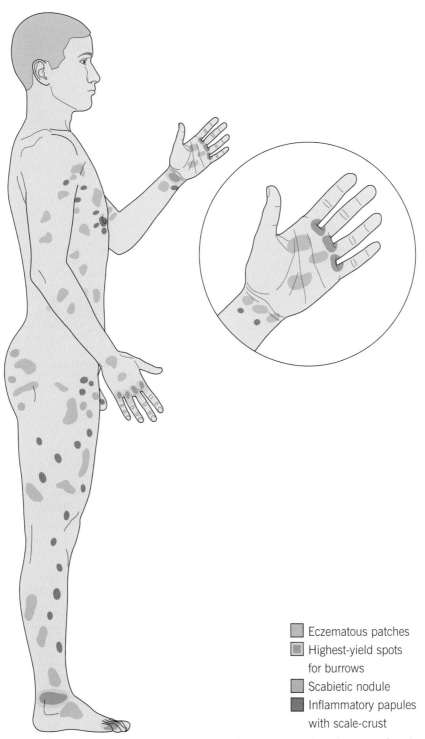

Eczematous patches

Highest-yield spots
for burrows

Scabietic nodule

Inflammatory papules
with scale-crust

Fig. 16.5 Range of cutaneous lesions in scabies. Crusted scabies may show prominent hyperkeratosis of acral sites. *From Bolognia JL, Schaffer JV, Duncan KO, Ko CJ. Dermatology Essentials, 1e. Philadelphia: Saunders, 2014, with permission.*

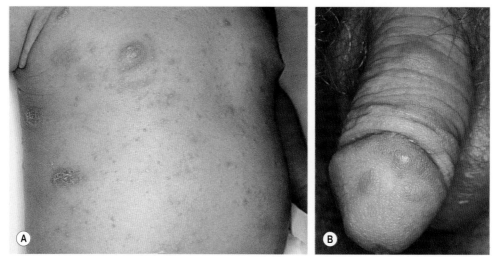

Fig. 16.6 Scabies infestation. A Eczematous patches and inflammatory papules. **B** Scabietic nodules. *A, Courtesy, Yale Dermatology Residents' Slide Collection. B, Courtesy, Robert Hartman, MD. A, From Bolognia JL, Jorizzo JL, Schaffer JV. Dermatology, 3e. London: Saunders, 2012, with permission. B, From Bolognia JL, Schaffer JV, Duncan KO, Ko CJ. Dermatology Essentials, 1e. Philadelphia: Saunders, 2014, with permission.*

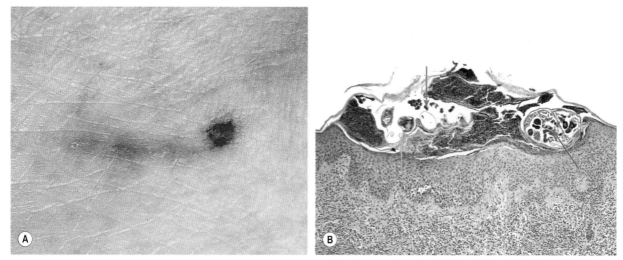

Fig. 16.7 Scabies. A Scabies linear burrow. **B** Microscopic mite (blue arrow), scybala (green arrow), and egg casings (orange arrow). *A, Courtesy, NYU Slide Collection. A, From Bolognia JL, Jorizzo JL, Schaffer JV. Dermatology, 3e. London: Saunders, 2012, with permission.*

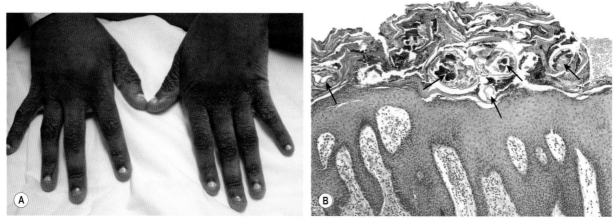

Fig. 16.8 Crusted scabies. The hyperkeratotic lesions, most typically on the hands, house numerous mites (arrows) and scybala (*). *Courtesy, Yale Dermatology Residents' Slide Collection.*

DEMODEX FOLLICULITIS

Due to *Demodex* spp.
Erythematous papules and/or pustules on the face
(Figs 16.9, 16.10)
Background of erythema and/or rosacea

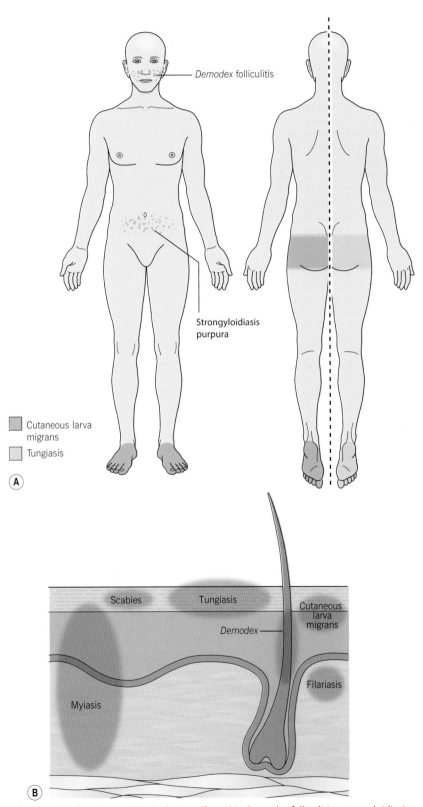

Fig. 16.9 Distribution of selected infestations. A Typical sites affected in *Demodex* folliculitis, strongyloidiasis, tungiasis, and cutaneous larva migrans. **B** Histopathologic location of selected arthropods/helminths. Microfilariae of filariasis are located in the dermis, but adult worms are in subcutaneous tissue or lymphatics.

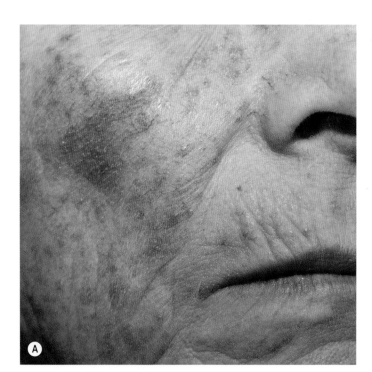

Fig. 16.10 *Demodex* **folliculitis.** *Demodex* mites are within follicles as well as in the dermis (arrow) surrounded by acute inflammation. *A, Courtesy, Kalman Watsky, MD.*

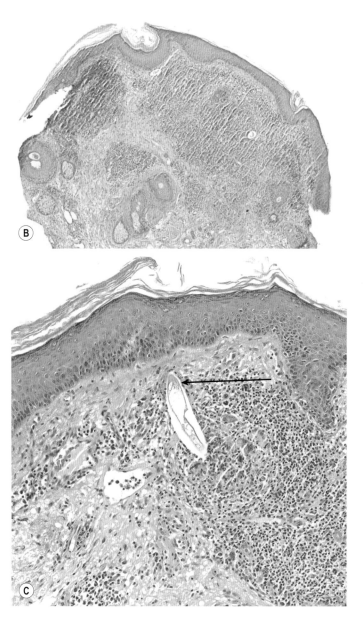

STRONGYLOIDIASIS

Due to *Strongyloides stercoralis*
Thumbprint purpura, typically on the abdomen of
immunocompromised hosts *(see Fig. 16.9; Fig. 16.11)*
Larva currens, serpiginous skin lesions, migrating up to
10 cm a day

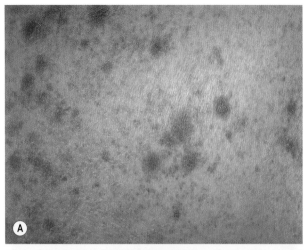

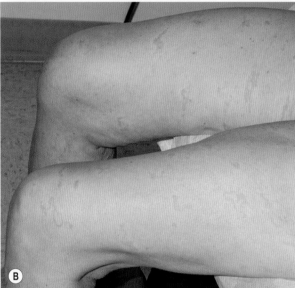

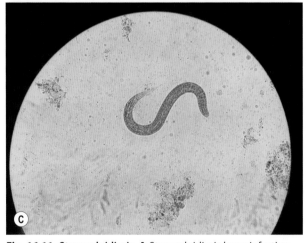

Fig. 16.11 Strongyloidiasis. A Strongyloidiasis hyperinfection.
B Larva currens. **C** *Strongyloides* larva isolated from the stool.
*A, Courtesy, Jean L Bolognia, MD. A, From Bolognia JL, Jorizzo JL,
Schaffer JV. Dermatology, 3e. London: Saunders, 2012, with
permission. B,C, From Pichard DC, Hensley JR, Williams E, et al. Rapid
development of migratory, linear, and serpiginous lesions in
association with immunosuppression. J Am Acad Dermatol.
2014;70:1130–4, © Elsevier.*

TUNGIASIS

Due to infestation by a burrowing flea, e.g. *Tunga penetrans*
Generally on the feet or the buttocks after contact with infested soil *(see Fig. 16.9; Fig. 16.12)*

CUTANEOUS LARVA MIGRANS (CREEPING ERUPTION)

Due to animal hookworm larvae (e.g. *Ancylostoma caninum*, *A. braziliense* and *Uncinaria stenocephala*)
Commonly on feet or other body sites that have contacted contaminated soil or sand (e.g. buttocks; *see Fig. 16.9*)
Serpiginous skin lesions *(Fig. 16.13)*, migrating 1–2 cm day

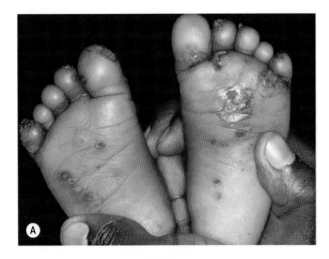

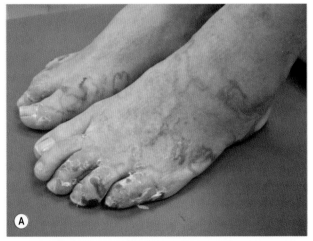

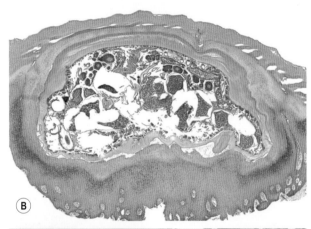

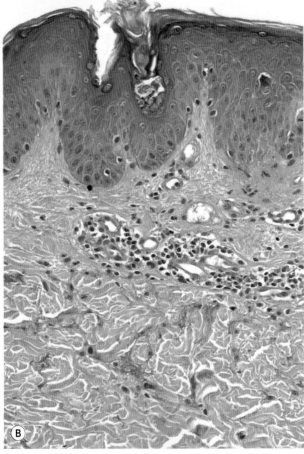

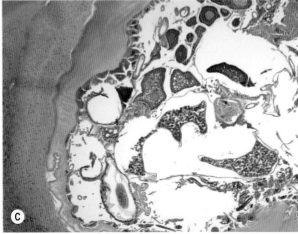

Fig. 16.12 Tungiasis. *A, Courtesy, Terri L Meinking, MD, Craig N Burkhart, MD, and Craig G Burkhart, MD. A, From Bolognia JL, Jorizzo JL, Schaffer JV. Dermatology, 3e. London: Saunders, 2012, with permission.*

Fig. 16.13 Cutaneous larva migrans. *A, Courtesy, Peter Klein, MD. A, From Bolognia JL, Jorizzo JL, Schaffer JV. Dermatology, 3e. London: Saunders, 2012, with permission.*

MYIASIS

Infestation by fly larvae, e.g. *Dermatobia hominis*
Presents as an erythematous nodule *(Fig. 16.14)* or as infestation of wounds

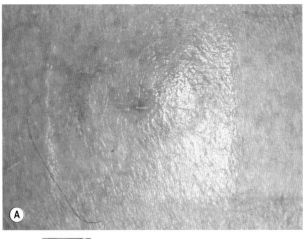

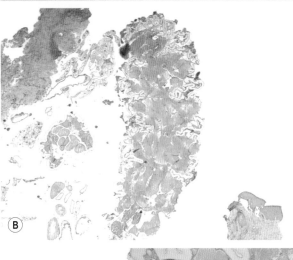

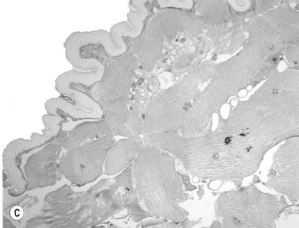

Fig. 16.14 Myiasis. *A, Courtesy, Yale Dermatology Residents' Slide Collection. A, From Bolognia JL, Schaffer JV, Duncan KO, Ko CJ. Dermatology Essentials, 1e. Philadelphia: Saunders, 2014, with permission.*

TICK BITES

Clinically, attached ticks *(Fig. 16.15)* may be mistaken for a nodular melanoma

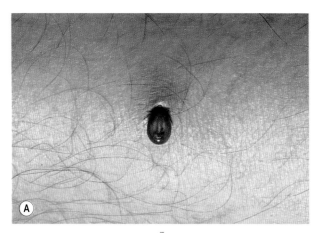

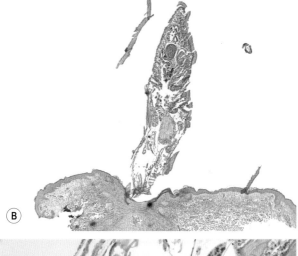

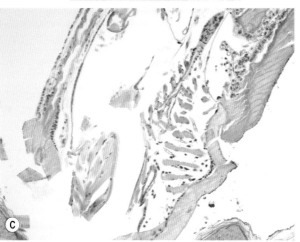

Fig. 16.15 Attached tick. *A, From James WD, Berger T, Elston D. Andrews' Diseases of the Skin, 11e. Edinburgh: Saunders, 2011.*

SUBCUTANEOUS FILARIASIS – ONCHOCERCIASIS (RIVER BLINDNESS)

Due to *Onchocerca volvulus*, transmitted by black flies
(*Simulium* spp.)
Various manifestations *(Figs 16.16–16.18)*

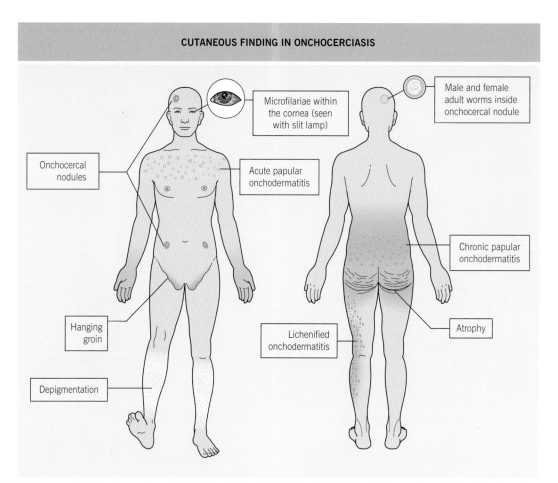

Fig. 16.16 Cutaneous findings in onchocerciasis. *From Bolognia JL, Jorizzo JL, Schaffer JV. Dermatology, 3e. London: Saunders, 2012, with permission.*

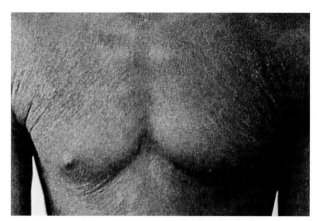

Fig. 16.17 Onchocerciasis. Diffuse lichenification, hyperpigmentation, and focal areas of leukoderma. *Courtesy, Omar P Sangüeza, MD. From Bolognia JL, Jorizzo JL, Schaffer JV. Dermatology, 3e. London: Saunders, 2012, with permission.*

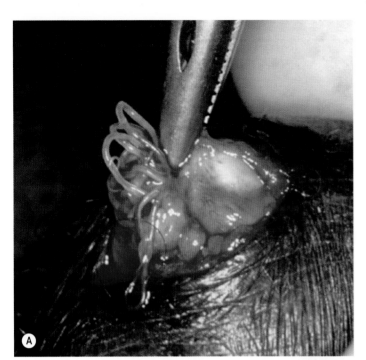

Fig. 16.18 Onchocercal nodule containing an adult worm. *A, Courtesy, Steven A Nelson, MD and Karen E Warschaw, MD. A, From Bolognia JL, Jorizzo JL, Schaffer JV. Dermatology, 3e. London: Saunders, 2012, with permission.*

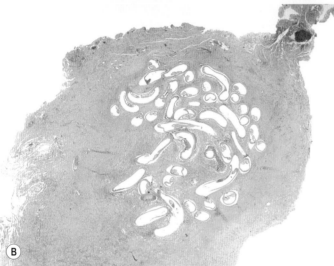

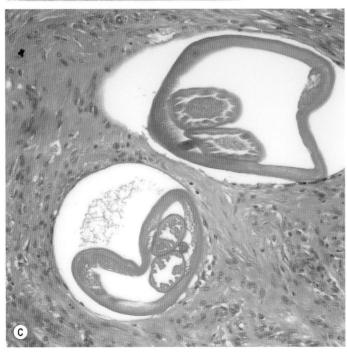

LYMPHATIC FILARIASIS

Due to infection by tissue nematodes, e.g. *Wuchereria bancrofti, Brugia* spp.

Lymphatics are occluded by adult worms, leading to chronic lymphedema, hanging groin, and elephantiasis (Fig. 16.19)

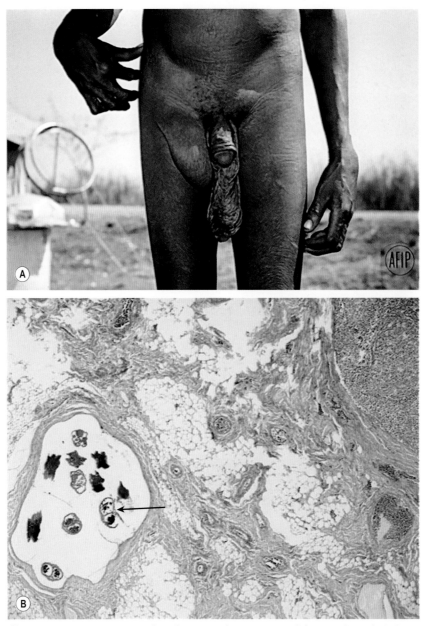

Fig. 16.19 Lymphatic filariasis. A Hanging groin. **B** A lymphatic vessel contains an adult worm (arrow). *A, Courtesy, Daniel Conner. A, From Tyring SK, Lupi O, Hengge UR. Tropical Dermatology. London: Churchill Livingstone, 2005. B, From Bolognia JL, Jorizzo JL, Schaffer JV. Dermatology, 3e. London: Saunders, 2012, with permission.*

Ulcers | 17

Three major types of ulcers occur on the legs (*Table 17.1*), and these ulcers are often diagnosed clinically. Histopathology can be helpful in diagnosing the cause of particular ulcers, for example, pyoderma gangrenosum (*Fig. 17.1*), infections (*Figs 17.2–17.4*), vasculitides (*Figs 17.5, 17.6*), vaso-occlusive processes (*Fig. 17.7*), or tumors (*Fig. 17.8*). Selected other causes of ulcers are depicted in *Figures 17.9–17.16*.

Table 17.1 Common leg ulcers – key differences

	Venous	Arterial	Neuropathic/mal perforans*
Location	Medial malleolar region	Pressure sites (lateral malleolar region) Distal points (toes)	Pressure sites
Morphology	Irregular borders Yellow fibrinous base	Dry, necrotic base Well-demarcated ("punched out")	"Punched out"
Surrounding skin	Yellow–brown to brown discoloration due to hemosiderin deposits Pinpoint petechiae ("stasis purpura") Lipodermatosclerosis	Shiny atrophic skin with hair loss	Thick callus
Other physical examination findings	Varicosities Leg/ankle edema ± Stasis dermatitis ± Lymphedema	Weak/absent peripheral pulses Prolonged capillary refill time (>3–4 seconds) Pallor on leg elevation (45° for 1 min) Dependent rubor	Peripheral neuropathy with decreased sensation ± Foot deformities

*Most commonly due to diabetes mellitus.

Images, Courtesy, David L Troutman Jr, DPM, Tammie C Ferringer, MD, Ariela Hafner, MD and Eli Sprecher, MD. Table adapted from Bolognia JL, Jorizzo JL, Schaffer JV. Dermatology, 3e. London: Saunders, 2012, with permission.

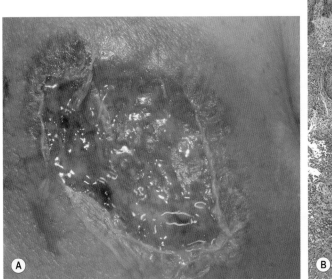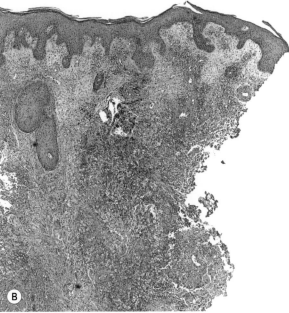

Fig. 17.1 Pyoderma gangrenosum. A Classic ulcerative pyoderma gangrenosum. The edge of this ulceration on the shin is undermined with a violet–gray color as well as an inflammatory rim. Note the central scarring. **B** In expanding untreated lesions, a diffuse infiltrate of neutrophils is present. *A, Courtesy, Yale Dermatology Residents' Slide Collection.*

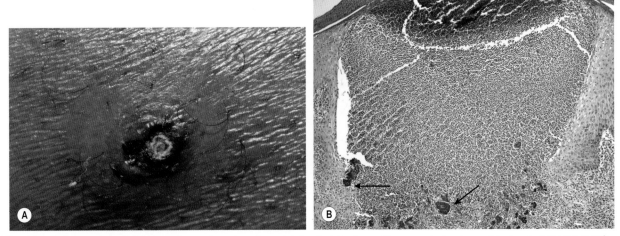

Fig. 17.2 Ecthyma. Superficial ulceration and crust on the wrist due to infection with group A streptococci (arrows). *A, Courtesy, Yale Dermatology Residents' Slide Collection.*

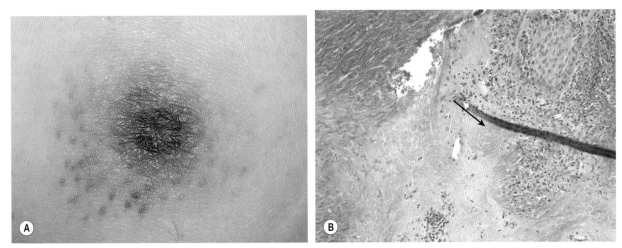

Fig. 17.3 Ecthyma gangrenosum. A Embolic lesion of *Pseudomonas aeruginosa* on the chest. Note the necrotic center and inflammatory border. **B** Histopathologic findings include dermal necrosis and a light blue haze of organisms (arrow). *A, Courtesy, Yale Dermatology Residents' Slide Collection.*

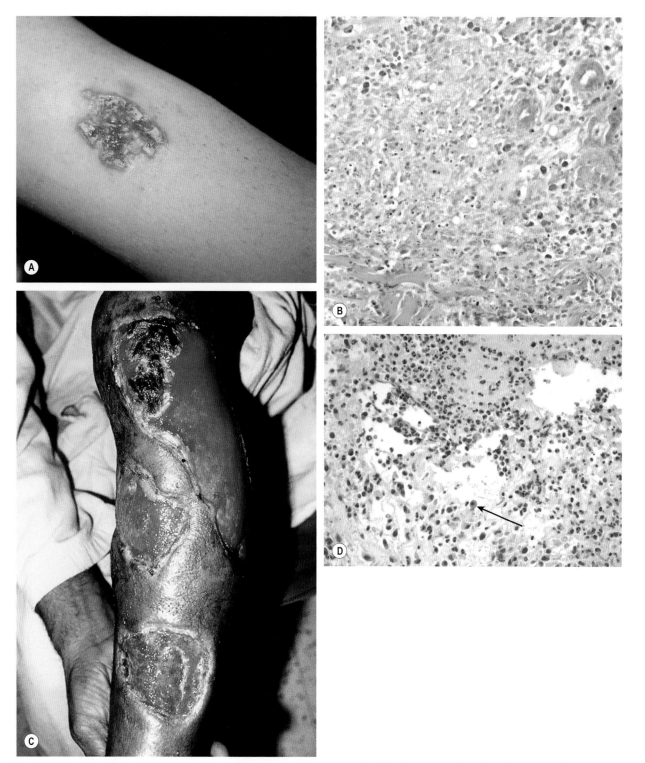

Fig. 17.4 Infectious ulcers. A,B Ulcerative form of cutaneous leishmaniasis. Multiple lower extremity ulcers in a rural worker.
C Amebiasis. Multiple large, destructive ulcers. **D** Mixed inflammation and rare trophozoites (arrow). *A, Courtesy, Yale Dermatology Residents' Slide Collection; B, Courtesy, Nemanja Rodic, MD, PhD; C, Courtesy, Omar P Sangüeza, MD. A–C, From Bolognia JL, Jorizzo JL, Schaffer JV. Dermatology, 3e. London: Saunders, 2012, with permission.*

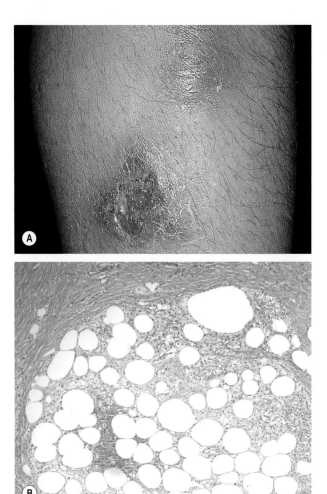

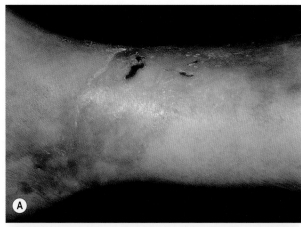

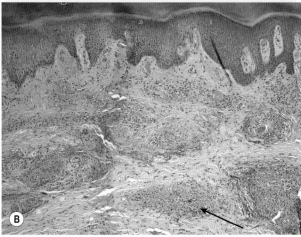

Fig. 17.5 Erythema induratum. A Nodular lesions on the lower leg, with evidence of ulceration. **B** Lobular panniculitis. The infiltrate is lymphocytic and granulomatous. *A, Courtesy, Kenneth E Greer, MD. A, From Bolognia JL, Jorizzo JL, Schaffer JV. Dermatology, 3e. London: Saunders, 2012, with permission.*

Fig. 17.6 Superficial ulcerating rheumatoid necrobiosis. A Shiny, yellow plaques with red–brown edges and areas of ulceration that clinically resemble necrobiosis lipoidica. **B** Vasculitis (fibrin and inflammation within vessel walls; arrow). *A, Courtesy, Kathryn Schwarzenberger, MD. A, From Bolognia JL, Jorizzo JL, Schaffer JV. Dermatology, 3e. London: Saunders, 2012, with permission.*

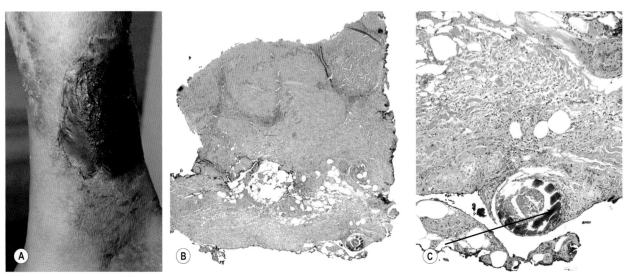

Fig. 17.7 Calciphylaxis. A Necrotic skin lesions in the setting of severe end-stage renal disease due to amyloidosis of the kidney. **B,C** Calcium within a vessel (arrow). *A, Courtesy, Yale Dermatology Residents' Slide Collection.*

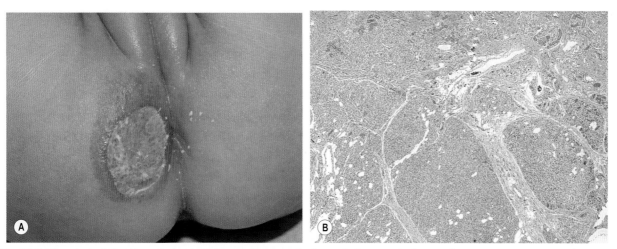

Fig. 17.8 Ulcerated minimal/arrested growth hemangioma on the buttock. Because the hemangioma component may not be obvious, this diagnosis should be considered when an infant presents with an ulcer in the diaper area. *Courtesy, Julie V Schaffer, MD. From Bolognia JL, Jorizzo JL, Schaffer JV. Dermatology, 3e. London: Saunders, 2012, with permission.*

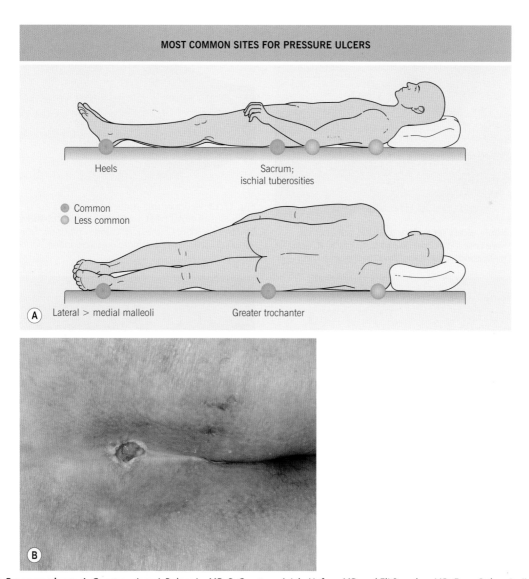

MOST COMMON SITES FOR PRESSURE ULCERS

Heels

Sacrum;
ischial tuberosities

● Common
● Less common

Lateral > medial malleoli   Greater trochanter

Fig. 17.9 Pressure ulcers. *A, Courtesy, Jean L Bolognia, MD. B, Courtesy, Ariela Hafner, MD and Eli Sprecher, MD. From Bolognia JL, Jorizzo JL, Schaffer JV. Dermatology, 3e. London: Saunders, 2012, with permission.*

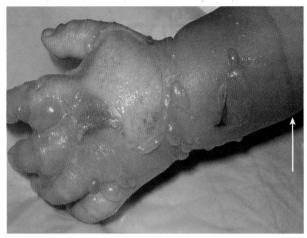

Fig. 17.10 Burn injury due to dunking in hot water. Note the sharp line of demarcation of the burn on the arm (arrow). *Courtesy, Sharon Ann Raimer, MD. From Bolognia JL, Jorizzo JL, Schaffer JV. Dermatology, 3e. London: Saunders, 2012, with permission.*

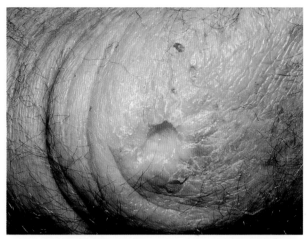

Fig. 17.11 Ulceration of the elbow in a patient with systemic sclerosis. *Courtesy, Joyce Rico, MD. From Bolognia JL, Jorizzo JL, Schaffer JV. Dermatology, 3e. London: Saunders, 2012, with permission.*

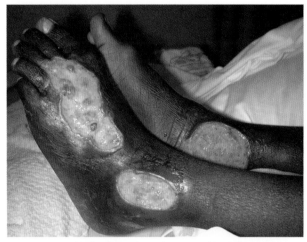

Fig. 17.12 Multiple ulcers secondary to sickle cell anemia. *Courtesy, NYU Slide Collection. From Bolognia JL, Jorizzo JL, Schaffer JV. Dermatology, 3e. London: Saunders, 2012, with permission.*

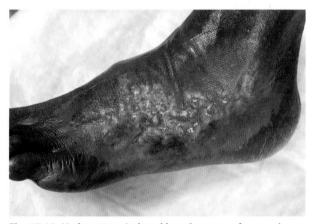

Fig. 17.13 Hydroxyurea-induced leg ulcers are often on the malleolus or tibial crest, exceedingly painful and surrounded by atrophic skin. *Courtesy, NYU Slide Collection. From Bolognia JL, Jorizzo JL, Schaffer JV. Dermatology, 3e. London: Saunders, 2012, with permission.*

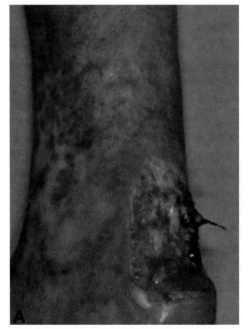

Fig. 17.14 Werner syndrome. Large deep ulcer with thick necrotic tissue near Achilles tendon on right posterior distal leg. *From Noda S, Asano Y, Masuda S, et al. Bosentan: a novel therapy for leg ulcers in Werner syndrome. J Am Acad Dermatol. 2011;65:e54–5, © Elsevier.*

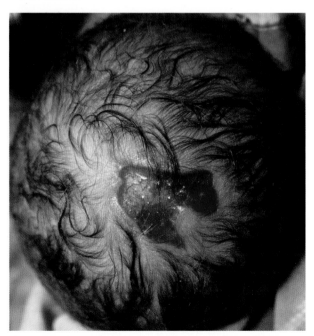

Fig. 17.15 Cutis aplasia on the scalp in a newborn. *Courtesy, Yale Dermatology Residents' Slide Collection.*

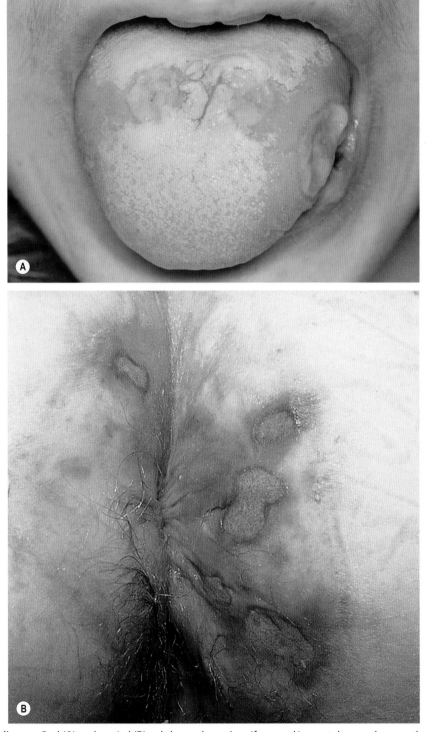

Fig. 17.16 Behçet's disease. Oral (**A**) and genital (**B**) aphthous ulcers. Acneiform and/or pustular papules are other skin manifestations of Behçet's disease. *A,B Courtesy, Samuel L Moschella, MD. From Bolognia JL, Jorizzo JL, Schaffer JV. Dermatology, 3e. London: Saunders, 2012, with permission.*

Purpura, Small Vessel Vasculitis, and Vascular Occlusion | 18

Purpura is a manifestation of extravascular erythrocytes. The morphology of purpura is important – flat vs raised and smooth vs irregular/retiform border/outline *(Fig. 18.1)*. The irregular/retiform pattern corresponds to the cutaneous network of small vessels that produces livedo reticularis *(see Fig. 1.22A,B)*. This chapter focuses on the distinction between palpable purpura and retiform purpura.

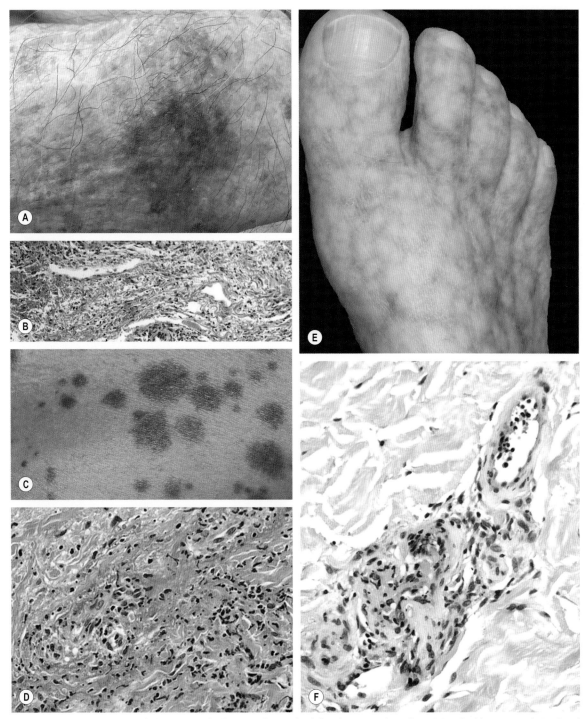

Fig. 18.1 Purpura. A,B Actinic (solar) purpura. The lesion is flat and solid with a smooth outline. **C,D** Palpable purpura (raised with a smooth outline). **E,F** Retiform purpura. The lesions are a flat network of interconnecting rings ("retiform"). Biopsy findings: solar purpura – extravasated erythrocytes (**B**); palpable purpura – leukocytoclastic vasculitis (**D**); retiform purpura – vascular occlusion with sparse perivascular inflammation (**F**). *C, Courtesy, Yale Dermatology Residents' Slide Collection. C, From Bolognia JL, Jorizzo JL, Schaffer JV. Dermatology, 3e. London: Saunders, 2012, with permission.*

PALPABLE PURPURA

Palpable purpura *(morphology: raised and solid with smooth borders; Fig. 18.1B)* is a common manifestation of cutaneous small vessel vasculitis. Causes are diverse and include Henoch–Schönlein purpura *(Fig. 18.2A)*, drug exposure, malignancies *(especially hematologic; Fig. 18.2B)*, systemic disease *(Fig. 18.2C–F)*, and infections. History, other clues on examination

(see rheumatoid nodules in Fig. 18.2F), and/or laboratory studies are necessary to ascertain the ultimate cause. Other diseases with underlying small vessel damage include acute hemorrhagic edema of infancy *(Fig. 18.3A–C)*, urticarial vasculitis *(Fig. 18.3D,E)*, and erythema elevatum diutinum *(Fig. 18.3F,G)*.

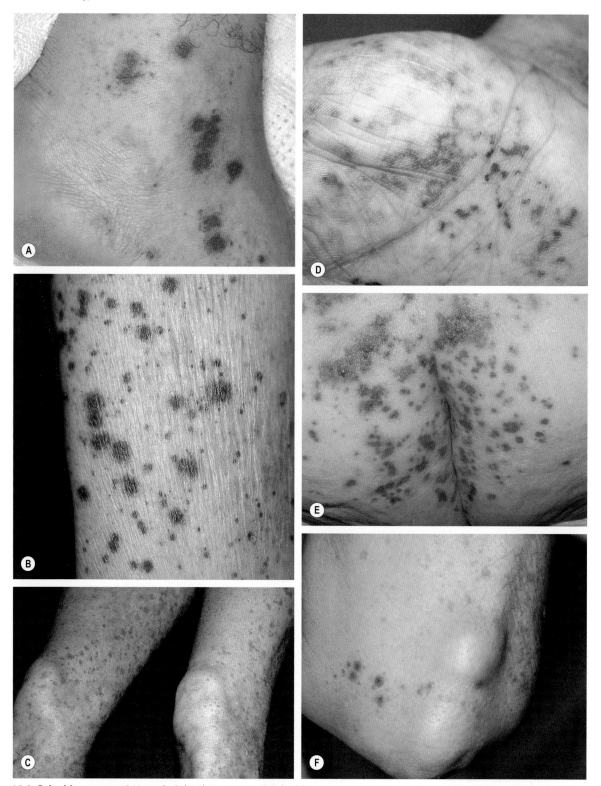

Fig. 18.2 Palpable purpura. A Henoch–Schönlein purpura. **B** Palpable purpura in a patient with myelodysplasia and relapsing polychondritis. **C** Mixed cryoglobulinemia. **D** Granulomatosis with polyangiitis (Wegener granulomatosis). **E** Eosinophilic granulomatosis with polyangiitis (Churg-Strauss syndrome). **F** Rheumatoid arthritis. *A,D,F, Courtesy, Yale Dermatology Residents' Slide Collection; B, Courtesy, Jean L Bolognia, MD. C, Courtesy, Lorinda Chung, MD, Bory Kea, MD and David F Fiorentino, MD. E, Courtesy, Kanade Shinkai, MD and Lindy P Fox, MD. A–C,E,F, From Bolognia JL, Jorizzo JL, Schaffer JV. Dermatology, 3e. London: Saunders, 2012, with permission.*

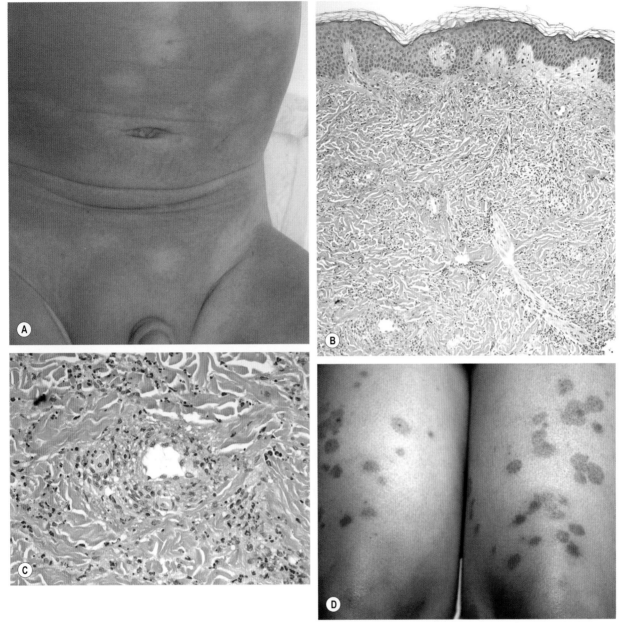

Fig. 18.3 Small vessel damage. A–C Acute hemorrhagic edema of infancy. **D,E** Urticarial vasculitis. *Continued*

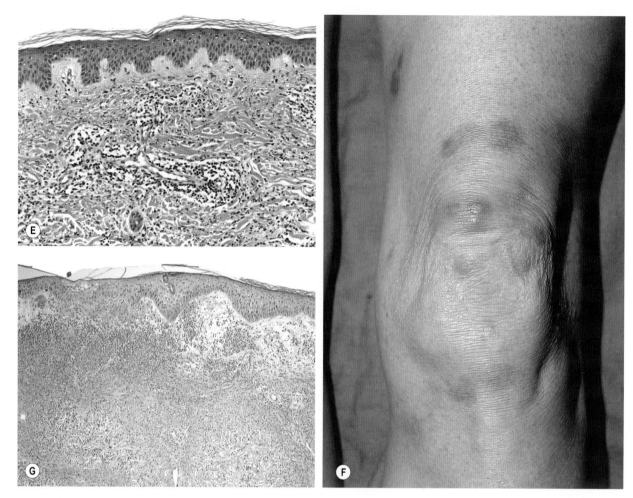

Fig. 18.3, cont'd F,G Erythema elevatum diutinum. In all three of these diseases, there is inflammation surrounding vessels; fibrinous change is not present in acute hemorrhagic edema of infancy or urticarial vasculitis. Erythema elevatum diutinum has a heavier inflammatory infiltrate that is neutrophil-predominant. *A,D,E, Courtesy, Yale Dermatology Residents' Slide Collection; F, Courtesy, Kenneth Greer, MD. F, From Bolognia JL, Jorizzo JL, Schaffer JV. Dermatology, 3e. London: Saunders, 2012, with permission.*

RETIFORM PURPURA

In retiform purpura, portions of the normal vascular network become fixed and visible *(see Fig. 18.1C)*. In later stages, centers of lesions are solid and/or necrotic, but the borders of lesions remain scalloped/irregular or "retiform" *(Fig. 18.4)*. Retiform purpura is generally due to vascular occlusion, especially when not preceded by clinical erythema. Retiform pupura that is preceded by clinical erythema may be secondary to occlusion *(Fig. 18.4A–G)* or vasculitis *(Fig. 18.4H–I)*.

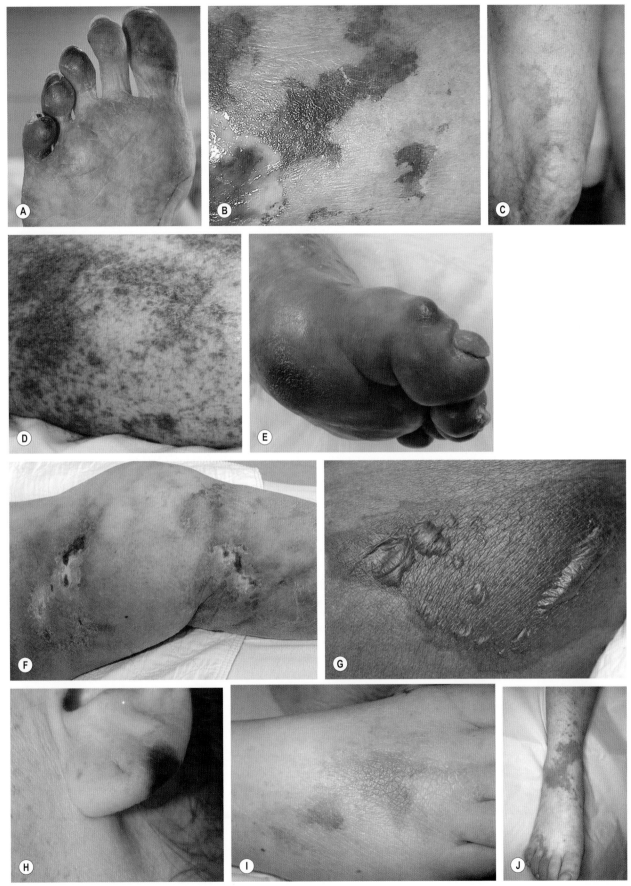

Fig. 18.4 Retiform purpura. A Antiphospholipid syndrome. **B** Calciphylaxis. **C** Cholesterol embolus. **D** Cryoglobulinemia, monoclonal.
E Disseminated intravascular coagulation. **F** Intravascular lymphoma. **G** Warfarin-induced necrosis. Tendency to affect fatty areas like
hips, abdomen, buttocks. **H** Levamisole-induced vasculitis. A typical site of involvement is the ear. **I** Polyarteritis nodosa. **J** Rocky
mountain spotted fever. *A,B,D,E,G–J, Courtesy, Yale Dermatology Residents' Slide Collection. C, Courtesy, Norbert Sepp, MD; F, Courtesy,
Lucinda Buescher, MD. B,C,F,I,J, From Bolognia JL, Jorizzo JL, Schaffer JV. Dermatology, 3e. London: Saunders, 2012, with permission.*

Epidermally-Based Lesions | 19

Epidermally-based lesions generally have a characteristic morphology and/or color *(Tables 19.1–19.4)*. Thickness of the tumor is reflected in the microscopic appearance (acanthosis). Other characteristic features are marked.

Table 19.1 Epidermally-based lesions: color – brown

Lesion	Appearance	Histopathology	Other clues
Seborrheic keratosis	• Various colors *(Fig. 19.1A)* but commonly tan to dark brown plaque • Horn cysts *(arrows; Fig. 19.1B,C)* • Stuck on appearance	• Several different subtypes, commonly acanthosis with pseudohorn cysts	**Dermoscopy** • Multiple milia-like cysts • Comedo-like openings
Solar lentigo *(Fig. 19.2)*	• Uniform macules • Sun-exposed skin	• Pigmented basal cell layer	**Dermoscopy** • Moth-eaten borders • Fingerprinting • Short, interrupted thin lines
Junctional melanocytic nevus *(Fig. 19.3)*	• Brown macule	• Regular distribution of melanocytes, often in nests	**Dermoscopy** • Regular pigment network
Melanoma *in situ*	• Asymmetry • Irregular borders • Variegate pigment *(Fig. 19.4)*	• Irregular confluent melanocytes	• On acral surfaces, pigment on the ridges is an important clue *(Fig. 19.5)* **Dermoscopy** • Asymmetry of color and structure • Atypical network • Blue–white structures • Black dots and globules

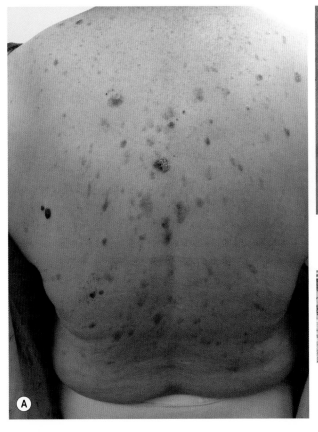

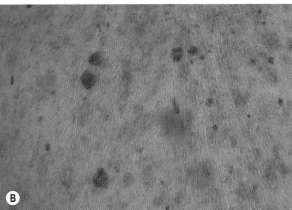

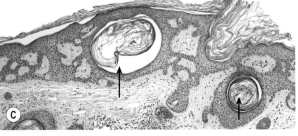

Fig. 19.1 Seborrheic keratosis.

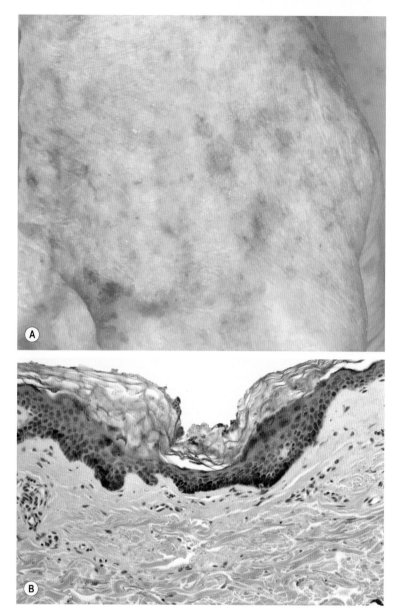

Fig. 19.2 Solar lentigo.

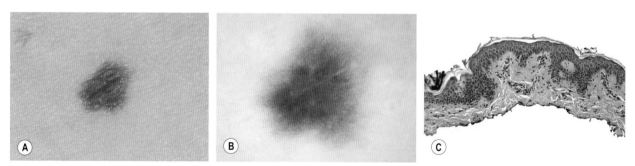

Fig. 19.3 Junctional melanocytic nevus. *A,B, Courtesy, Giuseppe Argenziano, MD, and Iris Zalaudek, MD. A,B, From Bolognia JL, Jorizzo JL, Schaffer JV. Dermatology, 3e. London: Saunders, 2012, with permission.*

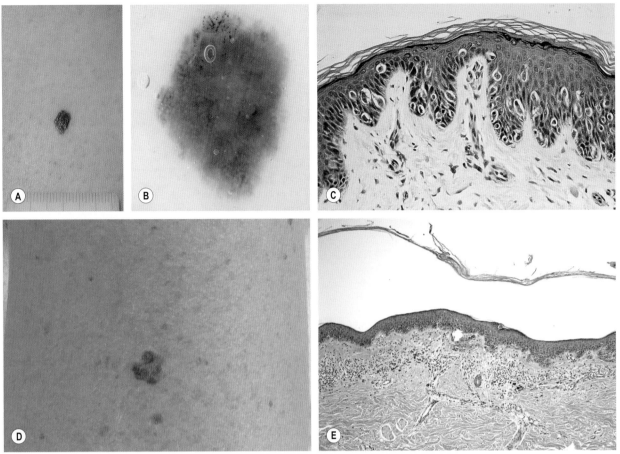

Fig. 19.4 Melanoma *in situ*. *A,B, Courtesy, Giuseppe Argenziano, MD, and Iris Zalaudek, MD. C, Courtesy, Helmut Kerl, MD. A–C, From Bolognia JL, Jorizzo JL, Schaffer JV. Dermatology, 3e. London: Saunders, 2012, with permission.*

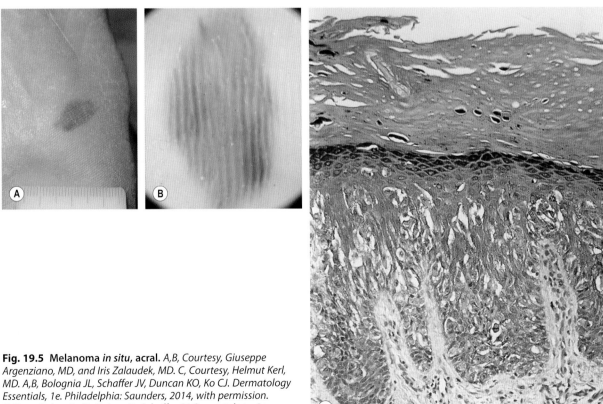

Fig. 19.5 Melanoma *in situ*, acral. *A,B, Courtesy, Giuseppe Argenziano, MD, and Iris Zalaudek, MD. C, Courtesy, Helmut Kerl, MD. A,B, Bolognia JL, Schaffer JV, Duncan KO, Ko CJ. Dermatology Essentials, 1e. Philadelphia: Saunders, 2014, with permission. C, From Bolognia JL, Jorizzo JL, Schaffer JV. Dermatology, 3e. London: Saunders, 2012, with permission.*

Table 19.2 Epidermally-based lesions: color – pink–red to tan

Lesion	Appearance	Histopathology	Other clues
Actinic keratosis (Fig. 19.6)	• Gritty white–yellow scale • Papule or plaque	• Atypical keratinocytes underlying parakeratosis	
Lichenoid keratosis (Fig. 19.7)	• Flat-surfaced pink plaque	• Band of dermal lymphocytes	
Disseminated superficial actinic porokeratosis	• Thin skin-colored to tan–pink papule or plaque • Raised, sharp double-edged rim (arrow; Fig. 19.8)	• Tiered parakeratosis above an abnormal granular layer	
Large cell acanthoma	• Thin pink to tan plaque (Fig. 19.9)	• Enlarged keratinocytes	
Squamous cell carcinoma in situ (Fig. 19.10)	• Scaly pink plaque	• Atypical cells throughout the entire epidermis	**Dermoscopy** • Glomerular vessels • Superficial scales
Superficial basal cell carcinoma (Fig. 19.11)	• Scaly pink plaque	• Basaloid islands off the base of the epidermis	**Dermoscopy** • Fine telangiectasias

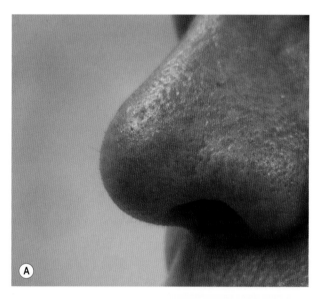

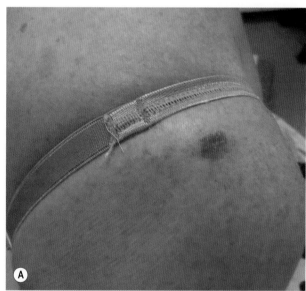

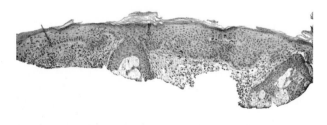

Fig. 19.6 Actinic keratosis, thin and subtle lesion that is better appreciated with palpation.

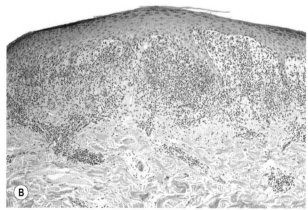

Fig. 19.7 Lichenoid keratosis.

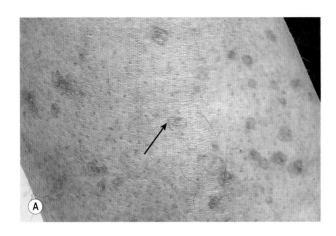

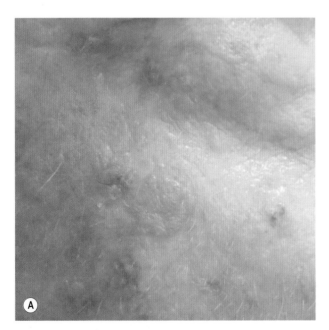

Fig. 19.8 Disseminated superficial actinic porokeratosis. *A, Courtesy, Yale Dermatology Residents' Slide Collection.*

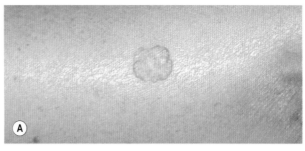

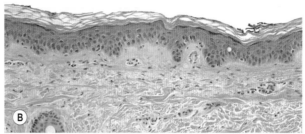

Fig. 19.9 Large cell acanthoma. *A, Courtesy, Luis Requena, MD. A, From Bolognia JL, Schaffer JV, Duncan KO, Ko CJ. Dermatology Essentials, 1e. Philadelphia: Saunders, 2014, with permission.*

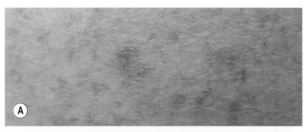

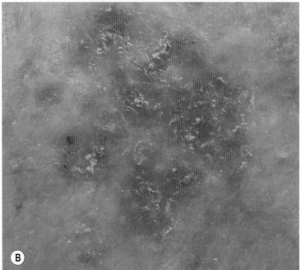

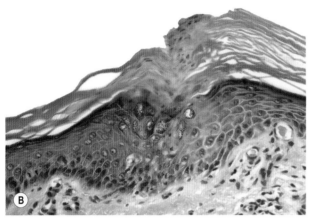

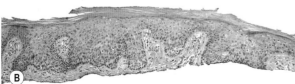

Fig. 19.10 Squamous cell carcinoma *in situ*.

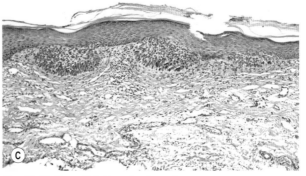

Fig. 19.11 Superficial basal cell carcinoma.

Table 19.3 Epidermally-based lesions: color – red–pink

Lesion	Appearance	Histopathology	Other clues
Clear cell acanthoma	• Well-demarcated, red, shiny papule; wafer-like collarette of scale *(Fig. 19.12)*	• Pale cells within the epidermis • Overlying parakeratosis	
Poroma	• Erythematous papule *(Fig. 19.13)*	• Monomorphous round to oval blue cells • Vascular stroma	
Paget disease *(Fig. 19.14)*	• Erythema, erosion, and scale	• Enlarged cells with abundant cytoplasm • Clusters of cells appear to surround a lumen	• Unilateral • Site: nipple/areola
Extramammary Paget disease *(Fig. 19.15)*	• Well-demarcated erythema with erosions and scale		• Site: groin

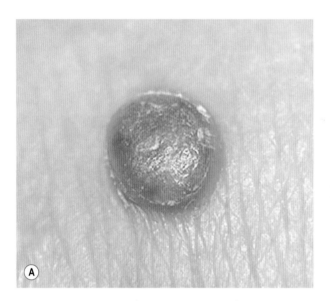

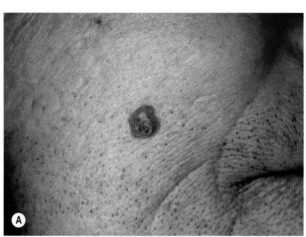

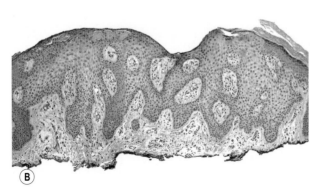

Fig. 19.12 Clear cell acanthoma. *A, Courtesy, Luis Requena, MD; B, Courtesy, Lorenzo Cerroni, MD. A, From Bolognia JL, Schaffer JV, Duncan KO, Ko CJ. Dermatology Essentials, 1e. Philadelphia: Saunders, 2014, with permission.*

Fig. 19.13 Poroma. *A, From Bolognia JL, Jorizzo JL, Schaffer JV. Dermatology, 3e. London: Saunders, 2012, with permission.*

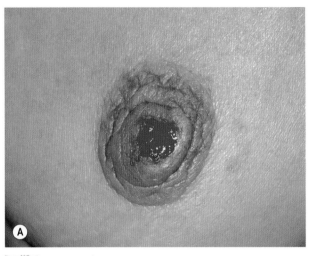

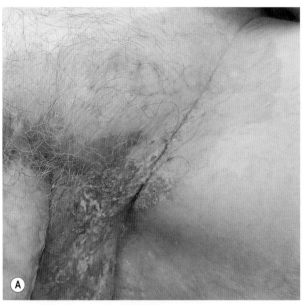

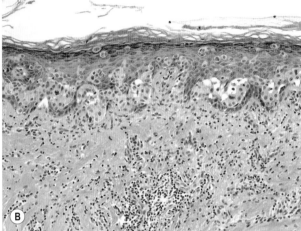

Fig. 19.14 Paget disease of the breast. *A, Courtesy, Robert Hartman, MD. A, From Bolognia JL, Jorizzo JL, Schaffer JV. Dermatology, 3e. London: Saunders, 2012, with permission.*

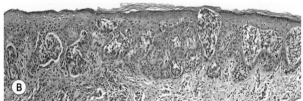

Fig. 19.15 Extramammary Paget disease.

Table 19.4 Epidermally-based lesions: color – white to skin-colored

Lesion	Appearance	Histopathology
Verruca vulgaris	• Finger-like projections • Punctate red–brown dots	• Papillomatosis *(arrows; Fig. 19.16)* • Koilocytes
Molluscum *(Fig. 19.17)*	• White to light pink, pearly papules • Often with central umbilication	• Oval to round large pink cytoplasmic inclusions
Trichilemmoma *(Fig. 19.18)*	• Verrucous to smooth yellow–white papule	• Lobules of pale cells
Tumor of the follicular infundibulum *(Fig. 19.19)*	• White thin papules	• Anastomosing columns of pale cells
Keratoacanthoma, regressing	• Crateriform lesion consisting mostly of a keratin *(arrow; Fig. 19.20)*	• Thinned epidermis in a cup-shape around keratin *(arrow; Fig. 19.20)*

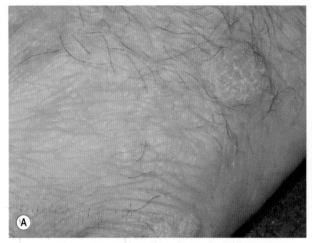

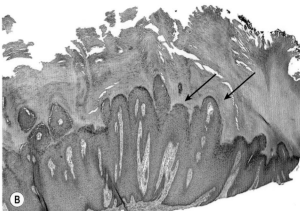

Fig. 19.16 Verruca vulgaris.

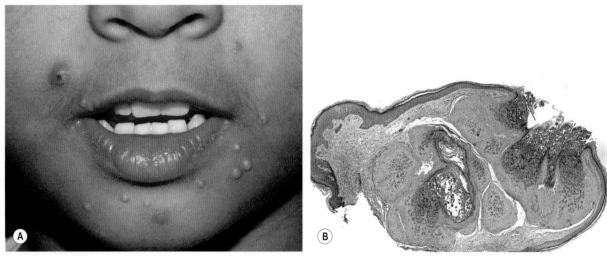

Fig. 19.17 Molluscum. *A, Courtesy, Julie V Schaffer, MD. A, From Bolognia JL, Schaffer JV, Duncan KO, Ko CJ. Dermatology Essentials, 1e. Philadelphia: Saunders, 2014, with permission.*

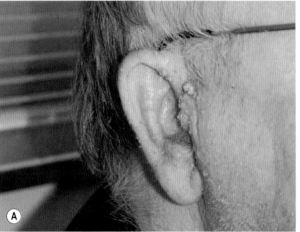

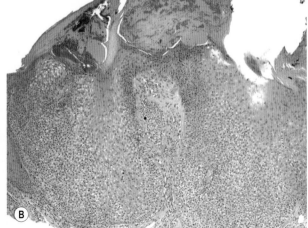

Fig. 19.18 Trichilemmoma. *A, Courtesy, Jennifer Choi, MD.*

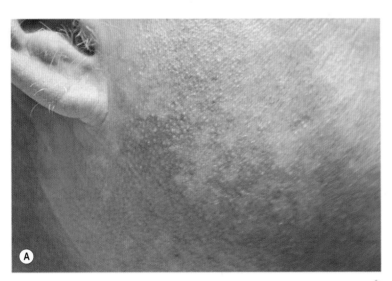

Fig. 19.19 Tumor of the follicular infundibulum.
A, Courtesy, Peter Heald, MD.

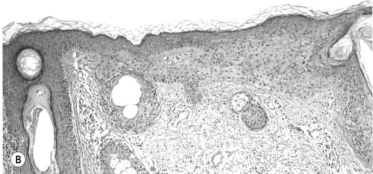

Fig. 19.20 Keratoacanthoma, regressing.
A, Courtesy, Jennifer Choi, MD.

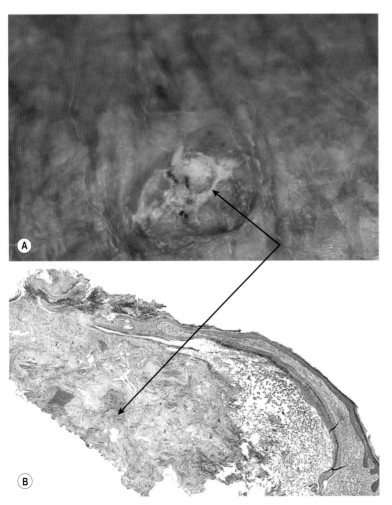

Dermally-Based Lesions | 20

While dermal tumors of different origins can have a similar appearance, with history and/or biopsy important for the correct diagnosis *(Fig. 20.1)*, this chapter focuses on characteristic presentations of dermally-based tumors *(Tables 20.1, 20.2)*.

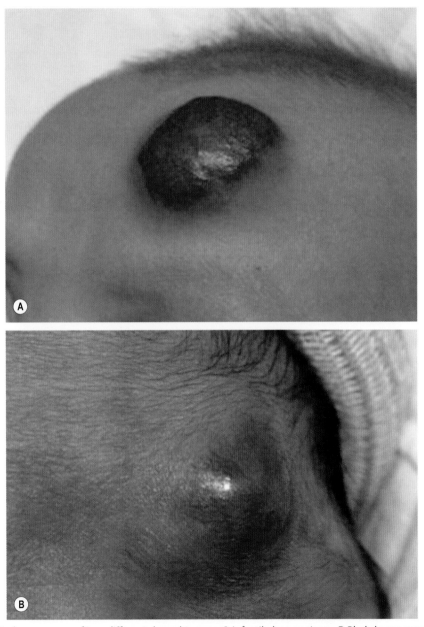

Fig. 20.1 Similar clinical appearance of two different dermal tumors. **A** Infantile hemangioma. **B** Rhabdomyosarcoma. *From Eichenfield LF, Frieden IJ, Zaenglein AL, Mathes E. Neonatal and Infant Dermatology, 3e. London: Saunders, 2014.*

Table 20.1 Dermally-based lesions

Entity	Classic morphologic clues*	Histopathology
Vascular tumors		
Infantile hemangioma	• **History:** Not present at birth, grows rapidly over first couple of months • Bright red nodule *(see Fig. 20.1A)*	• Lobules of small capillaries (GLUT-1-positive) • Often extends into the subcutaneous
Congenital hemangioma	• **History:** Present at birth • **Site:** Predilection for pressure points • Oval shape • Blue–red nodule with white–green halo *(Fig. 20.2)*	• Lobules of small capillaries (GLUT-1-negative)
Tufted angioma	• Mottled to solid red patches and red papules *(Fig. 20.3A,B)*	• Small lobules (tufts) of small capillaries • Dilated lymphatic spaces
Glomuvenous malformation (glomangioma)	• May be autosomal dominant inheritance, particularly if multiple lesions • Clustered blue papules *(Fig. 20.3C,D)*	• Dilated spaces lined by one to two layers of monomorphous cells with round blue nuclei
Fibrous tumors		
Myofibroma	• **Site:** Often on the head/neck or trunk • Firm or rubbery nodule or infiltrative plaque • Skin-colored to red–purple • May be multiple *(see Fig. 20.4)*	• Biphasic with increased vascularity and spindle cells (myofibroblasts)
Infantile digital fibroma	• **Site:** Typically on the 2nd toe • Firm, pink nodule *(Fig. 20.5)*	• Elongated spindle cells with cytoplasmic pink inclusions
Hematologic processes		
Mastocytoma	• **History:** Intermittent blistering • Brown–pink to red papulonodule • Leathery surface *(Fig. 20.6)*	• Fried-egg-shaped cells with granular cytoplasm

*Not every case will have these features.

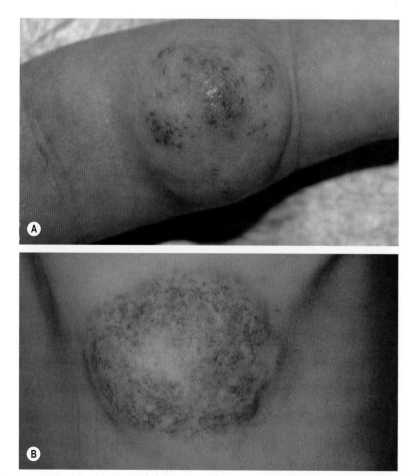

Fig. 20.2 Congenital hemangioma. A Rapidly involuting congenital hemangioma. **B** Non-involuting congenital hemangioma. These lesions are distinguished by clinical course. *From Eichenfield LF, Frieden IJ, Zaenglein AL, Mathes E. Neonatal and Infant Dermatology, 3e. London: Saunders, 2014.*

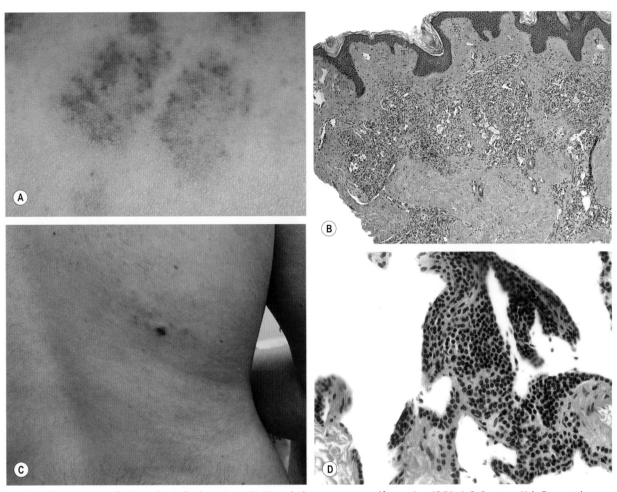

Fig. 20.3 Characteristic findings for tufted angioma (A,B) and glomuvenous malformation (C,D). *A,C, Courtesy, Yale Dermatology Residents' Slide Collection; D, Courtesy, Nemanja Rodic, MD, PhD.*

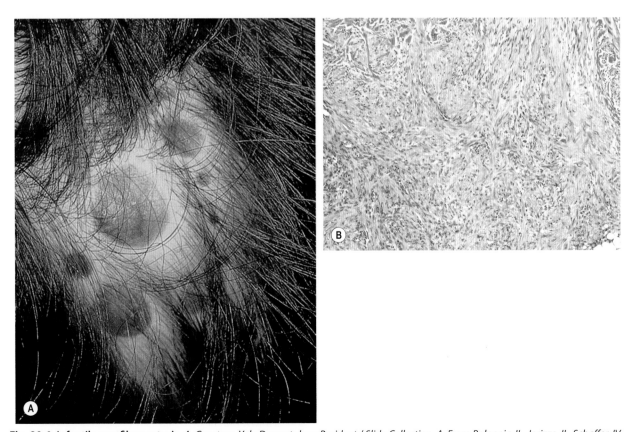

Fig. 20.4 Infantile myofibromatosis. *A, Courtesy, Yale Dermatology Residents' Slide Collection. A, From Bolognia JL, Jorizzo JL, Schaffer JV. Dermatology, 3e. London: Saunders, 2012, with permission.*

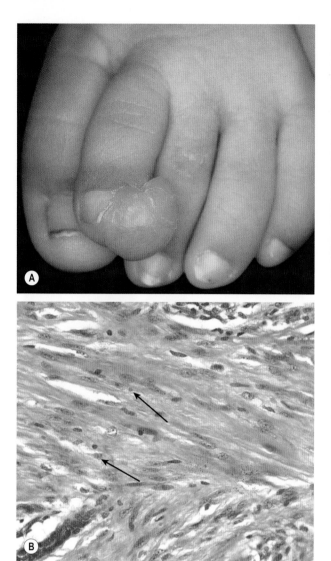

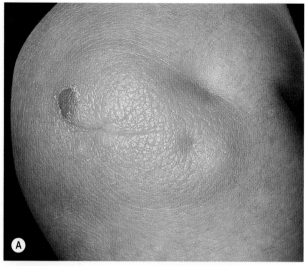

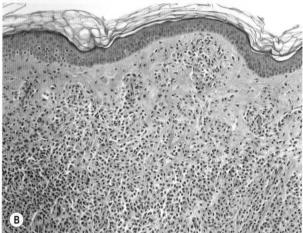

Fig. 20.5 Infantile digital fibroma. *A,Courtesy, Yale Dermatology Residents' Slide Collection. A, From Bolognia JL, Schaffer JV, Duncan KO, Ko CJ. Dermatology Essentials, 1e. Philadelphia: Saunders, 2014, with permission.*

Fig. 20.6 Mastocytoma. *Courtesy, Michael Tharp, MD. A, From Bolognia JL, Schaffer JV, Duncan KO, Ko CJ. Dermatology Essentials, 1e. Philadelphia: Saunders, 2014, with permission.*

Table 20.2 Characteristic papulonodules in children/adults

Entity	Classic morphologic clues*	Histopathology
Adnexal tumors		
Pilomatricoma *(Fig. 20.7)*	• Bluish tinge • Firm to hard plate-like papulonodule • Lesion will "teeter-totter" with pressure on one side or another	• Shadow cells within butterscotch-colored keratin
Apocrine hidrocystoma *(see Fig. 21.4)*	• **Site:** Eyelid • Bluish, translucent papule	• Cuboidal cells lining a lumen
Syringoma *(see Fig. 2.1D)*	• **Site:** Eyelids • Flesh-colored papules	• Tadpole-shaped epithelium with clear cells and ductal differentiation
Sebaceous hyperplasia *(see Fig. 2.1E)*	• **Site:** Face • Yellow papule with central dell	• Dilated follicular infundibulum surrounded by sebaceous glands
Vascular tumors		
Cherry angioma *(Fig. 20.8)*	• Bright red papule	• Clusters of dilated spaces lined by endothelial cells
Pyogenic granuloma *(Fig. 20.9)*	• **Site:** Predilection for head/neck, fingers • History of rapid growth • Eroded red papule, often pedunculated	• Polypoid • Lobules of small vessels
Hobnail hemangioma *(targetoid hemosiderotic hemangioma; Fig. 20.10)*	• 3-colored zones	• Dilated vessels superficially and centrally • Slit-like vessels deeper • Hemosiderin at periphery
Neural tumor		
Neurofibroma *(Fig. 20.11)*	• Soft, compressible pink papule	• Delicate spindle cells with pink stroma
Plexiform neurofibroma *(Fig. 20.12)*	• Bag-like mass with patchy hyperpigmentation	• Multiple separate cords of spindle cells with pink stroma
Fibrous tumors		
Fibrous papule *(Fig. 20.13)*	• **Site:** Commonly on the nose • Firm skin-colored to pink papule	• Dense pink collagen • Dilated vessels • Stellate fibroblasts
Dermatofibroma *(Fig. 20.14)*	• **Site:** Often on the lower legs • Various colors • Firm papule • Becomes slightly depressed with lateral pressure • **Dermoscopy:** delicate peripheral pseudonetwork	• Busy dermis filled with spindle cells • Collagen entrapment
Keloid *(Fig. 20.15)*	• **Site:** Favors the upper trunk/proximal arms • Firm dark pink papulonodule • May be in linear configurations	• Thickened "bubble-gum" collagen
Malignant tumors of epidermal origin		
Basal cell carcinoma, pigmented *(Fig. 20.16)*	• Translucent papule with globules of dark pigment	• Basaloid islands with brown pigment
Basal cell carcinoma, nodular *(Fig. 20.17)*	• Light pink translucent nodule • Telangiectasias	• Large basaloid islands
Squamous cell carcinoma *(Fig. 20.18)*	• Indurated nodule with overlying keratin	• Keratin overlying atypical islands of keratinocytes
Melanocytic tumors		
Blue nevus	• **Site:** Predilection for the hands/feet, but also the face, scalp and other sites • Blue–black papule • **Dermoscopy:** uniform blue–gray color	• Spindled, pigmented cells
Malignant melanoma, nodular *(Fig. 20.19)*	• Rapidly growing black nodule	• Large melanocytes in irregular nests
Lymphoma		
Patch/plaque-stage mycosis fungoides *(Fig. 20.20)*	• **Site:** Double-covered skin *(see Fig. 1.16B)* • Annular to solid deeply pink plaques • Wrinkled surface and dry scale	• Atypical lymphocytes within the epidermis and in a dermal band

*Not every case will have these features.

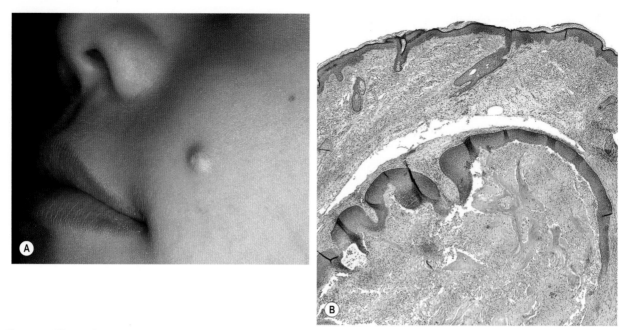

Fig. 20.7 Pilomatricoma. *A, Courtesy, Yale Dermatology Residents' Slide Collection. A, From Bolognia JL, Schaffer JV, Duncan KO, Ko CJ. Dermatology Essentials, 1e. Philadelphia: Saunders, 2014, with permission*

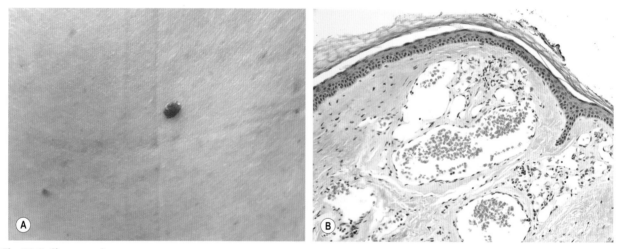

Fig. 20.8 Cherry angioma.

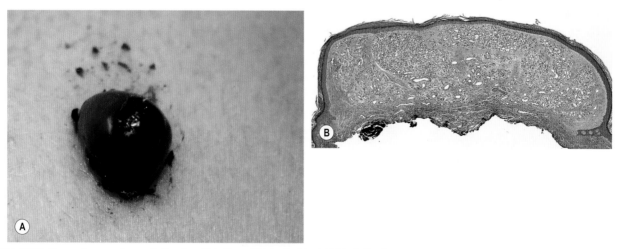

Fig. 20.9 Pyogenic granuloma. *A, Courtesy, Yale Dermatology Residents' Slide Collection.*

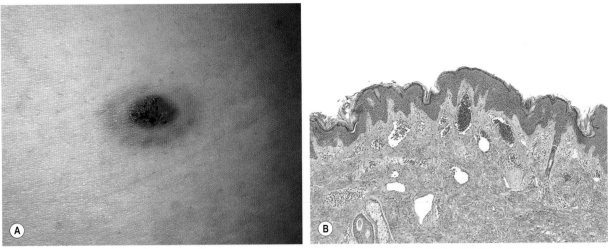

Fig. 20.10 **Hobnail hemangioma (targetoid hemosiderotic hemangioma).** *A, Courtesy, Ronald P Rapini, MD. A, From Bolognia JL, Jorizzo JL, Schaffer JV. Dermatology, 3e. London: Saunders, 2012, with permission.*

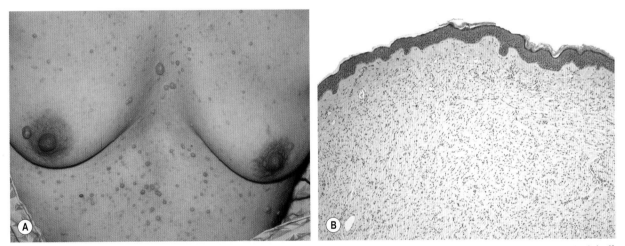

Fig. 20.11 **Neurofibromas in a patient with neurofibromatosis.** *A, Courtesy, Julie V Schaffer, MD. A, From Bolognia JL, Jorizzo JL, Schaffer JV. Dermatology, 3e. London: Saunders, 2012, with permission.*

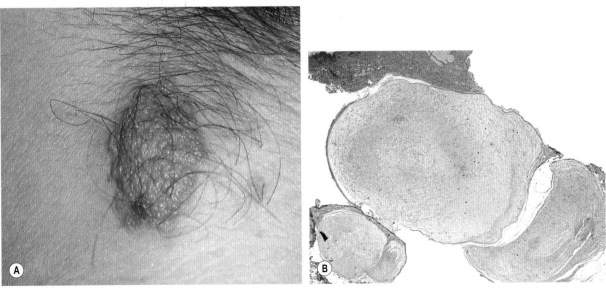

Fig. 20.12 **Plexiform neurofibroma.** *A, Courtesy, Yale Dermatology Residents' Slide Collection.*

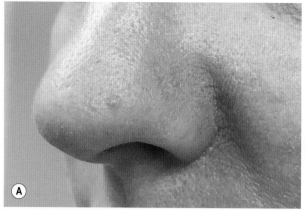

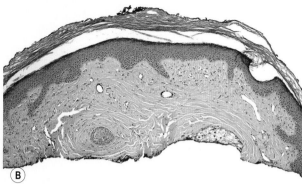

Fig. 20.13 Fibrous papule.

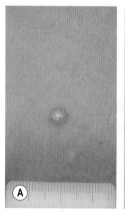

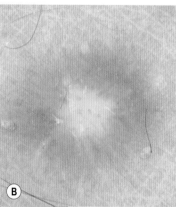

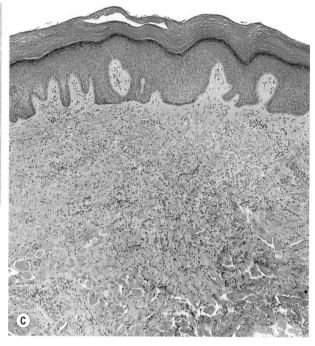

Fig. 20.14 **Dermatofibroma.** *A,B, Courtesy, Giuseppe Argenziano, MD, and Iris Zalaudek, MD. A, B, From Bolognia JL, Schaffer JV, Duncan KO, Ko CJ. Dermatology Essentials, 1e. Philadelphia: Saunders, 2014, with permission.*

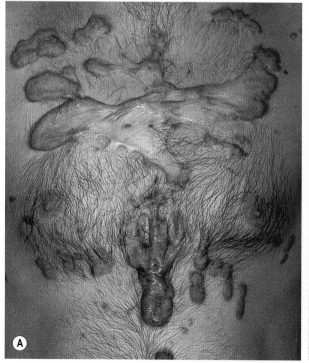

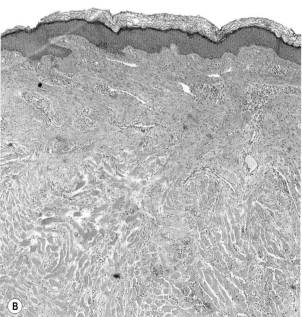

Fig. 20.15 **Keloid.** *A, Courtesy, Yale Dermatology Residents' Slide Collection. A, From Bolognia JL, Jorizzo JL, Schaffer JV. Dermatology, 3e. London: Saunders, 2012, with permission.*

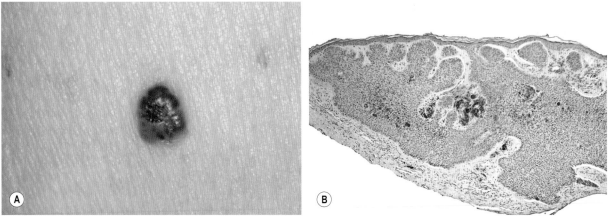

Fig. 20.16 Basal cell carcinoma, pigmented. *Courtesy, H. Peter Sawyer, MD. A, From Bolognia JL, Schaffer JV, Duncan KO, Ko CJ. Dermatology Essentials, 1e. Philadelphia: Saunders, 2014, with permission.*

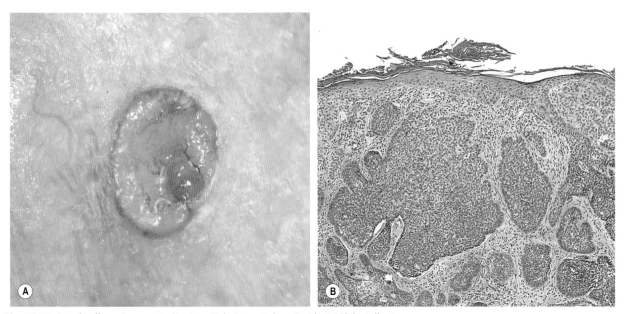

Fig. 20.17 Basal cell carcinoma. *A, Courtesy, Yale Dermatology Residents' Slide Collection.*

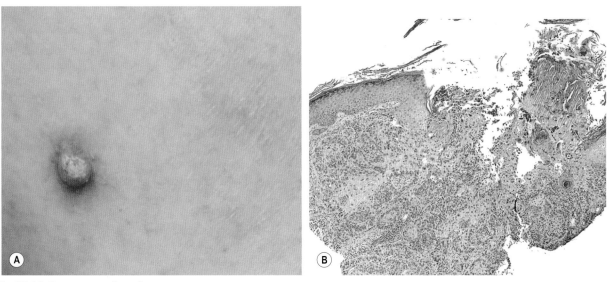

Fig. 20.18 Squamous cell carcinoma.

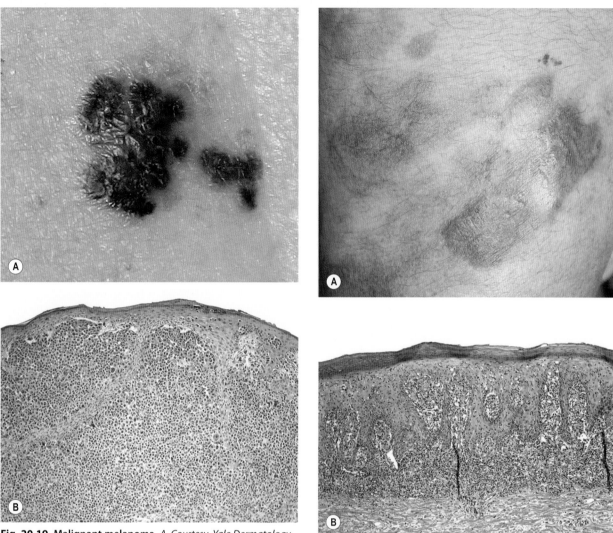

Fig. 20.19 Malignant melanoma. *A, Courtesy, Yale Dermatology Residents' Slide Collection.*

Fig. 20.20 Patch/plaque-stage mycosis fungoides. *A, Courtesy, Yale Dermatology Residents' Slide Collection.*

CONGENITAL/INFANTILE NODULES

Causes of congenital nodules include vascular tumors *(see Figs 20.1, 20.2, 20.3)* and malformations, solid tumors (e.g. myofibroma *[Fig. 20.4]*, rhabdomyosarcoma *[see Fig. 20.1B]*), hematologic processes (e.g. mastocytoma, leukemia cutis, dermal erythropoiesis), and developmental anomalies (see Chapter 21).

Dermal Cysts/Developmental Anomalies

21

Although the most common cyst, the epidermoid cyst, may be located anywhere, most cysts/tracts and developmental anomalies have characteristic locations *(Fig. 21.1)* and presentations *(Fig. 21.2 – distinctive punctum; Figs 21.3–21.8 – typical location)*. For midline lesions, the clinical presentation can be similar for different entities (i.e. dermoid cyst vs encephalocele), and imaging may be indicated. A combination of site and histopathology are useful for cysts located on the neck *(see Fig. 21.1B and Figs 21.9–21.11)*; other anomalies have characteristic clinical presentations *(Figs 21.12–21.15)*. Over the lumbosacral spine, clues for an underlying spinal defect include segmental hemangiomas, a deep dimple, a pseudotail, and/or a deviated gluteal cleft *(Figs 21.16–21.17)*.

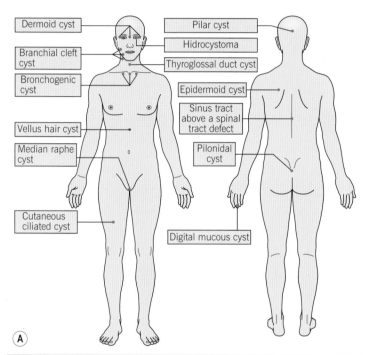

(A)

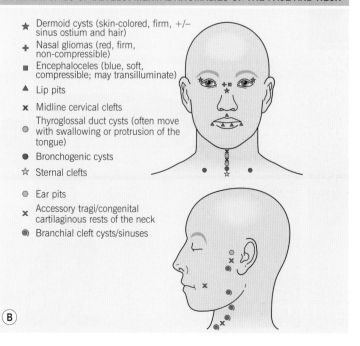

COMMON SITES OF DEVELOPMENTAL ANOMALIES OF THE FACE AND NECK

★ Dermoid cysts (skin-colored, firm, +/– sinus ostium and hair)

✚ Nasal gliomas (red, firm, non-compressible)

■ Encephaloceles (blue, soft, compressible; may transilluminate)

▲ Lip pits

✕ Midline cervical clefts

◦ Thyroglossal duct cysts (often move with swallowing or protrusion of the tongue)

● Bronchogenic cysts

☆ Sternal clefts

◦ Ear pits

✕ Accessory tragi/congenital cartilaginous rests of the neck

◉ Branchial cleft cysts/sinuses

(B)

Fig. 21.1 Common sites of cysts (A), and developmental anomalies of the face and neck (B). *B, From Bolognia JL, Jorizzo JL, Schaffer JV. Dermatology, 3e. London: Saunders, 2012, with permission.*

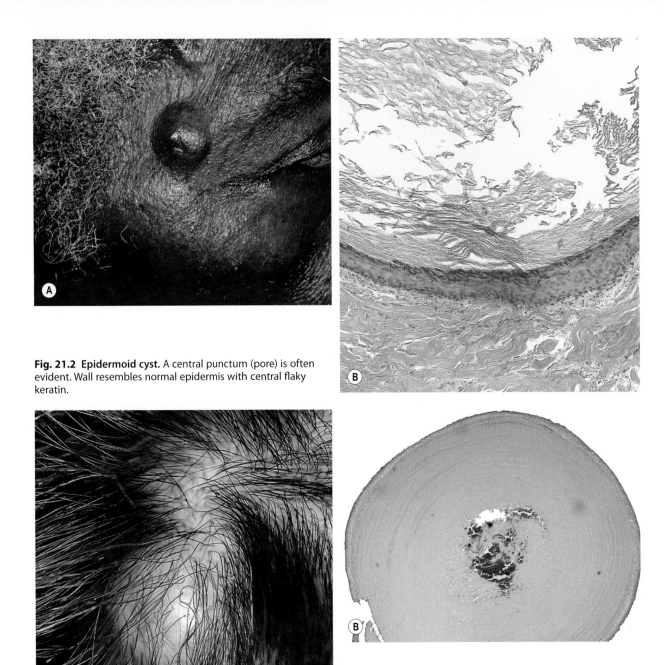

Fig. 21.2 Epidermoid cyst. A central punctum (pore) is often evident. Wall resembles normal epidermis with central flaky keratin.

Fig. 21.3 Pilar cyst. This cyst is most common on the scalp. Wall lacks a granular layer and surrounds dense keratin. *A, Courtesy, Mary Stone, MD. A, From Bolognia JL, Schaffer JV, Duncan KO, Ko CJ. Dermatology Essentials, 1e. Philadelphia: Saunders, 2014, with permission.*

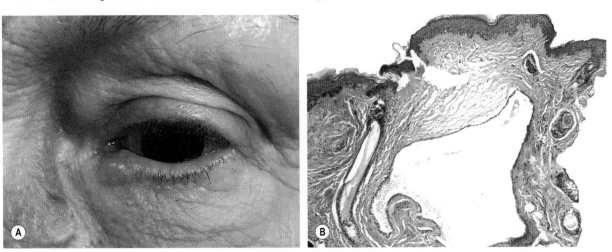

Fig. 21.4 Hidrocystoma. Translucent to blue papule, often on the eyelid margin. Double-layered epithelium with "snouts" on the cell surface at lumen.

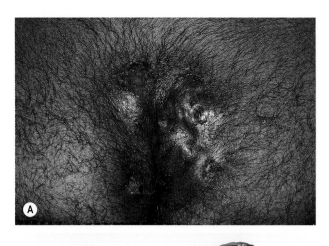

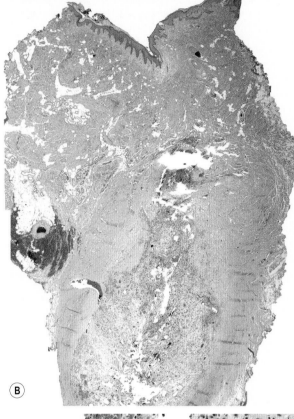

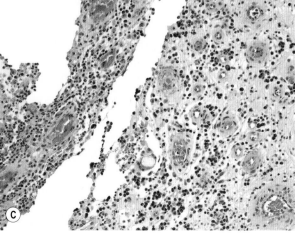

Fig. 21.5 Pilonidal sinus tracts. Biopsy findings include epithelial lined tracts (not shown), acute and chronic inflammation, and free hair shafts. The most common location is the sacral area. *Courtesy, Kalman Watsky, MD.*

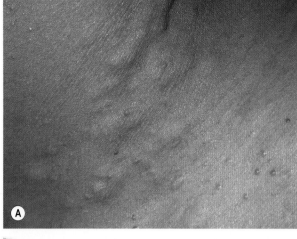

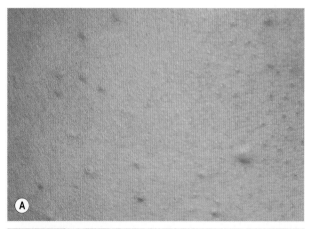

Fig. 21.6 Steatocystoma multiplex. This cyst can develop on any site; when multiple, lesions are typically larger than vellus hair cysts and present on the trunk. Wall with sebaceous glands and an inner rim that is bright pink and undulating. *A, Courtesy, Yale Dermatology Residents' Slide Collection.*

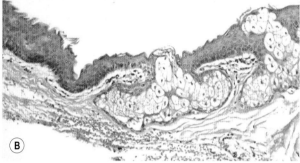

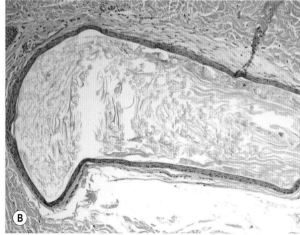

Fig. 21.7 Vellus hair cysts. Multiple lesions characteristically affect the trunk. *A, Courtesy, Yale Dermatology Residents' Slide Collection.*

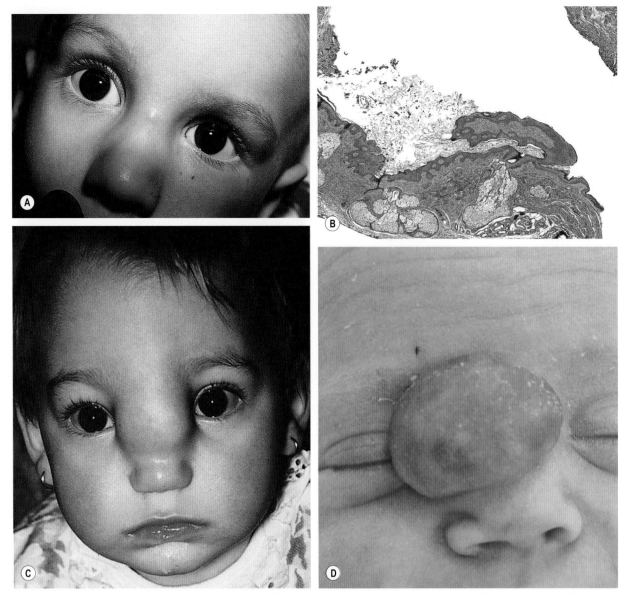

Fig. 21.8 Midline glabellar lesions. A,B Dermoid cyst. Wall contains adnexal structures. **C** Frontal encephalocele. **D** Nasal glioma. *C, Courtesy, Odile Enjolras, MD; D, Courtesy, Mary Chang, MD. A,C, From Schachner LA, Hansen RE. Pediatric Dermatology, 4e. London: Mosby, 2011, with permission. D, From Bolognia JL, Schaffer JV, Duncan KO, Ko CJ. Dermatology Essentials, 1e. Philadelphia: Saunders, 2014, with permission.*

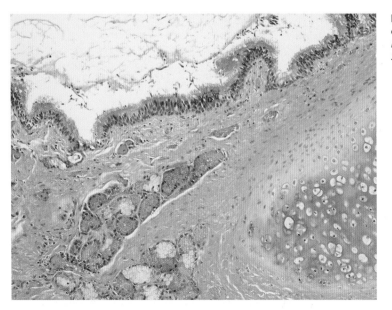

Fig. 21.9 Bronchogenic cyst. Wall is columnar; cartilage often present. *From Husain A. Thoracic Pathology. High Yield Pathology series. Philadelphia: Saunders, 2012.*

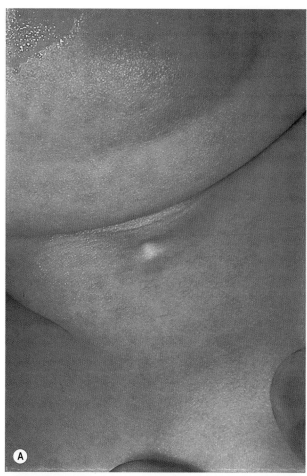

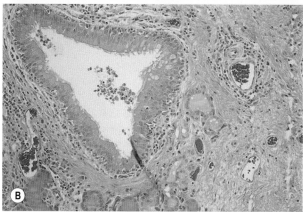

Fig. 21.10 Thyroglossal duct cyst. Wall with thyroid follicles. *B, Courtesy, Mary Stone, MD. A, From Schachner LA, Hansen RE. Pediatric Dermatology, 4e. London: Mosby, 2011. B, From Bolognia JL, Jorizzo JL, Schaffer JV. Dermatology, 3e. London: Saunders, 2012, with permission.*

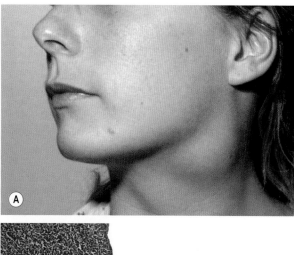

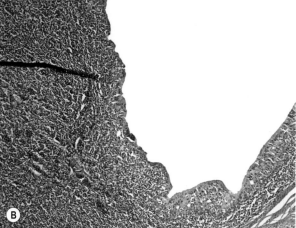

Fig. 21.11 Branchial cleft cyst. Columnar epithelium with dense inflammation. *A, From Myers EN. Operative Otolaryngology: Head and Neck Surgery, 2e. Philadelphia: Saunders, 2008.*

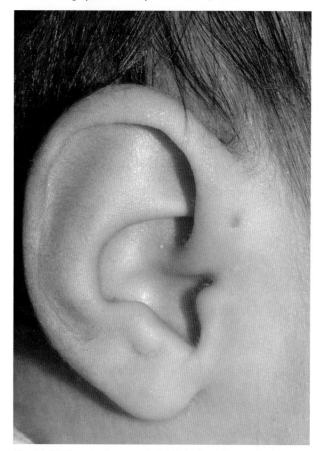

Fig. 21.12 Ear pit. *Courtesy, Julie V Schaffer, MD. From Bolognia JL, Jorizzo JL, Schaffer JV. Dermatology, 3e. London: Saunders, 2012, with permission.*

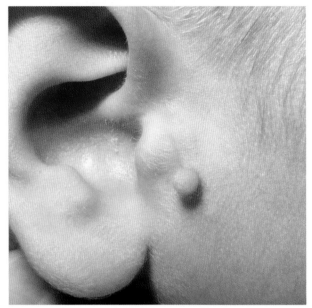

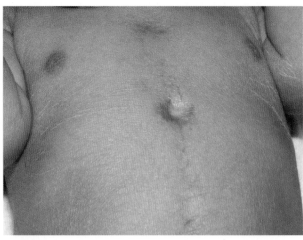

Fig. 21.15 Sternal cleft. *Courtesy, Julie V Schaffer, MD. From Bolognia JL, Jorizzo JL, Schaffer JV. Dermatology, 3e. London: Saunders, 2012, with permission.*

Fig. 21.13 Accessory tragus. *Courtesy, Antonio Torrelo, MD. From Schachner LA, Hansen RE. Pediatric Dermatology, 4e. London: Mosby, 2011.*

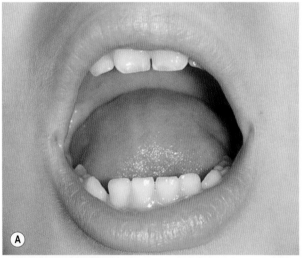

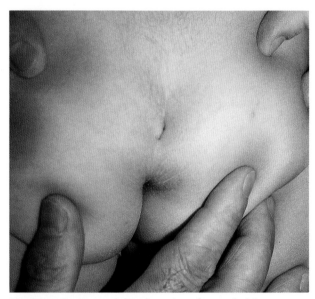

Fig. 21.16 Deep sacral dimple, a sign of an underlying myelomeningocele. *Courtesy, Seth J Orlow, MD, PhD. From Bolognia JL, Jorizzo JL, Schaffer JV. Dermatology, 3e. London: Saunders, 2012, with permission.*

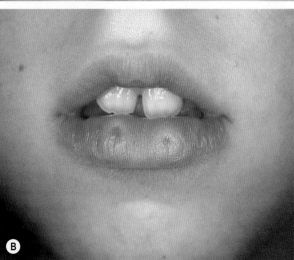

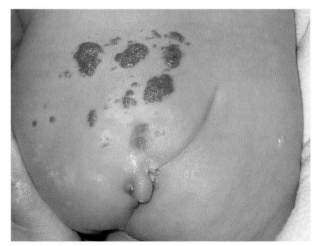

Fig. 21.14 Lip pit. *A, Courtesy NYU. B, Courtesy, Richard Antaya, MD and Julie V Schaffer, MD. A,B, From Bolognia JL, Jorizzo JL, Schaffer JV. Dermatology, 3e. London: Saunders, 2012, with permission.*

Fig. 21.17 Multiple midline cutaneous stigmata overlying a lipomeningomyelocele. *Courtesy, Richard Antaya, MD. From Bolognia JL, Jorizzo JL, Schaffer JV. Dermatology, 3e. London: Saunders, 2012, with permission.*

Dermal Change Due to Deposition 22

Certain materials, when deposited in the dermis, have a characteristic clinical presentation, with particular histopathologic findings. Mucin deposition can be seen in a variety of different disorders with a more variable clinical presentation. Deposition may manifest as a broad, textural change or as papulonodules.

BROAD, TEXTURAL CHANGE

Macular/Lichen/Biphasic Amyloidosis

Site:
Predilection for the upper back (macular amyloidosis) and shins (lichen amyloidosis)
Rippled, hyperpigmented plaques composed of linear arrays of monomorphous papules *(Figs 22.1, 22.2)*

Histopathology:
Light pink, smooth deposits in the papillary dermis, often with associated pigment incontinence; deposits are larger and associated with epidermal hyperplasia in lichen amyloidosis
Deposits stain with cytokeratins

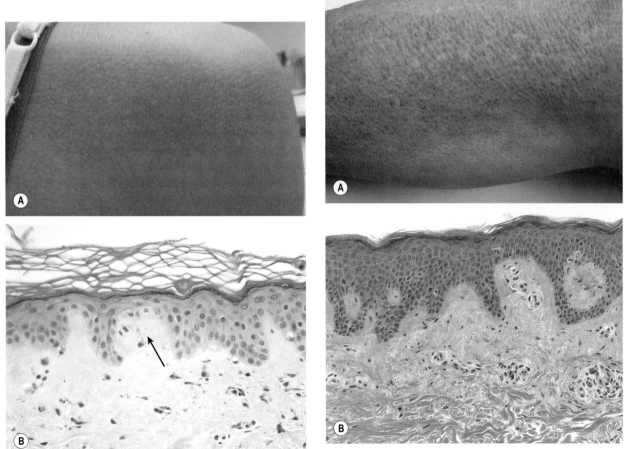

Fig. 22.1 Macular amyloidosis.

Fig. 22.2 Lichen amyloidosis. *A, Courtesy, Sean Christensen, MD PhD.*

Pretibial Myxedema *(Fig. 22.3)*

Pink plaque(s) that are nodular in later stages, especially on the lower extremity

Histopathology:
Mucin throughout the reticular dermis

Adult Colloid Milium *(Fig. 22.4)*

Brown to yellow translucent papules, especially on chronically sun-damaged skin of the face and/or hands but other sites may be affected

Histopathology:
Nodules of pink, fissured material

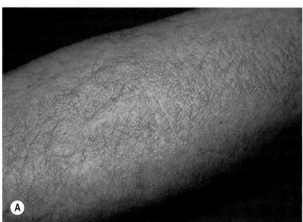

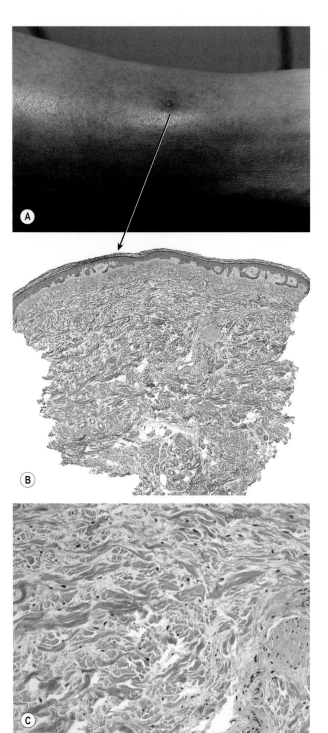

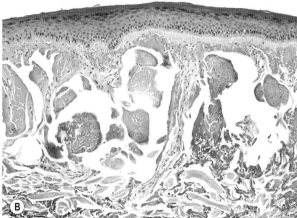

Fig. 22.4 Colloid milium. *A, From Lewis AT, Le EH, Quan LT, et al. Unilateral colloid milium of the arm. J Am Acad Dermatol. 2002;46:S5–7, © Elsevier.*

Fig. 22.3 Pretibial myxedema. A shows an early lesion of indurated erythema with a biopsy site. *A, Courtesy, Kalman Watsky, MD.*

Lipoid Proteinosis *(Fig. 22.5)*

Genodermatosis with mutations in *ECM1*
Waxy papules and plaques on extensor surfaces and face with scarring

Histopathology:
Pink dermal material, sometimes with a vertical orientation in the upper dermis; material may be accentuated around adnexal structures

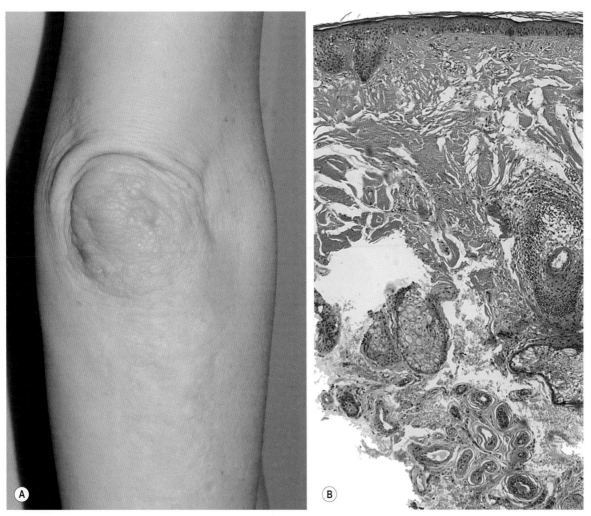

Fig. 22.5 Lipoid proteinosis. *A, Courtesy, Julie V Schaffer, MD. A, From Bolognia JL, Jorizzo JL, Schaffer JV. Dermatology, 3e. London: Saunders, 2012, with permission.*

Erythropoietic Protoporphyria *(Fig. 22.6)*

Genodermatosis, mutation in ferrochelatase
Sun-exposed skin is affected, especially the nose, cheeks, and dorsal hands
Erythema, erosions, waxy scarring

Histopathology:
Pink dermal material around vessels (early lesions) and/or filling the upper dermis (later lesions)

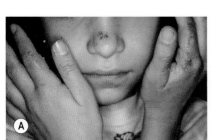 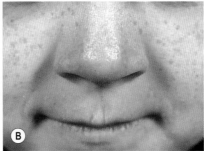 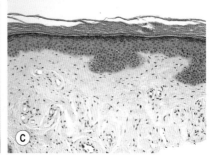

Fig. 22.6 Erythropoietic protoporphyria. *A, Courtesy, Yale Dermatology Residents' Slide Collection. B, Courtesy, Gillian Murphy, MD. From Bolognia JL, Jorizzo JL, Schaffer JV. Dermatology, 3e. London: Saunders, 2012, with permission.*

PAPULONODULES

Nodular Amyloidosis *(Fig. 22.7)*

Variably sized pink–orange papulonodule(s)

Histopathology:
Light pink material filling the dermis, interspersed plasma cells may be evident

Systemic Amyloidosis *(Fig. 22.8)*

Multiorgan disorder (e.g. kidneys, gastrointestinal tract, heart) with deposition of AL protein (immunoglobulin light chain fragment)

Enlargement of the tongue
Waxy papules/plaques, commonly on the face
Periorbital purpura

Histopathology:
Perivascular light pink, smooth deposits; apple-green birefringence with polarization

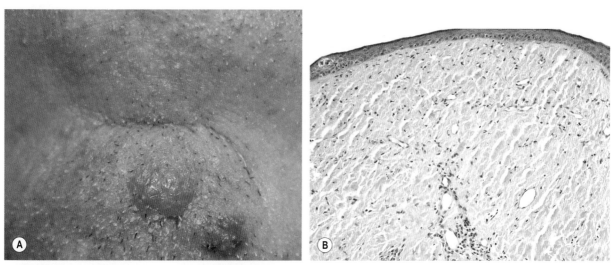

Fig. 22.7 Nodular amyloidosis. *A, Courtesy, Yale Dermatology Residents' Slide Collection.*

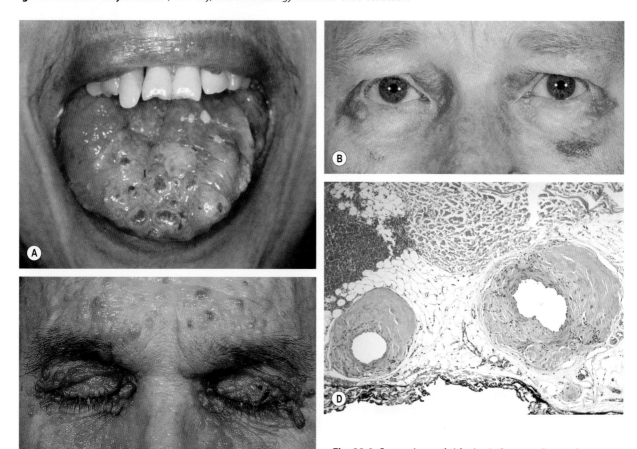

Fig. 22.8 Systemic amyloidosis. *A, Courtesy, Dennis Cooper, MD; B, Courtesy, M Joyce Rico, MD; C, Courtesy, Jean L Bolognia, MD. A–C, From Bolognia JL, Jorizzo JL, Schaffer JV. Dermatology, 3e. London: Saunders, 2012, with permission.*

Osteoma Cutis

May be a manifestation of a genodermatosis

Miliary type:

Multiple, small skin-colored to blue papules – often on the face *(Fig. 22.9)*

Histopathology:
Dense pink material with small lacunae containing nuclei

Chronic Tophaceous Gout *(Fig. 22.10)*

Predilection for the ear or periarticular foci
Firm dermal/subcutaneous, variably colored papulonodules

Histopathology:
Needle-like or feathery spaces within light blue–pink material surrounded by histiocytes

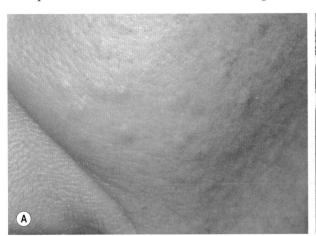

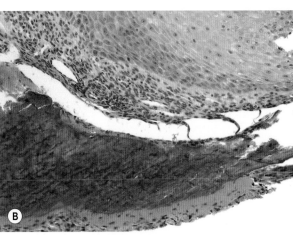

Fig. 22.9 **Osteoma cutis.** *A, Courtesy, Yale Dermatology Residents' Slide Collection. A, From Bolognia JL, Jorizzo JL, Schaffer JV. Dermatology, 3e. London: Saunders, 2012, with permission.*

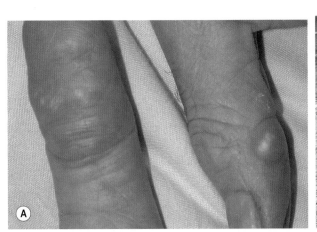

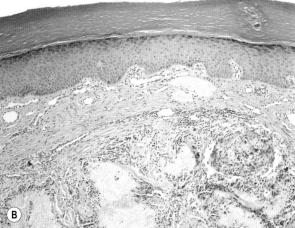

Fig. 22.10 **Gout.** Tophi on the digits. *A, Courtesy, Yale Dermatology Residents' Slide Collection.*

Calcinosis Cutis *(Fig. 22.11)*

Calcification can be the sequelae of a tissue injury
Calcium deposits in the skin are associated with limited systemic sclerosis and dermatomyositis

Histopathology:
Bluish, chunky (sometimes granular) material

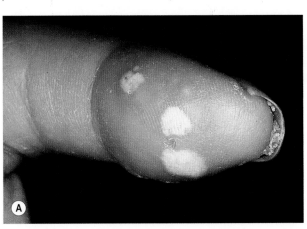

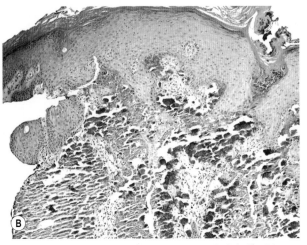

Fig. 22.11 **Calcinosis cutis.** *A, Courtesy, Yale Dermatology Residents' Slide Collection. A, Courtesy, Bolognia JL, Jorizzo JL, Schaffer JV. Dermatology, 3e. London: Saunders, 2012, with permission.*

Eruptive Xanthoma *(Fig. 22.12)*

Associated with high lipid levels, uncontrolled diabetes mellitus, and thyroid disorders
Favors the extensor surfaces, especially the buttocks/thighs

Red to yellow papules

Histopathology:
Intra- and extracellular lipid

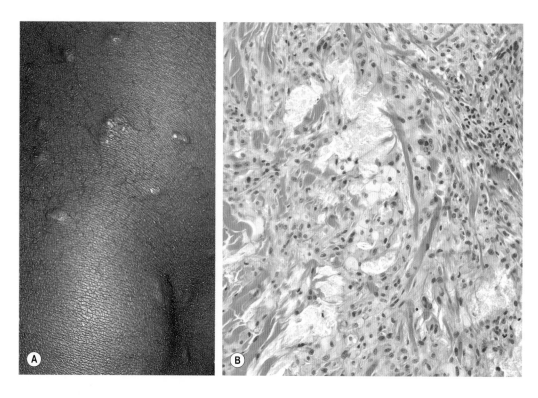

Fig. 22.12 Eruptive xanthomas.
A, Courtesy, Yale Dermatology Residents' Slide Collection.

Xanthelasma *(Fig. 22.13)*

Yellowish papules and plaques on the eyelids

Histopathology:
Foamy cells in the dermis; typical features of eyelid with thin epidermis and vellus hairs

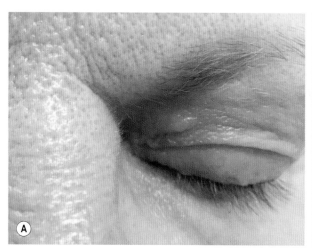
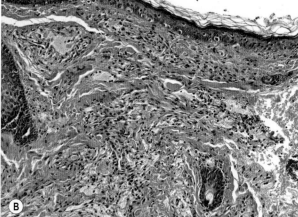

Fig. 22.13 Xanthelasma.

Digital Myxoid Cyst *(Fig. 22.14)*

Near a joint space of the finger
Bluish to skin-colored slightly translucent papulonodule

Histopathology:
No epithelial lining (not a true cyst), increased dermal mucin, keratin typical of an acral site (stratum lucidum)

Focal Cutaneous Mucinosis *(Fig. 22.15)*

Localized flesh-colored to pink papule

Histopathology:
Mucin in the dermis

Follicular Mucinosis *(see Fig. 9.11)*
Erythema Elevatum Diutinum, Late Stage *(Fig. 22.16)*

Symmetric, on extensor surfaces
Red–brown to purplish, soft to firm papulonodules
Associated with HIV infection

Histopathology:
Fibrosis with or without vasculitis, intracellular lipid ("extracellular cholesterolosis")

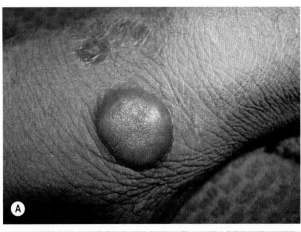

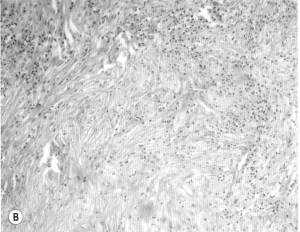

Fig. 22.16 Erythema elevatum diutinum, late stage.
A, Courtesy, Rachel Moore, MD. A, From Bolognia JL, Jorizzo JL, Schaffer JV. Dermatology, 3e. London: Saunders, 2012, with permission.

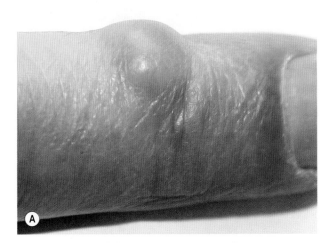

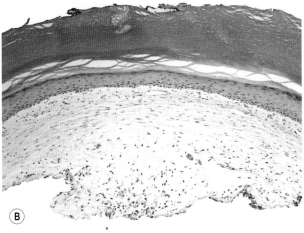

Fig. 22.14 Digital myxoid cyst with mucin in the dermis.
A, Courtesy, Yale Dermatology Residents' Slide Collection.

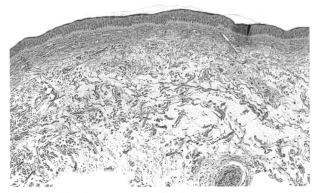

Fig. 22.15 Focal cutaneous mucinosis.

Deep Soft Tissue Disorders: Panniculitis and Others | 23

This chapter addresses disorders that primarily affect tissue below the dermis *(Table 23.1; Figs 23.1–23.4)*.

Inflammation may affect the fat and/or fascia *(Fig. 23.3)*.

Table 23.1 Common panniculitides			
Entity	**Clinical**		**Histopathology**
	Site *(Fig. 23.1)*	**Morphology**	
Erythema nodosum	• Especially on shins • Also thighs, forearms	• Bilateral, tender erythematous nodules *(Fig. 23.2A)*	• Septal fibrosis (blue arrow) and inflammation (orange arrow) *(Fig. 23.2B)*
Erythema induratum	• Posterior lower legs	• Erythematous nodules • May ulcerate *(Fig. 23.2C)*	• Lobular panniculitis with mixed inflammation, sometimes granulomatous, +/– vasculitis *(Fig. 23.2D)*
Lipodermatosclerosis	• Favors the lower medial legs	• Indurated pink to red–brown plaques *(Fig. 23.2E,F)*	• Lipomembranous change within fat lobules *(Fig. 23.2G)*
Lupus panniculitis	• Proximal extremities/hips • Upper trunk/face	• May have overlying changes of discoid lupus and/or skin may be tethered down *(Fig. 23.2H)*	• Hyaline necrosis of fat with lymphoid follicles (blue arrow) *(Fig. 23.2I)*

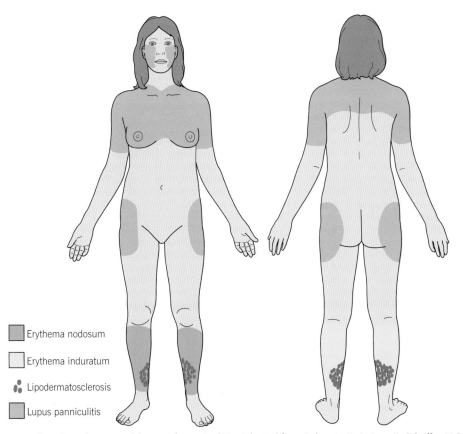

- Erythema nodosum
- Erythema induratum
- Lipodermatosclerosis
- Lupus panniculitis

Fig. 23.1 Most common locations for several forms of panniculitis. *Adapted from Bolognia JL, Jorizzo JL, Schaffer JV. Dermatology, 3e. London: Saunders, 2012, with permission.*

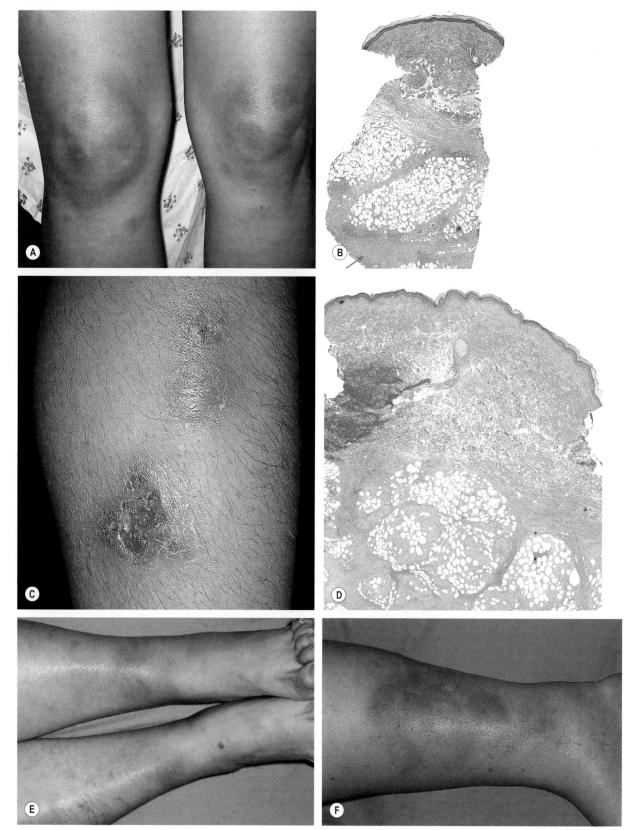

Fig. 23.2 Common forms of panniculitis. A,B Erythema nodosum. **C,D** Erythema induratum. **E–G** Lipodermatosclerosis.

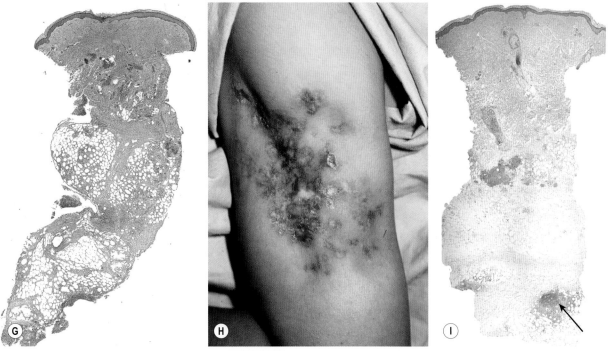

Fig. 23.2, cont'd H,I Lupus panniculitis. *A, Courtesy, Yale Dermatology Residents' Slide Collection. C,F,H, Courtesy, Kenneth E Greer, MD. E, Courtesy, James Patterson, MD. C,E,F,H, From Bolognia JL, Jorizzo JL, Schaffer JV. Dermatology, 3e. London: Saunders, 2012, with permission.*

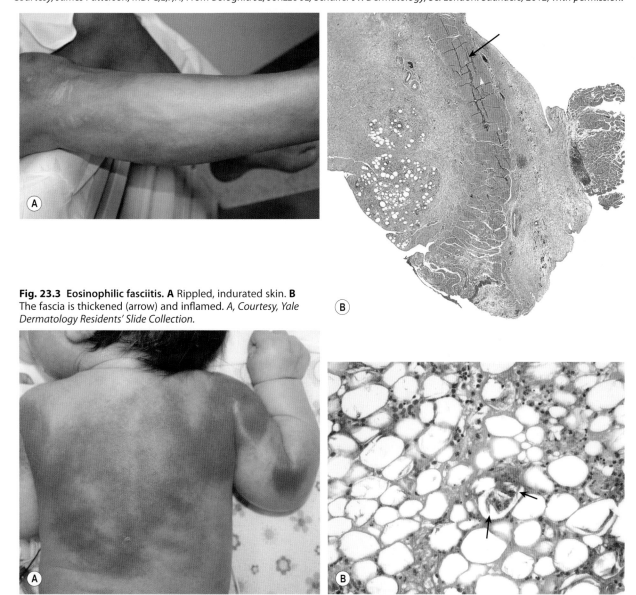

Fig. 23.3 Eosinophilic fasciitis. A Rippled, indurated skin. **B** The fascia is thickened (arrow) and inflamed. *A, Courtesy, Yale Dermatology Residents' Slide Collection.*

Fig. 23.4 Subcutaneous fat necrosis of the newborn. Erythematous, indurated plaques with inflammation and crystals (arrows) in the fat. *A, Courtesy, Yale Dermatology Residents' Slide Collection.*

Case Reviews | 24

The focus of this chapter is to build on the major aims of this atlas – 1) visually analyzing something you may have never seen before, and 2) teaching the brain to "see" in a more educated manner, thus enhancing observational skills. The following brief case reviews are of presentations that may be classic, rare, or visually similar to another entity. Careful observation of clinical and histopathologic findings, as well as the course of the disease, led to a working diagnosis on which to base management.

For a given patient, many of the principles and concepts in previous chapters come into consideration *(Table 24.1)*, and this will happen seamlessly and automatically with greater experience. The process may be primarily epidermal or dermal, and the inflammatory cell type may be predictable from the clinical appearance. Importantly, while not stressed in other chapters, in some situations, the clinical history and course are key elements.

Table 24.1 Clinical principles and concepts to consider when evaluating a case

History *(i.e. acute vs. chronic; past medical history; medications; recent procedures)*

Distribution *(i.e. generalized, intertriginous)*

Pattern *(i.e. annular, linear)*

Where is the action? *(i.e. epidermal, dermal)* Is there scale?

Is it inflamed? If so, the predominant cell type? *(i.e. lymphocytic, neutrophilic, granulomatous)*

Associated clues *(i.e. nail changes, oral lesions)*

Pertinent negatives

Course of disease

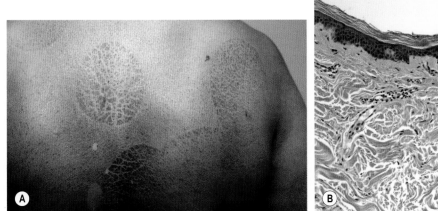
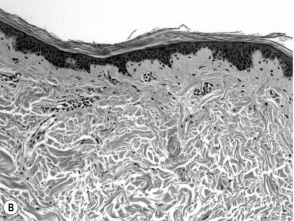

Fig. 24.1 Pityriasis rotunda. 63-year-old female with thyroid storm secondary to amiodarone, treated with thyroidectomy. There are circular thin plaques of scale on the back. Biopsy findings include epidermal changes (slight hyperkeratosis and focal hypogranulosis) and minimal inflammation. The lesions spontaneously resolved. *A, Courtesy, Brittany Craiglow and Leon Luck.*

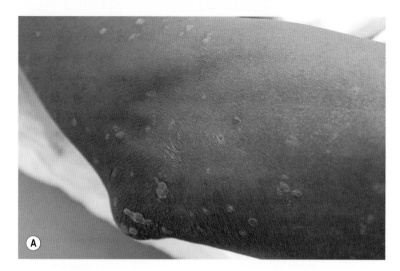

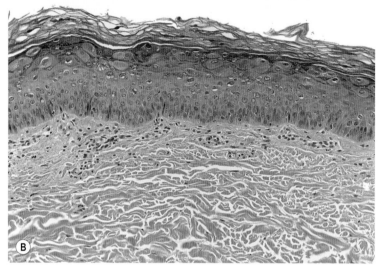

Fig. 24.2 Epidermodysplasia verruciformis. This HIV-negative male developed hypopigmented, flat-topped papules on the extremities in early adulthood. Clinically, the changes appear to be in the epidermis, and this corresponds to the biopsy findings of hyperkeratosis and altered cells (keratinocytes with expanded light pink–purple cytoplasm) in the granular layer. *A,B, Courtesy, Yale Dermatology Residents' Slide Collection.*

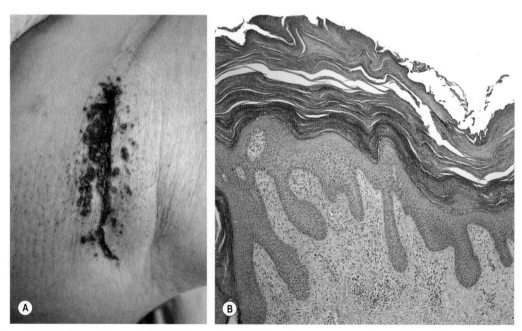

Fig. 24.3 Axillary granular parakeratosis. Keratotic papules, centrally confluent, correspond to epidermal hyperplasia with prominent hyperkeratosis. The stratum corneum contains retained keratohyaline granules. *A,B, Courtesy, Yale Dermatology Residents' Slide Collection.*

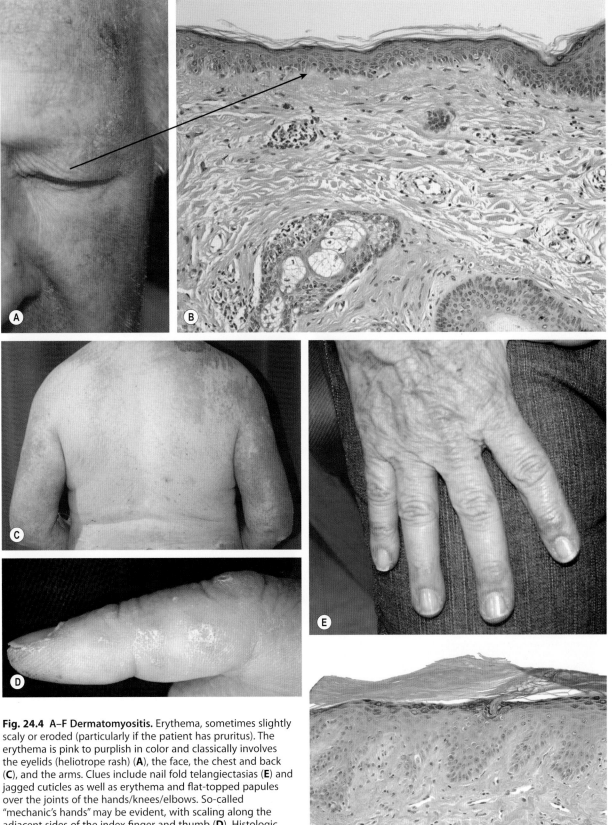

Fig. 24.4 A–F Dermatomyositis. Erythema, sometimes slightly scaly or eroded (particularly if the patient has pruritus). The erythema is pink to purplish in color and classically involves the eyelids (heliotrope rash) (**A**), the face, the chest and back (**C**), and the arms. Clues include nail fold telangiectasias (**E**) and jagged cuticles as well as erythema and flat-topped papules over the joints of the hands/knees/elbows. So-called "mechanic's hands" may be evident, with scaling along the adjacent sides of the index finger and thumb (**D**). Histologic findings include subtle interface vacuolar change, often with minimal inflammation (**B,F**). *A,C,D,E, Courtesy, Yale Dermatology Residents' Slide Collection.*

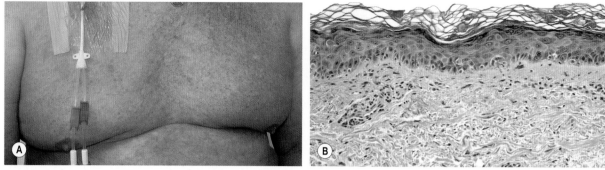

Fig. 24.5 Acute graft-versus-host disease. The clinical findings alone are non-specific and can closely simulate a maculopapular drug eruption. Clues include gastrointestinal symptoms/signs (i.e. diarrhea, liver function abnormalities). Classic histopathologic findings include interface vacuolar change with necrotic keratinocytes, sometimes extending into follicular epithelium. *A, Courtesy, Yale Dermatology Residents' Slide Collection.*

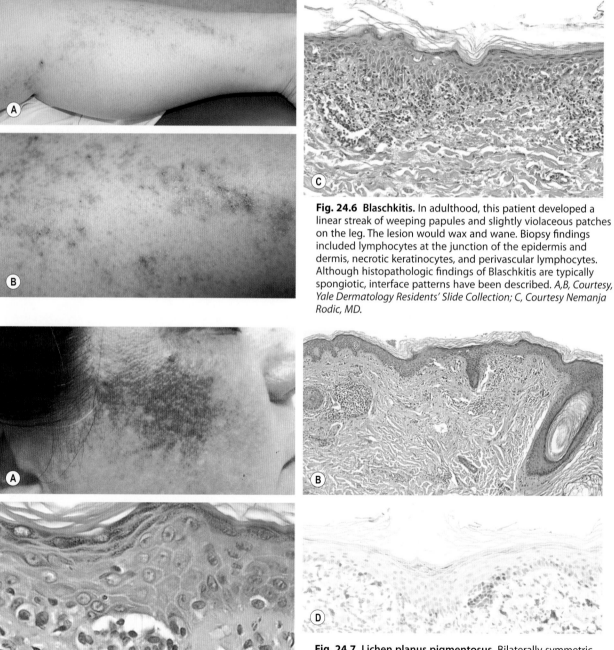

Fig. 24.6 Blaschkitis. In adulthood, this patient developed a linear streak of weeping papules and slightly violaceous patches on the leg. The lesion would wax and wane. Biopsy findings included lymphocytes at the junction of the epidermis and dermis, necrotic keratinocytes, and perivascular lymphocytes. Although histopathologic findings of Blaschkitis are typically spongiotic, interface patterns have been described. *A,B, Courtesy, Yale Dermatology Residents' Slide Collection; C, Courtesy Nemanja Rodic, MD.*

Fig. 24.7 Lichen planus pigmentosus. Bilaterally symmetric hyperpigmented patches on the cheeks (**A**). Biopsy findings alone have some resemblance to melanoma in situ (**B**), with small cells clustered in nests and arranged singly at the dermal–epidermal junction (**C**). Some of these cells are positive with MITF (**D**), but correlation with the clinical findings avoids misdiagnosis as a melanocytic process.

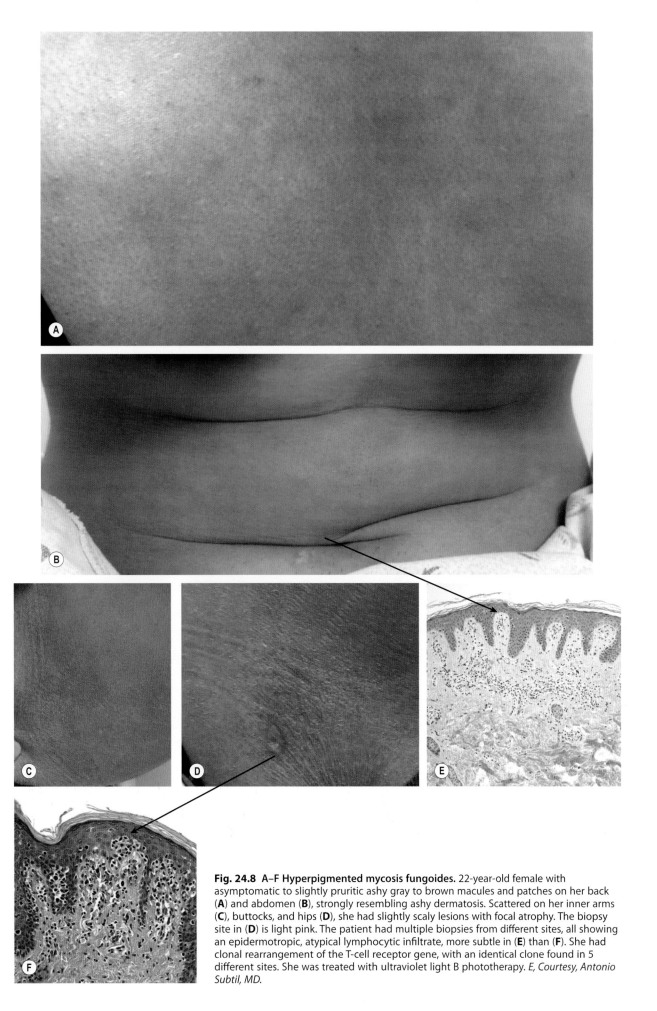

Fig. 24.8 A–F Hyperpigmented mycosis fungoides. 22-year-old female with asymptomatic to slightly pruritic ashy gray to brown macules and patches on her back (**A**) and abdomen (**B**), strongly resembling ashy dermatosis. Scattered on her inner arms (**C**), buttocks, and hips (**D**), she had slightly scaly lesions with focal atrophy. The biopsy site in (**D**) is light pink. The patient had multiple biopsies from different sites, all showing an epidermotropic, atypical lymphocytic infiltrate, more subtle in (**E**) than (**F**). She had clonal rearrangement of the T-cell receptor gene, with an identical clone found in 5 different sites. She was treated with ultraviolet light B phototherapy. *E, Courtesy, Antonio Subtil, MD.*

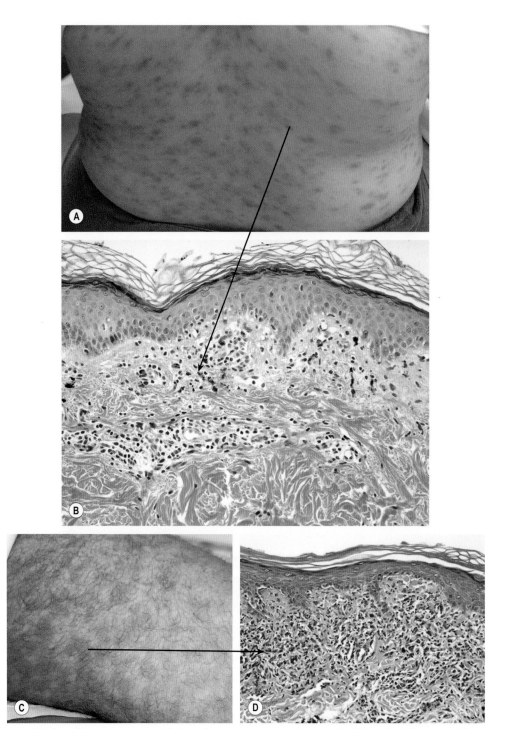

Fig. 24.9 Erythema dyschromicum perstans and lichen planus pigmentosus (inversus). Although erythema dyschromicum perstans (**A,B**) may have a thin pink border to the gray–brown oval lesions, as in this patient, such a border is more typically absent. The lesions often involve the trunk and upper arms and can be arranged in a distribution similar to pityriasis rosea. Lichen planus pigmentosus (**C,D**) is more brown in color, may involve intertriginous sites (so-called inversus, as in this patient with inner thigh lesions) and/or the face and neck, and may be associated with typical flat-topped, purplish lesions of lichen planus. Erythema dyschromicum perstans is typically less inflamed than lichen planus pigmentosus, with interface change and pigment incontinence (**C**). While lichen planus pigmentosus sometimes shows only pigment incontinence, this example shows lichenoid inflammation as well (**D**).

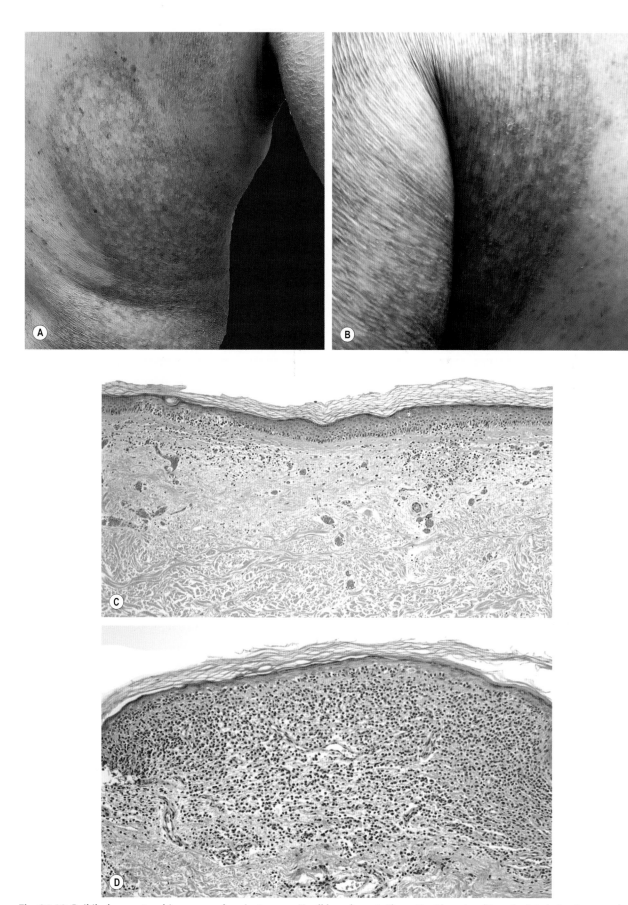

Fig. 24.10 Poikiloderma atrophicans vasculare (cutaneous T-cell lymphoma). The patient has atrophic, reticulated, dyspigmented patches over his flanks (**A**) and the inner arms (**B**). An initial biopsy was suggestive, but not fully diagnostic, of the diagnosis, with epidermal atrophy, patchy lymphocytic inflammation, and dilated vessels (**C**). A second biopsy was taken due to high clinical suspicion and showed a dense lymphocytic infiltrate, with epidermotropic CD4+, CD5−, CD7− cells (**D**). *A,B, Courtesy, Jeffrey Alter, MD and Antonio Subtil, MD.*

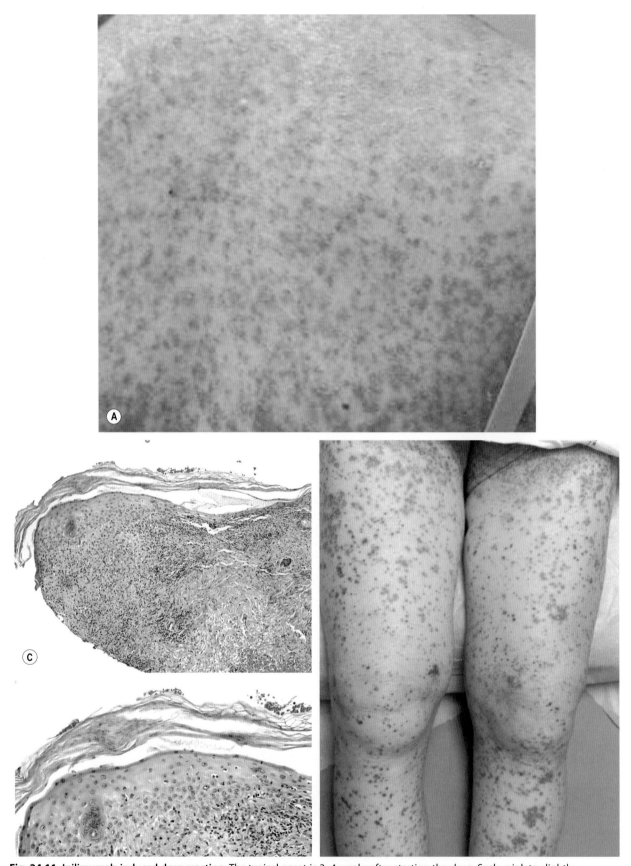

Fig. 24.11 Ipilimumab-induced drug reaction. The typical onset is 3–4 weeks after starting the drug. Scaly, pink to slightly violaceous, eroded papules, becoming confluent in some areas (**A,B**) over the back and the extremities. Parakeratosis, interface change, and dermal lymphocytic inflammation (**C,D**). *A,B, Courtesy, Jennifer N Choi, MD.*

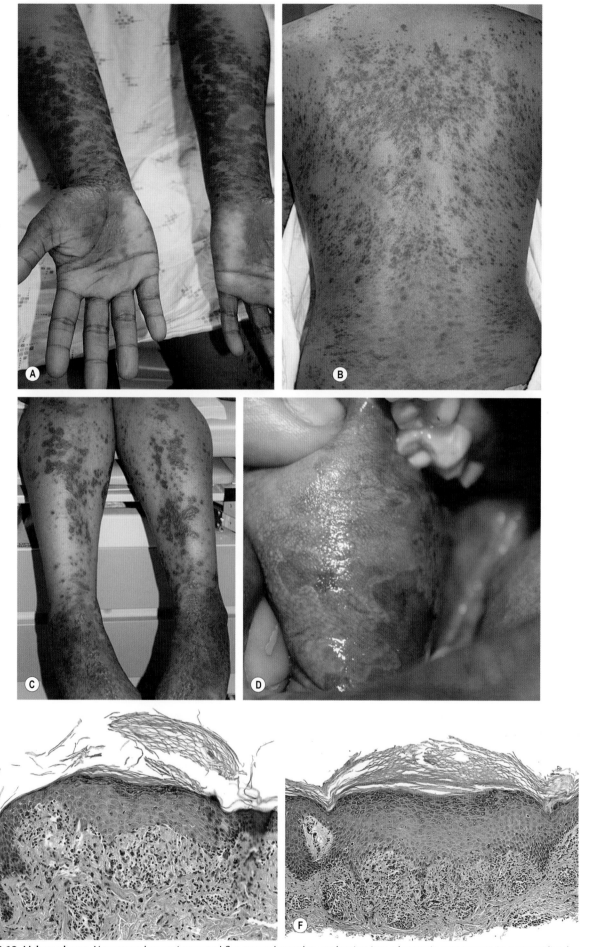

Fig. 24.12 Lichen planus. Numerous hyperpigmented flat-topped papules, coalescing into plaques in some areas, in a generalized distribution. A clue to the diagnosis includes lacy, focally eroded plaques on the buccal mucosa. Biopsy findings from the shoulder (**E**) and wrist (**F**) showed similar features, with hyperkeratosis, hypergranulosis, lichenoid inflammation, and pigment incontinence. *A–F, Courtesy, Yale Dermatology Residents' Slide Collection.*

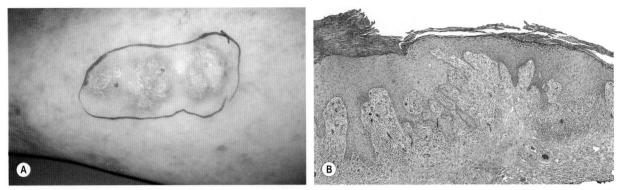

Fig. 24.13 Hypertrophic lichen planus. Individual lesions of hypertrophic lichen planus can mimic squamous cell carcinoma clinically and histopathologically; lesions have a predilection for the lower extremities. Clinical clues include multiple lesions and Wickham's striae (**A**). Biopsy clues include hypergranulosis and lichenoid inflammation accentuated at the tips of elongated rete (**B**). *A, Courtesy, Yale Dermatology Residents' Slide Collection.*

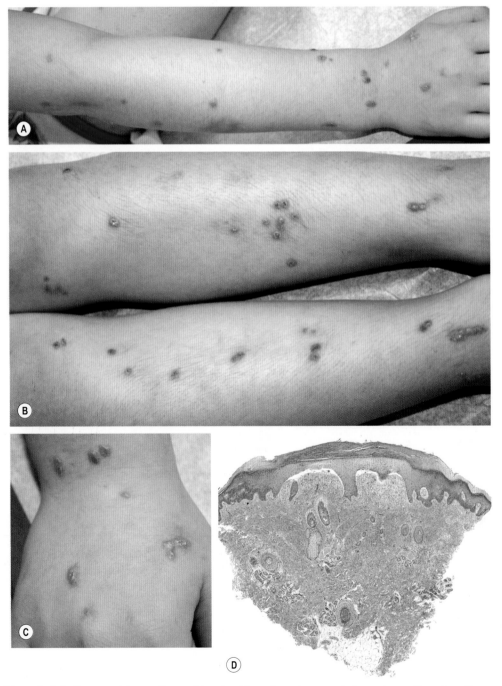

Fig. 24.14 Epidermolysis bullosa pruriginosa. 7-year-old male with erythematous, eroded papules on the extremities, resembling prurigo nodules. Biopsy findings included hyperkeratosis and acanthosis, but also a subepidermal split. Other potential clinical clues are a history of spontaneous blistering and nail atrophy/dystrophy. *A–C, Courtesy, Richard Antaya, MD.*

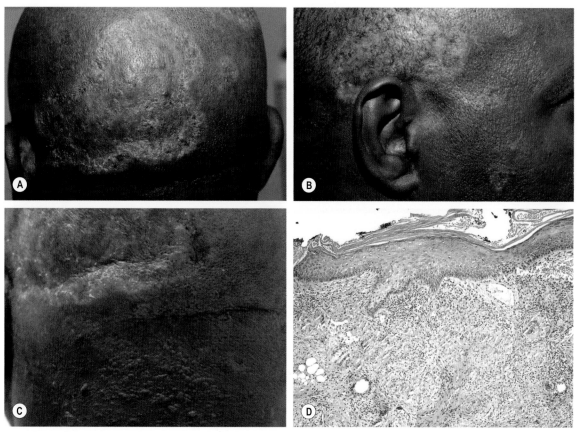

Fig. 24.15 Sarcoidosis. 58-year-old male with indurated, dyspigmented plaques on the scalp that had clinical resemblance to discoid lupus erythematosus. Clinical clues to the diagnosis included raised papules at the borders of the plaques, annular flesh-colored papules on the cheek (**B**), and papules on the occipital scalp (**C**). The conchal bowl is spared, a pertinent negative. Biopsy findings: granulomatous inflammation. *A,C, Courtesy, Yale Dermatology Residents' Slide Collection; B, Courtesy, Kalman Watsky, MD.*

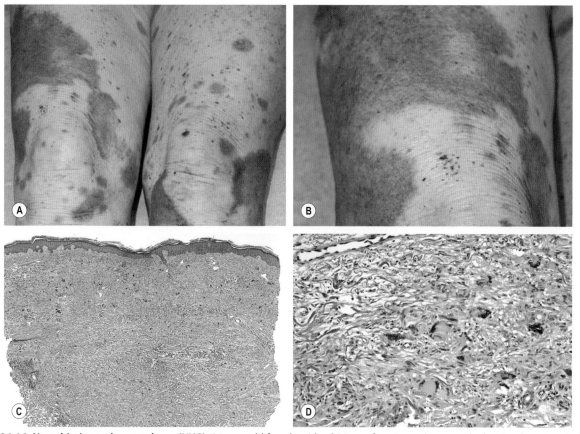

Fig. 24.16 Necrobiotic xanthogranuloma (NXG). 84-year-old female with a history of acute myelogenous leukemia who presented with somewhat annular red–brown, indurated plaques on the extremities. Biopsy findings were in the dermis and included foci of altered collagen surrounded by numerous bizarre giant cells, histiocytes, and lymphocytes. Although NXG is classically periorbital, it can affect other sites.

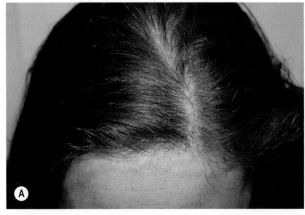

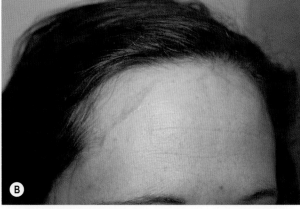

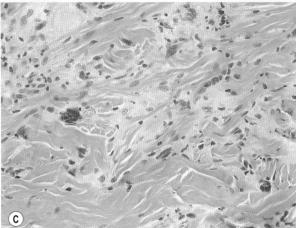

Fig. 24.17 Annular elastolytic giant cell granuloma. Although some consider this a variant of granuloma annulare, the clinical presentation is classically annular plaques on the forehead/scalp and/or other sun-exposed sites. There is minimal epidermal change clinically. Histologic findings are based in the dermis and include giant cells with elastophagocytosis. *A–C, Courtesy, Yale Dermatology Residents' Slide Collection.*

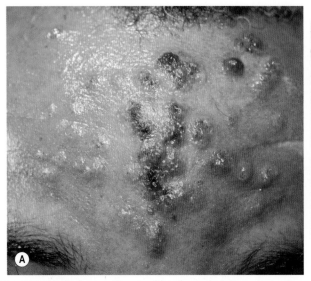

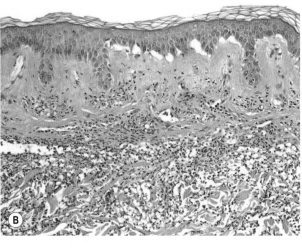

Fig. 24.18 Iododerma. 62-year-old male, several days status post multiple procedures using IV contrast, with numerous raised, somewhat translucent papules on his forehead (**A**) as well as scattered over his body. Biopsy findings included a dermal infiltrate of neutrophils (**B**). The lesions spontaneously resolved. *A, Courtesy, Yale Dermatology Residents' Collection.*

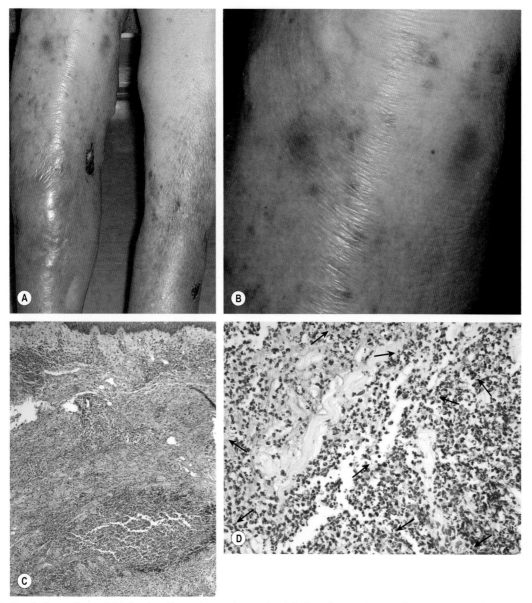

Fig. 24.19 Atypical mycobacterial infection. Purpuric papules on the right leg; the scar is secondary to excision of a squamous cell carcinoma (**A,B**). The patient had been soaking the right leg wound from the surgical excision in a water bath. Biopsy findings were based in the dermis and included extravasated erythrocytes as well as neutrophilic abscesses (**C**) with rare acid-fast bacteria (arrows) (**D**).

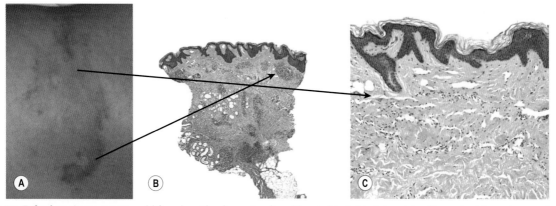

Fig. 24.20 Tufted angioma. 14-year-old female with a long-standing, blanchable light pink patch with a raised, irregular purplish red border (**A**). The raised border corresponded to "cannonballs" or "tufts" of small capillaries in the dermis (**B**). The flat pink portion correlated with dilated lymphatic vessels in the dermis (**C**). *A, Courtesy, Richard Antaya, MD. Reported in Am J Dermatopathol 2012; 35:400.*

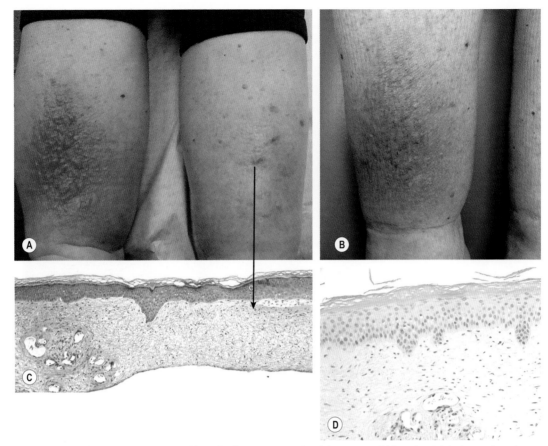

Fig. 24.21 Stasis mucinosis (obesity-associated lymphedematous mucinosis). 74-year-old female with indurated erythema, right > left leg, studded with raised firm, pseudovesicular papules (**A**). She had no thyroid abnormality, a pertinent negative. Follow-up with compression alone showed marked improvement (**B**). Biopsy of a raised papule with dermal edema, clustered vessels, and slightly increased dermal mucin (**C,D**). *A,B, Courtesy, Ronnie Klein, MD.*

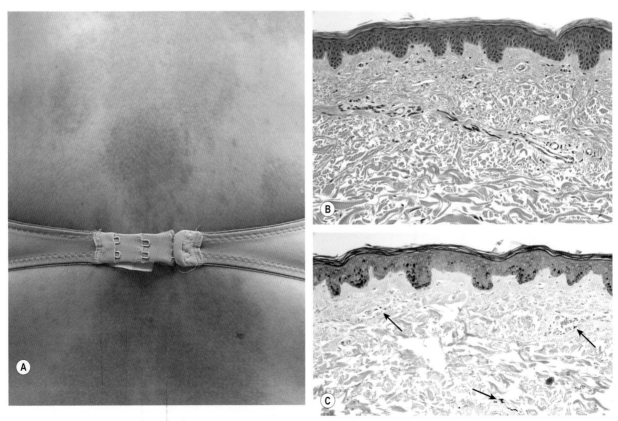

Fig. 24.22 Hydroxychloroquine-induced pigmentation. 44-year-old female with history of mixed connective tissue disorder, on hydroxychloroquine for several years. Acquired, grey patchy pigmentation was scattered on her extremities and back. Biopsy findings included yellow–brown pigment in macrophages in the dermis, particularly around vessels. The dermal pigment stained with Fontana Masson (arrows) and did not stain with Perls' stain for iron. Hydroxychloroquine-related pigmentary change has a predilection for the shins; the pigment may stain with Fontana Masson alone or also stain with Perls' stain for iron. *A, Courtesy Jennifer M McNiff, MD.*

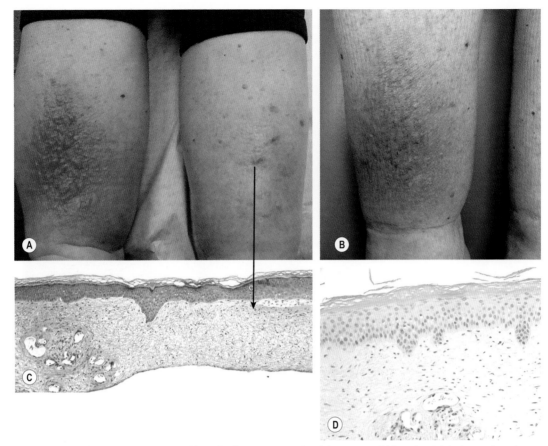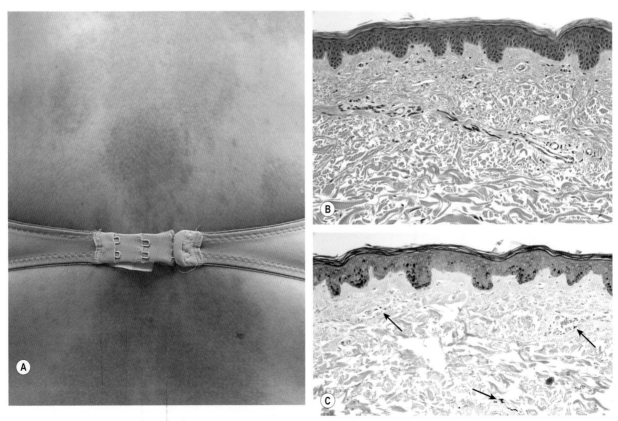

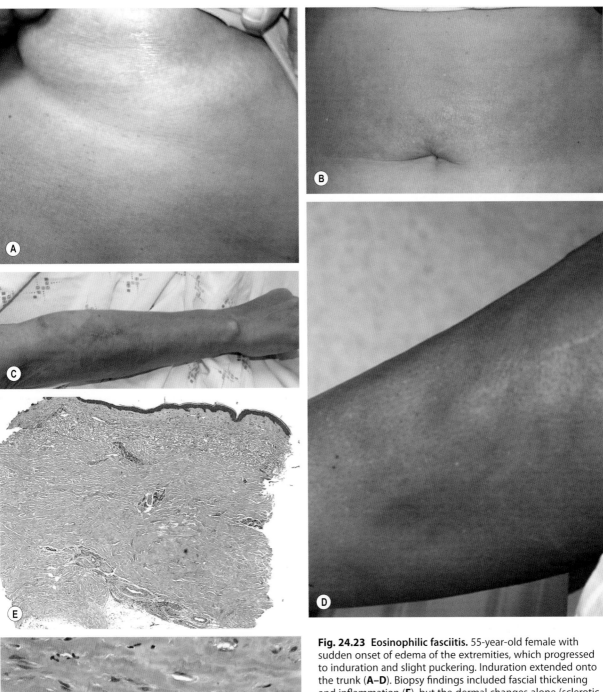

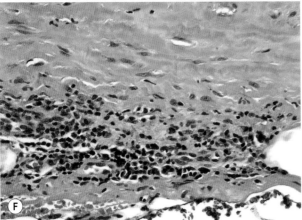

Fig. 24.23 Eosinophilic fasciitis. 55-year-old female with sudden onset of edema of the extremities, which progressed to induration and slight puckering. Induration extended onto the trunk (**A–D**). Biopsy findings included fascial thickening and inflammation (**F**), but the dermal changes alone (sclerotic collagen) resembled morphea (**E**). *A–D, Courtesy, Yale Dermatology Residents' Slide Collection.*

Page numbers followed by "*f*" indicate figures, "*t*" indicate tables, and "*b*" indicate boxes.